THE PATIENT'S PLAYBOOK

THE
PATIENT'S
PLAYBOOK

LESLIE D. MICHELSON

VINTAGE BOOKS

A DIVISION OF PENGUIN RANDOM HOUSE LLC   NEW YORK

The Library of Congress has cataloged the Knopf edition as follows:

Michelson, Leslie D.

The patient's playbook : how to save your life and the lives of those you love / by Leslie D. Michelson

pages cm

1. Patient advocacy. 2. Patient education. 3. Medical errors—Prevention.
4. Medicine—Decision making. 5. Self-care, Health.

I. Title.

R727.45.M53 2015

610.69'6—dc23   2015014325

Vintage Trade Paperback ISBN: 978-0-8041-7043-7
eBook ISBN: 978-0-385-35229-1

Designed by Claudia Martinez

www.vintagebooks.com

Printed in the United States of America
10 9 8 7 6 5 4 3 2 1

IN MEMORY OF
Erwin Michelson, my father, whose integrity, courage, and leadership
set the bar high, and whose boundless love and confidence
gave me everything I needed to reach for it.

WITH GRATITUDE TO
The many people who have trusted me to help manage their medical care,
enabling me to learn the lessons in this book.

IN HONOR OF
The countless physicians, nurses, aides, and other caregivers
who work tirelessly in the face of formidable obstacles
to provide their patients with the very best care.

CONTENTS

FOREWORD   XI

INTRODUCTION: HOW TO SAVE A LIFE   3

PART I   HOW TO BE PREPARED

The way you interact with doctors and hospitals could be dangerous to your health. Here are your take-charge steps: Find and partner with a good primary care physician, complete your personal health binder, and round up your wellness team.   19

1   WHY HAVING THE RIGHT PRIMARY CARE PHYSICIAN WILL CHANGE YOUR LIFE: How to view this essential relationship—and what your doctor should be doing for you   21

2   HOW TO FIND THE BEST PRIMARY CARE PHYSICIAN FOR YOU: . . . or develop a better relationship with the one you have. Plus: advice from doctors on dealing with them   37

3   THREE THINGS YOU CAN DO RIGHT NOW TO BE BETTER PREPARED: Write your family's medical memoir, collect your records, and take inventory.   63

4   DEVELOP A SUPPORT TEAM: Why you need to recruit an effective health care quarterback—and how to ask   77

PART II   EXPERTS AND EMERGENCIES

When a potential health crisis looms, how to get to the bottom of the problem and the top tier of medical care. Plus: how to handle yourself in an emergency (room).   87

5   OVERTREATMENT CAN BE AS DANGEROUS AS UNDERTREATMENT: How to find the right level, no matter your condition   89

6 HOW TO FIND AND INTERVIEW THE MEDICAL EXPERTS YOU NEED: Don't just Google it—here are smarter ways to get the right specialists. 107

7 EMERGENCY ROOM 101: The four most common mistakes made in the first twenty-four hours of a medical emergency 139

PART III WHAT TO DO WHEN SERIOUS ILLNESS STRIKES

Get to the No-Mistake Zone by following the four steps of Intensive Case Management. 165

8 PATIENT, M.D.: You've got a major health problem. Approach it like a pro. 167

9 STEP 1—IMMERSION: Learn everything you can about your illness and the doctors who are passionate about it. 175

10 STEP 2—DIAGNOSIS: How to be sure you've been correctly diagnosed? Follow the carpenter's rule: Measure twice, cut once. 197

11 STEP 3—TREATMENT: How to identify the right treatment plan—and the best doctor for you 213

12 STEP 4—COORDINATION: How to make sure your doctors are performing like a team 245

13 COMPETENCE AND COURAGE: Now that you've got it, lead the way. 269

ONE FINAL THOUGHT 273

ACKNOWLEDGMENTS 277
APPENDIX 283
NOTES 309
INDEX 337

FOREWORD

As the chief of surgery of a major hospital, I find I spend more and more of my time helping people navigate the health care system. I've been practicing medicine for more than forty years, my father was a surgeon, and I come from a family of doctors. So when someone asks, "Who should I see for my medical problem?," I'm in a good position to guide them. But even with all of my contacts, I sometimes find it very hard to come up with the right answer. It often requires a considerable amount of research and persistence on my part. It can be especially frustrating when a close friend or family member is struggling with a health problem. So I can certainly imagine how scary and puzzling it is for the majority of patients who must confront serious medical issues without the benefit of insider knowledge.

Leslie Michelson captures this dilemma with great insight in *The Patient's Playbook: How to Save Your Life and the Lives of Those You Love.* Successfully steering a serious health problem through the medical system can be a challenge. In *The Patient's Playbook,* Michelson gives away secrets of the trade—lessons he's learned from more than thirty years of helping people get better outcomes—that you can use yourself. He levels the playing field by providing average patients who have ordinary health insurance and Internet access (or an Internet savvy friend) with the resources, advice, and tools they need to make better medical decisions and achieve optimal results.

I found *The Patient's Playbook* to be enlightening, helpful, and full of sound recommendations. The guidance Michelson offers is well-documented and expertly informed, based on the latest evidence from outcomes research and comparative-effectiveness studies. And to this he adds good old common sense. *The Patient's Playbook* is engrossing, suspenseful, exciting, and reassuring. It grabs your attention with compelling stories that at times read like a detective thriller. Those stories yield practical ideas that show you how to prepare for a life of better care. And you don't have to be wealthy or connected to get there.

My surgeon father used to say that the cheapest medicine is the best medicine. In other words, getting the diagnosis and the treatment right is the least expensive way to take good care of patients and get the best results in the long run. Michelson follows this same mantra. Throughout *The Patient's Playbook,* he provides instructions for obtaining high-quality care on the first try. For example, he points out that the first step in any treatment decision is making sure you have the correct diagnosis. This is crucial. As an oncologist at a major cancer center, I see patients come in all the time with a diagnosis and set of treatment recommendations that I find, upon my own review, just don't fit. Occasionally, we find their disease is much worse than was thought. But most often we find that people don't need as much treatment or surgery as they were initially told. These experiences affirm something the author emphasizes in the book: be cautious, consult with experts, and think twice before you dive into treatment. None of us are perfect, and physicians can make mistakes or overlook things, but the majority of us try to do our very best every day. Still, the idea of accepting whatever your doctor says without question makes no sense. I've always considered it perfectly appropriate for my patients to ask questions, challenge statements, and seek out second opinions. *The Patient's Playbook* walks you through this process, demonstrating how to partner with your physician in an empowering and respectful way.

In fact, one of the most important things that Michelson points out is that most of the major medical centers and doctors who are the prominent leaders in their fields take insurance and Medicare. If you need an operation and you're covered by Medicare, for essentially no cost out of your pocket you can go to one of the most distinguished surgeons in your field of need. So why wouldn't you go to the best? This is a mistake that many people are prone to make. A case comes to mind of a patient who suffered from an abnormal heartbeat, a complicated arrhythmia. When he had to be admitted to the local community hospital several times, I encouraged him to come to the medical center in Houston, where I was working, to see a world-class cardiologist. He refused. He was comfortable with his hometown doctors, who were friendly and attentive, and he didn't see the point. He eventually had another arrhythmia and died at his small-town hospital because his doctors couldn't manage it. This was a man who had his own plane and wouldn't think anything of flying his family to France for a week's vacation. Yet he wouldn't go the distance to see the best physician for his condition. Michelson implores readers to bring the same scrutiny and judgment to a medical decision that they would to buying a car, finding a good place to live, or selecting the right school for their children. If you, like the arrhythmia patient, are facing a serious illness, the decisions you make about your medical care will have a profound impact on you and your family's life—and they deserve at least as much attention and consideration.

Some patients take their responsibility very seriously, examining every possible option. But when it's time to make a decision about treatment, they become extremely anxious. They worry, "Am I getting this right? Have I done everything I need to do?" *The Patient's Playbook* gives you the power to take a deep breath, do your research very carefully, and then break down what seems like a complicated, hopeless problem into a series of steps that you can tackle in a reasonable amount of time with a reasonable amount of effort. As a patient, you have more power than you think. This book will help you find that power and use it to maximum advantage. Don't underestimate the impact you can have on the health care system. You have a profound influence on the system every time you choose a physician network to be involved in, a specialist to see, or a hospital to visit. You have life-defining choices and a proactive part to play. But it takes becoming an informed medical consumer to get it right. You can do it. And you don't have to be wealthy or have a doctor in your family or close connections in the medical field. Keep this book close at hand as a family medical reference. I think you'll find it helpful, as I certainly have, in navigating your way through the system. It is a wonderful guide to help you make wise, well-informed decisions that will lead to a life of better health.

—*Peter T. Scardino, M.D.*
Chair, Department of Surgery
Memorial Sloan Kettering Cancer Center

THE PATIENT'S PLAYBOOK

➤ *How to Save a Life*

By the time Catherine* came to me for help, in the spring of 2012, the health care system had pretty much destroyed her health.

"I've been diagnosed with this . . . condition," she began. "It's called Churg-Strauss. They want to do surgery in a few weeks to confirm that I have it."

Normally, this fifty-three-year-old management professional lights up a room with her grace and vitality. Today was different: three different doctors had just told her that she likely had a rare and fatal autoimmune condition.

Churg-Strauss Syndrome typically develops in three stages, starting with severe asthma and allergies. Next, the immune system fails, manifesting as fatigue, coughs, abdominal pain, and gastrointestinal bleeding. In the third phase, the arteries and veins become so inflamed that blood can't get to vital organs, causing all sorts of nasty symptoms: nausea, vomiting, chest pain, shortness of breath, and numbness in the toes and fingers so bad that you can't walk. All the major organs (lungs, skin, heart, kidneys), muscles, and joints are attacked. Researchers aren't sure what causes Churg-Strauss, and

*Not her real name. Patients' names and some identifying characteristics have been changed throughout the book.

there is no cure, but treatment—corticosteroids to start and, if it progresses, chemotherapy—can help keep the final stage at bay.

Catherine had long suffered from asthma, fatigue, and coughing, but recent bouts of pneumonia, urinary tract infections, and gastroesophageal reflux disease (searing heartburn so bad she couldn't eat or sleep) set off alarms for her doctors, who now suspected advanced Churg-Strauss.

Sitting across from me that day, she seemed confused and exhausted, uncertain of what to do, and fought back tears every time she said the words *Churg-Strauss*. The process of trying to get better had only made her feel worse.

It was clear that Catherine required more than just medical advice; she needed the courage to take charge of her own health care. Her history would provide the important clues we needed to get her back on track. "Tell me everything," I said. "Start from the beginning."

"It's the most peculiar thing. At about the age of thirty, when my son was nine months old, I got a really bad cold that turned into bronchitis." At the time, Catherine was breastfeeding and was advised against taking antibiotics. Six months later she was still sick. Her doctors diagnosed her with late-onset asthma.

As the daughter of a physician, Catherine tended to follow orders. She took her medications, adapted to her symptoms, and learned to live as if deep, full breaths were a gift. Over the years, she struggled with increasing tightening in her chest and a painful cough that got worse in cold air. One evening she fractured four ribs from coughing. Another time she awoke in the middle of the night short of breath and grabbed for the inhaler on her bedside table. It didn't open her airways. She took a shower, hoping that the hot steam would loosen things up. But her gasping only intensified. She roused her husband, barely able to get out the words: *Take me to the emergency room.*

"It was a twenty-minute drive, and I started to get desperate," she recalled. "It felt like I was drowning." At the hospital, Catherine was put on an IV of adrenaline and cortisone to stabilize her breathing. She slowly recovered. "There may have been some trigger that day. Who knows? I can never tell what the trigger is."

In her twenty-three-year quest to feel better, Catherine had endured a battery of tests prescribed by countless well-meaning doctors. (Actually, I did count: ten specialists, not including the physicians who treated her during hospital stays.) She underwent numerous CT scans of her lungs and sinuses. She was pinpricked for food, mold, roach, and dust mite allergies, and she was tested some more for fungal infections, cystic fibrosis, and even the inherited condition alpha-1 antitrypsin deficiency, which can cause severe lung damage. She spent roughly ten thousand dollars a year in out-of-pocket health care costs and thousands more pulling up carpets and remodeling her home to minimize allergens.

All her doctors could tell for sure was that she had a slight allergic reaction to dust. That, and her asthma was getting worse. But there was an additional issue that went undiagnosed: treatment fatigue.

Catherine's physicians meant well, but no one was *coordinating* her care. As a result, she was pursuing a try-it-and-see-what-happens approach with each new doctor. Over the years, she had taken an array of steroids, bronchodilators, and antibiotics—adding more drugs to mitigate the side effects of the ones she was already on, which, at various times, included Advair, Didronel, Fosamax, Medrol, prednisone, Qvar, Rhinocort, Singulair, Spiriva, theophylline, Ventolin, Xolair, Zyflo, long-term antibiotics, and dust mite shots.

Catherine had spent two decades on anywhere from 10 to 60 milligrams a day of prednisone, a corticosteroid that helped her breathe. But prednisone at such high doses can cause terrible side effects: bloating, bone deterioration, hyperactivity, insomnia, thinning of the skin. Her legs were covered in scars. If she so much as bumped into a chair, she'd develop purple bruises and gaping cuts that couldn't be stitched because her skin was too fragile. She donned soccer-style shin guards under her pants and never wore skirts.

One morning in late 2011, to her horror, as she was flushing her sinuses with a neti pot, which she does twice a day, a blob of tissue tumbled out. An ear, nose, and throat doctor shined a light up her nostrils, discovered her septum had perforated, and proclaimed that it must have been caused by one of three things.

"He said to me," Catherine recalled, "'You're either a past or current cocaine user'—and I've never done drugs—'or the Rhinocort inhaler thinned your skin. Or *it could be* Wegener's.'"

Wegener's is a potentially fatal vascular disease that can lead to serious lung and kidney damage. To Catherine, her ENT sounded a little too enthusiastic about the possibility of such a rare diagnosis. But doctors are imperfect like us, and when they have to see twenty to forty patients a day just to maintain their practice, sensitivity can fall by the wayside.

She next went to a rheumatologist who, thankfully, ruled out Wegener's. But he was concerned about her recent history of urinary tract infections, pneumonia, and reflux disease—and especially her CT scans, which showed that her lungs were functioning at about 50 percent. He asked Catherine if she had ever heard of Churg-Strauss Syndrome.

Next stop: a pulmonologist. He was fascinated by Catherine's symptoms, telling her, "You know, you so seldom see Churg-Strauss, but I've just had a patient who went from having her asthma under control into serious Churg-Strauss. Now she has renal failure, and she's on dialysis."

To test this hunch, Catherine was referred to another ENT. He advised that she undergo sinus-scrape surgery to look for signs of eosinophilia—an abundance of a type of white blood cell that multiplies in force when the body is under attack—which, he said, would certainly point to a diagnosis of Churg-Strauss. The doctor proposed going up Catherine's nose with an endoscope and stainless steel tools to scrape away bone and blockages (chisel, hammer, suction is the general idea), collecting enough tissue for a proper analysis. Catherine would have to endure two black eyes, severe pain, and several weeks of recovery.

Her story horrified me, for a number of reasons. "Stop," I said. "You've been through enough already. Don't do anything right now. I'm going to help you."

While Catherine's diagnosis was very rare, her feelings of helplessness and defeat were not. I see this all the time: before we get sick, we believe that there is a health care "system" out there that will help us navigate whatever ails us. But when illness strikes, the journey to wellness is terribly confusing: a different language, contradictory signals, rapidly changing science, and no one to copilot. We quickly discover there is no map. It's no wonder that so often we let go of the wheel and place our fate in the hands of doctors, no questions asked.

When you or someone you care for is sick and you don't know what to do, it's easy to become paralyzed, as Catherine did. Whether the flashpoint is a child's allergic reaction, a parent's stroke, a diagnosis of cancer, or a car accident—in that moment of anxiety and vulnerability, there are critical choices we must make. Yet all too often we don't know how to collect the right information, frame our options, and ensure that we're making the best decisions. We don't even know that we are in serious danger, as Catherine was, of becoming a patient safety statistic.

In 1999, a groundbreaking Institute of Medicine (IOM) report, titled *To Err Is Human*, revealed the dirty secret that our system can be extremely harmful to our health. It estimated that at least 44,000 and up to 98,000 people in the United States were dying each year as a result of medical error—things like inaccurate diagnoses, the wrong drugs or treatments, and equipment failures. In 1998, as its authors noted, more people had died as a result of medical error than from car accidents (43,458), breast cancer (42,297), or AIDS (16,516).

But those figures didn't tell the whole story.

A year later, in a 2000 *Journal of the American Medical Association* (*JAMA*) article, a distinguished professor at the Johns Hopkins School of Medicine combined patient deaths from medical error with an even-larger number of deaths that were due to adverse events—unnecessary surgeries, fatal infections, and the like. She discovered that the *actual* number of Americans who needlessly died every year at the hands of those tasked with saving their lives was closer to 225,000. That's akin to a jumbo jet crashing and killing everyone on board once a day, 365 days a year. And it makes medical error the third leading cause of death in the United States today, just behind heart disease and cancer.

These startling reports, picked up by every major media outlet, sent shock waves through the medical community. Congress unanimously passed the Patient Safety and Quality Improvement Act, which allowed for the creation of patient safety organizations, tasked with collecting and analyzing medical error data, looking for patterns that could explain mishaps, and proposing solutions. Numerous hospitals incorporated checklists to avoid missteps in patient care, and they spent millions of dollars on computerized drug-dispensing systems. Sleep-deprived residents' work shifts were soon limited to sixteen consecutive hours.

And yet . . . we are still no safer.

"Despite all the focus on patient safety, it seems we have not made much progress at all," says Dr. Ashish Jha, a professor of health policy and management at Harvard's School of Public Health and one of several experts who testified in the summer of 2014 at a congressional hearing titled *More Than 1,000 Preventable Deaths a Day Is Too Many: The Need to Improve Patient*

Safety. The hearing was inspired by a 2013 study in the *Journal of Patient Safety,* authored by a scientist who, after tragically losing his teenage son to medical error, vowed to take a closer look at the problem, given that the IOM numbers were based on thirty-year-old medical records. His analysis revealed that preventable adverse events actually contribute to the death of *more than 400,000 Americans a year.*

"The IOM probably got it wrong. It was clearly an underestimate of the toll of human suffering that goes on from preventable medical errors," Dr. Jha testified. "If I walk into an American hospital today, am I demonstrably, clearly safer than I was fifteen years ago? The unfortunate answer is, No. We have not moved the needle in any meaningful, demonstrative way."

Have no doubt—you are still at great risk whenever you blindly place yourself or loved ones in the hands of a fragmented health care system.

After meeting with Catherine, my team and I went into action, collecting her complete history: every lab test, X-ray, medical record, and scribbled doctors' note we could muster from the last twenty-three years of her life—the length of time she had been struggling with her illness.

Compiled in a four-inch white binder and topped with a bulleted summary of her medical milestones, Catherine's dossier was sent to Dr. Michael Wechsler, at the time a pulmonologist at Brigham and Women's Hospital at Harvard and an authority on Churg-Strauss Syndrome. Dr. Wechsler has published extensively on the presentation and treatment of this disease, and he's on the medical advisory board of the Churg-Strauss Syndrome Association. When we reached out to him by e-mail, he was happy to review her case.

A week later Catherine got a phone call that changed her life. "You must be somebody important. I've never seen a presentation folder like this," Dr. Wechsler said.

He began by asking questions about her current health status: "Do you have any neuropathy, any tingling or numbness? Any history of kidney issues?" She mentioned her urinary tract infections, the only symptom matching his concerns.

"Based on your records and what you're telling me, I wouldn't do the sinus surgery," Dr. Wechsler told her. "Churg-Strauss is a difficult disease to diagnose definitively. Doing a biopsy just to get a diagnosis, at this point, is not going to be helpful. Also, all these medications you are on will obfuscate any results."

Furthermore, he told her, until her kidneys or other organs were affected, or until she developed peripheral neuropathy, "I can't say that you have Churg-Strauss."

Dr. Wechsler believed that Catherine could have chronic eosinophilic pneumonia, or possibly a nasty case of worsening asthma with something called remodeling of the lungs. Her respiratory organs had been in a hypersensitive state for so long that they might have been permanently damaged.

She was also on too many medications. Catherine's hamster wheel of a drug regimen had led to a tolerance of some prescriptions (which didn't work for her anymore) and allergic reactions to others. The urinary tract infections that led her doctors to believe her kidneys were under attack? Those were probably exacerbated by the high levels of antibiotics she had taken for the pneumonia. Likewise, the bronchodilators contributed to her reflux disease.

But here's the scariest part: If Catherine had undergone sinus surgery, her physicians would have found what they were looking for, because her blood tests over the years had already shown increasing levels of eosinophils. Never mind that, as Dr. Wechsler explained to her: eosinophilia can be caused by a number of other factors, such as worsening asthma and lung remodeling, and by itself is *not* a definitive indicator of Churg-Strauss.

Yet Catherine's doctors surely would have declared a verdict, diagnosed her with Churg-Strauss Syndrome, and begun treatment for a disease she didn't have. Her story is a stark reminder of why it's so important to consult an expert—a medical professional with enough deep experience that he or she has probably seen almost every iteration of your specific illness—before taking action.

Catherine felt as if someone had just led her out of a dark cave where she'd spent years running into walls. Instead of the nightmare she'd anticipated—continuing physical and mental deterioration and eventually death—her future was bright again, with a few tolerable limitations. She now had the courage and competence to tell her doctors that she was canceling her surgery and changing to a course of *less* treatment.

A year later Catherine was flourishing on just 2.5 to 5 milligrams per day of prednisone, plus the use of her inhaler. Her reflux was gone, and she was under the care of excellent allergists in Los Angeles who were monitoring her condition. She rode her electric bike to work on sunny days. Catherine had finally regained peace of mind and was in control of her own health.

Everybody knows that health care in America is broken, yet we have been brought up to passively follow doctors' orders rather than partner with them. I'd go so far as to say we treat doctors and caregivers like clergy: they wear the white lab coats of their institution, signaling their authority; they speak a confusing language that excludes you, the layperson. More important, and curiously, we don't hold them accountable for outcomes. Certainly that makes sense for religious leaders (that's why it's called faith!), but for physicians? And to add insult to injury,* when you're terribly sick and feeling vulnerable, sitting naked in a flimsy paper gown on a cold examination table, and your doctor gives you fifteen, maybe twenty minutes of his time before moving to the next exam room—that's often when you are asked to make clear, rational decisions about treatment.

Now, to turn the tables, think about what it's like for doctors. A typical primary care physician manages two thousand to four thousand patients, and sees anywhere from twenty to forty patients a day. Why? One reason is that they have to work harder than ever before to meet the demands of higher office management costs and educational loans, while at the same time receiving lower reimbursements for their services from health insurers. I'm a pretty hard-working guy, but I can't imagine seeing twenty clients a day, five days a week. How do you think clearly and carefully about each one? No matter how charismatic, empathetic, and effective a doctor is, he or she cannot care for a human being in fifteen minutes.

As that landmark IOM report and subsequent studies prove, we have to be proactively engaged with our doctors in our own care, because the consequences of simply accepting whatever we are given can mean the difference between life and death.

Of course, not all medical mistakes are fatal. Many patients are poked, prodded, and subjected to unnecessary surgeries and treatments, just as Catherine was. In fact, one of the biggest dangers we face is a medication foul-up. In 2007 the IOM estimated that every hospital patient is subjected

---

*Just to be clear, doctors today don't have enough time to spend with patients because our reimbursement system doesn't pay them for the extra hours in a day it would take to stop and think, do more research, sit with you for as long as you need, and be even more thoughtful about your care. Virtually every physician I know wishes they could practice like that.

to at least one medication error per day. One a day! That's 1.5 million *preventable* adverse drug events per year. On one end of the spectrum, that's a nurse administering a little too much pain-killer, causing the patient to feel nausea or confusion; but on the other, it's a doctor accidentally prescribing penicillin for someone who is deathly allergic, or a new drug that has dangerous interactions with a patient's existing regimen. To put it in perspective, the Dallas Cowboys' AT&T Stadium can accommodate eighty thousand seated football fans. Subject every single man, woman, and child in that packed stadium to a medication foul-up—and you'd still have nineteen more packed-stadium games to go before you reached the number of people harmed every year.

It's easy to get lost in such large numbers, so let's bring it down to one famous and frightening case, when actor Dennis Quaid and his wife Kimberly Buffington almost lost their newborn twins. In November 2007 the couple welcomed home Thomas Boone and Zoë Grace. Days later the babies fell ill with staph infections, and the Quaids brought them to Cedars-Sinai Medical Center in Los Angeles, where they were admitted and put on intravenous antibiotics. As is common practice, the IV catheter that carried the medicine to their tiny bodies was flushed at regular intervals with a drug called Hep-Lock, to prevent clots from forming in the line. (Hep-Lock is a very weak form of the adult blood thinner heparin.) The twins seemed to be doing well. But then that night they turned purple.

The Quaids arrived early the next morning to discover that their twins were supposed to have received 10 units of Hep-Lock, but instead they had received 10,000 units of full-blast heparin—and not once but twice. Buffington later described the babies to Oprah Winfrey as appearing black and blue and bleeding out from their IVs, their blood the consistency of water.

The error chain had begun when a pharmacy technician put the 10,000-unit doses of heparin in the same bin as the 10-unit doses of Hep-Lock. Then the nurse who administered the drugs didn't double-check the bottle labels, which looked very similar. The Quaids would later say that they were in the room when the nurse administered the heparin, yet they had failed to oversee what she was doing. (But who does, really? We trust hospital workers with our lives, forgetting that they are only human.)

The infants, thankfully, pulled through. And Cedars-Sinai's response was swift and strong: the hospital underwent major staff retraining and invested $100 million in new technology, including bar-code scanners and multiple computer-assisted checks of medication. It was also transparent about its role in the mix-up, even inviting *The Oprah Winfrey Show* in to discuss the terrifying incident and share the safety measures it enacted.

Shaken by the ordeal, Dennis Quaid testified before Congress, and the couple started a foundation to raise awareness about the dangers of medication error, fully aware of the fact that theirs was just one story out of 1.5 million a year.

Helping people get the best possible health outcomes is my life's passion, but I am not a physician. I didn't go to medical school, and you won't see me balancing a stethoscope around my neck. I have been collaborating with doctors, patients, and policy makers for three decades, advising people from all walks of life when they need medical guidance.

In the 1970s, at age twenty-nine, I went to work as a special assistant to the general counsel of the U.S. Department of Health and Human Services, serving in both the Carter and Reagan administrations. I've been a founder, CEO, investor, adviser, and/or director for a variety of entrepreneurial health care and health technology companies. Before founding my own company, I was CEO of the Prostate Cancer Foundation (set up by Michael Milken after his successful battle against the disease), the world's largest philanthropic source of funding for prostate cancer research.

Today my official title is CEO of Private Health Management, but I'm really more of a health care quarterback, guiding clients through a wide range of ailments, from bunions and back pain to serious heart conditions and deadly cancers. My team and I have helped hundreds of private individuals, and thousands of corporate clients, achieve better care—and avoid medical error—by digging deep into their cases to ensure they are getting the right diagnoses, seeing the best doctors, and receiving the most effective treatments for their specific illnesses.

Everything I've learned from more than thirty years of experience helping others, I'm sharing here for the first time so that *you* can do it too, for yourself and your loved ones.

The actions I'm asking you to take in preparation (find and forge a relationship with a sharp primary care physician, take inventory of your family's health history, collect your medical records, and appoint someone to be your health care quarterback) will lay a strong foundation for the new patient-empowered approach I want you to take. Next, we'll focus on how to protect yourself from overtreatment, how to find and interview the right specialists when you are facing an unexpected illness or medical problem, and why you must prepare now for potential emergency room visits in the future. Finally, we'll turn to the question of serious illnesses. Whether it's cancer, an auto-immune disorder, or some other potentially life-changing disease, you will learn how to move forward using the same four-step process of Intensive Case Management (Immersion, Diagnosis, Treatment, and Coordination) that I've used to help many others get better care and live the longest, fullest life possible.

By the time you finish reading this book, you will have completely rethought the way you interact with caregivers and hospitals. You will have the confidence to make better decisions when you or someone you love gets sick and needs help. I know that these lessons work, because I've been putting them in action almost my entire life. In fact, how I *really* got my start as a patient advocate is another story, one that I've shared with only a few people until now.

After I was born, in 1951, my mother went into a major postpartum depression. For the first six months of my life, she couldn't get out of bed, leaving me in the care of my father and maternal grandmother. I actually didn't learn about this until I was forty-five, and someone casually mentioned it at a party. Sadly, the stigma of psychiatric illness was so great at the time (and still can be today) that families touched by chronic depression often had to carry the burden in silence. My parents had been counseled by doctors that they shouldn't discuss it, so they didn't.

My mother eventually recovered, but then she became bipolar, which meant there were days, months, and years when she'd be fine, and then long periods when she was incapable of getting up, making dinner, or holding a conversation. During her manic phases, she'd be on a high for days or weeks, talking nonstop and sometimes being cruel to me and others I know she loved. I couldn't predict when her disease would take control of her. Coming home from school, I never knew if I'd be greeted by a fire-breathing dragon or a smiling mother with a glass of milk and a plate of cookies. I had to feel around the edges of the door for danger, the way they teach you in fire safety training.

When I was ten, my mother screamed at me for forty-five minutes because I left a sneaker on the steps. The only ten-year-old who hasn't left a sneaker on the steps is a ten-year-old who doesn't have sneakers or steps.

During an ugly scene when I was twelve or thirteen, I physically held my mother down in a chair and told her, "You will stop yelling at my brother *right now*." That moment changed everything between us. She was my mother, and I loved her, but her disease was dangerous, and I had to be assertive.

Although my mother's illness was hard on me, it had to have been worse for my father. The instant I was born, he lost his wife. And yet he remained extraordinarily positive and strong. He was a genuine role model, the moral center of gravity for every community that he was in—whether it was our larger family, the synagogue, the Boy Scouts, his business, or his trade association. He was the guy who would solve other people's problems. I could talk to Dad for hours.

By my early teens, I was actively involved in helping with my mother's care. That was when she received her first electroshock therapy treatment for recurring depression. Later, we had her on daily lithium, a mood stabilizer. I had to grow up and become a responsible caregiver at a very young age.

And here's where the story gets complicated. When I was in high school, my father came home one evening, clearly agitated. For me, the sun came up at night when my father walked through the door. As tired as he was, those hours with him were absolutely precious. If he came home anxious or upset, that was a big deal.

He had gone for his annual physical that day with his primary care physician, a man with whom he'd attended high school in Newark, New Jersey. The doctor had recommended that my father see a certain cardiologist. A week or two later Dad came home even more rattled than before. The cardiologist had told him he needed to have open-heart surgery.

I was overcome with worry. Was my dad going to die? Losing him wouldn't just mean I'd be an orphan, practically speaking; it would mean I'd have to take full responsibility for my mother. That was not a reality I could handle.

That night I couldn't sleep. The next day I couldn't concentrate at school. I got home that afternoon and picked up the phone to dial Lenox Hill Hospital in New York. Although we lived in suburban Union, New Jersey, I read *The New York Times* every night, and somehow I recalled "Lenox Hill" always being mentioned. I knew that when you wanted to go to a nice restaurant, see a good play, or go to a top hospital—you went to New York.

"Can I please speak to the head of cardiology?" I asked. I'm sure my teenage voice must have cracked on the line as I spoke, but I wasn't going to aim low.

"Dad," I announced when my father got home, "I set up an appointment for you to get a second opinion from the chairman of cardiology at Lenox Hill."

"You know, that's a good idea," he said. "I'm gonna do it."

And that was that.

On the day of his appointment, I waited at home in agony. This had to go right. I couldn't imagine a future without him. I was seeing the walls coming down.

It was all I could do not to knock him over when he walked in the door. "What did he say, Dad? What did he say?"

"He said, 'There's nothing wrong with your heart, and the doctor who recommended surgery should be shot in a public square.'"

Exact words. He was ecstatic. And I still remember where I was standing in the kitchen when he said it. I remember this better than I remember what I had for breakfast today.

My father never had any heart problems. No high blood pressure, no calcium in his coronaries, no leaky valves. He passed away in 2007, succumbing to something totally unrelated to his heart. But back in 1988, when I was building my first company, I met Dr. Robert H. Brook, who was then the vice president and director of RAND Health, a health policy think tank. He had just published research showing that many of the major surgical procedures being done in the United States were harming rather than helping patients. In fact, when it came to coronary artery bypass graft surgeries—what my father was told he needed—14 percent were done for "inappropriate reasons," and 30 percent were done for "equivocal" reasons. I thought, *My God, this doctor has found scientific evidence of what I suspected was going on some twenty years ago.*

I still think of my father every day and how his "case" ignited my passion for helping people to get better care. Managing serious illness is not easy, but armed with the knowledge in this book, and the support of a trusted primary care doctor, I truly believe that everyone can—and must—become a more powerful and effective health care *consumer*.

In every realm but medicine, Americans are very good at effecting change with their wallets. We are more satisfied than ever with the cars we drive and the smartphones in our pockets because we influence and inspire the market. But the very fact that you have either employer- or government-funded insurance writing a check for your medical care changes the equation. You're not feeling like the consumer.

Further, you don't have information about quality and prices. You may know, thanks to a 2013 investigative series in *The New York Times,* that the cost of a routine colonoscopy in the New York area can range from $740 to $8,500. But when was the last time you asked your doctor, *How much is this going to cost?* (Chances are, because of our convoluted payment system, he or she couldn't even tell you.)

What if you had to buy a car without knowing how it fared against other cars when it came to performance, crash test safety, or miles per gallon? That's what we do when it comes to medicine. We undergo major procedures without getting expert opinions or even inquiring what past patients' experiences were like. But just as you shoulder the responsibility for buying a safe car, finding a good place to live, or selecting the right school for your child, you need to do your homework when it comes to your health care. The chasm between just taking what you are given and making sure you get the best is widening by the day.

On three occasions in our country's history, government action significantly transformed health care. The first was during World War II, when regulatory agencies capped wage increases but ruled that fringe benefits like sick leave and health insurance were not capped or taxable, giving employers a way to reward and attract talent with perks other than higher wages. For better or worse, this evolved into our present-day employer-based health insurance system.

The second event was in 1965 with the establishment of Medicare and Medicaid, ensuring health coverage for the elderly, injured, and impoverished. Today we are living in the age of a third major transformation: the Patient Protection and Affordable Care Act.

The Affordable Care Act is unquestionably one of the most sweeping and important pieces of health care legislation ever enacted. It guarantees that health insurance companies can no longer deny coverage for preexisting conditions, cancel coverage when you get sick, or impose annual or lifetime limits. It requires them to pay for preventive services and coverage for children up to the age of twenty-six. Yet at the same time, the Affordable Care Act significantly amplifies the power insurance companies have over physicians.

Normal businesses must be responsive to the needs of their customers or they will fail. But when it comes to health care, the insurance companies pay our doctors and our hospitals—they have the financial whip-handle. Physicians are caught between serving the patients they treat and the companies that compensate them. We're still stuck with a fractured, slow-to-move, convoluted process that doesn't meet our needs as consumers, or doctors' needs as caregivers. Decades later the words of legendary journalist Walter Cronkite still hold true: "America's health care system is neither healthy, caring, nor a system."

So it comes down to this. *You* have two choices, either take charge of your own care or wait for our fragmented system to get fixed. But guess what? There's no reason to believe it's going to get any better, and more important, you don't have time to wait because you don't know if there's a cell dividing in your body right now that will develop into cancer. You don't know if your immune system is starting to attack the cartilage in your knees and you'll need a knee replacement. You don't know if that car racing behind you on the freeway is going to stop before it meets your bumper.

Here's a real-life scenario that always troubles me. A patient who is dying decides to end therapeutic interventions. He just wants to be as comfortable as he can during his final days. The family turns to hospice care. One of the first questions a hospice worker asks the patient is "What are your goals and objectives? What are you looking for from us?" Tragically, this is frequently the *first* time anyone has asked the patient what *he or she* wants. You are the consumer, and it is your preferences and desires that matter most. Let's resolve now that whenever you interact with the medical community, even if no one ever asks what you want, you will have the courage and the competence to assert yourself—to make the health care delivery system respond to your needs and goals.

Millions of previously uninsured individuals now have coverage. Baby boomers are aging and demanding more medical attention just as we are facing a doctor shortage. Thankfully, the United States has some of the most advanced medical technologies, distinguished hospitals, and skilled practitioners in the world. Patients just don't know how to seek them out. But I'm going to show you how.

Now more than ever, we need to be effective consumers to get the best that we can out of a dysfunctional system. It's not easy. It will be a challenging commitment. But the rewards are enormous. This book will give you the tools, the competency, and the courage to do it well.

PART I

➤ *How to Be Prepared*

The way you interact with doctors and hospitals could be dangerous to your health. Here are your take-charge steps: Find and partner with a good primary care physician, complete your personal health binder, and round up your wellness team.

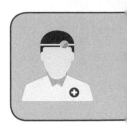

WHY HAVING THE RIGHT PRIMARY CARE PHYSICIAN WILL CHANGE YOUR LIFE

How to view this essential relationship—and what your doctor should be doing for you

Jennifer, a fifty-five-year-old attorney, came to me complaining of debilitating fatigue and chronic pain. She had been seeing the same primary care physician, or PCP, for the last seven years and found him to be thoughtful, not too rushed, and a good listener. But he was stumped by her symptoms, which had started in her late twenties as an unexplained "achy, deep bone pain" that waxed and waned. By her fifties, it had become unbearable and she was completely exhausted.

"It's almost flu-like. As if someone pulled the plug and I no longer have any power," she said. Her pain was the worst culprit in a slew of offenders that included depression, migraines, mild sleep apnea, psoriasis, fibroid disease, high cholesterol, and high blood pressure.

In her late forties, desperate for relief, Jennifer had enrolled in a pain-management program at a major teaching hospital. (The course had been recommended to her by a physician there after several doctors examined her and couldn't pinpoint a physical problem.) For three weeks, five days a week, she was schooled in the art of relaxation, positive self-talk, visualization, and the cardinal rule of the program: Do not discuss your pain. (Their theory was that verbalizing physical discomfort lights up sensors in the brain that reinforce one's *experience* of it.) She was also encouraged to stop taking her sleeping pills and to engage in spontaneous laughter as an endorphin-building exercise.

None of this really worked.

"My psychiatrist thought it was the stupidest thing she had ever heard of," she recalled. "But when you're desperate for help, you take desperate measures."

Shortly after Jennifer turned fifty-one, in 2009, she began to feel deep throbbing in her right hip, and a terrible stiffness when she sat for long periods. Her primary care physician ordered X-rays, diagnosed her with mild arthritis, and told her to take ibuprofen. When that didn't assuage the shooting pain, he told her to take more, until she was up to 600 milligrams of ibuprofen a day. He referred her to a podiatrist when her feet began to hurt, and to an orthopedic surgeon when her shoulders ached, but they offered her no new answers.

"Every time you go to a doctor, you have hope that *this* will be the person who figures it out," she said. "You go through more tests, they still can't figure it out, and it's just one more person telling you nothing's wrong."

The old "there's nothing wrong" diagnosis really troubles me. As a patient, you know when something is *really* wrong. But eventually Jennifer began to doubt her own experience of pain.

"I wondered if maybe I was a hypochondriac," she said. She devoted her limited energy to her private law practice and her teenage son, whom she raised alone. And she took antidepressants to help deal with her feelings of frustration and isolation.

By the spring of her fifty-fourth year, she was completely wiped out and sleeping like a teenager, up to twelve hours a day. Her left shoulder became a constant distraction, assaulting her with sharp jabs, like the sensation of a pinched nerve. She was losing range of motion. When she sent her son off to college that summer, she couldn't lift a single suitcase. The littlest things became big problems.

At dinner one night with friends, she said out loud to no one in particular, "Oh no, it's Wednesday—garbage night," and then had to explain that rolling her cans to the street was terribly difficult, like pushing a boulder up a mountain.

"You know, you said the same thing to us last Wednesday," someone said.

Jennifer cringed in embarrassment. *I sound like an old lady*, she thought. *Always complaining about how tired I am and how much I hurt.*

She decided to start working out, thinking, *If I just get in shape like everybody else, I'm going to feel better.* She treated herself to a week at a spa in New Mexico, where she ate healthy and participated in daily yoga, walks, and swimming. Her pain got worse.

By the time she came home, she couldn't touch her head or reach behind her back to unsnap her bra. Her orthopedist diagnosed her with "frozen shoulder," a condition whereby the capsule in the shoulder joint, which holds the bones, tendons, and ligaments together, thickens and causes restriction of movement. He gave her steroid shots and referred her to a physical therapist.

Despite the pain, Jennifer continued to eat her fruits and vegetables and go to the gym, because that's what healthy people do. She even lost weight. But she didn't feel any better. Soon her right shoulder began to throb. Her orthopedist gave her another steroid shot and said it wasn't out of the ordinary for both shoulders to freeze up. But her physical therapist insisted she get a second opinion.

Jennifer knew instinctively that all her health problems couldn't be separate issues. There had to be a connection. But she wasn't a doctor and couldn't connect the dots medically. That was her PCP's job. Yet by now she had lost faith in her PCP's guidance, so she came to me for help.

Forging a strong partnership with a caring and committed primary care physician is one of the most important first steps you can take in protecting your health. Unfortunately, Jennifer and her doctor had no such relationship. He gave up on the hard work of investigating the root cause of her pain, declared her to be an arthritis sufferer, ordered her to take ibuprofen, and then referred her to others who also gave best-guess diagnoses and Band-Aid treatments. Nobody was digging deep into her collection of symptoms to study the big picture. And Jennifer, lacking a health care partner, gave up her primary goal, which should have been to figure out the nature of her condition—*what was causing all this agony?*—and then seek out the best specialists and therapies for her illness.

The first thing we did was collect her medical records and imaging and send it with a summary of her condition to Dr. Robert R. Simon, former executive chair of emergency medicine for Cook County hospitals and a professor of emergency medicine at Rush University Medical Center in Chicago. Dr. Simon literally wrote the books used in standard practice for orthopedic emergencies and surgical procedures, and he's our go-to Sherlock Holmes for complex cases involving chronic pain and orthopedic issues. (Don't worry—in Chapter 6, I'm going to teach you ways to seek out the medical expert you need.)

Dr. Simon sent Jennifer pictures of various arm movements and asked her to describe what she was feeling as she went through them. "Jennifer, you do not have frozen shoulder," he said. "But I think you might have a connective tissue disorder." He believed her problem was a rheumatologic issue.

Jennifer seemed tentative when we got off the call. She'd been at this juncture before—a new doctor, a new hypothesis. She expected to be disappointed again but held out hope that this time would be different. In fact, she wouldn't have needed a detective like Dr. Simon if her PCP had taken the time to collect and study her records, to ensure that she was with the right specialist.

In addition to her phone consult with Dr. Simon, Jennifer also visited a top orthopedic surgeon in Los Angeles, who ordered new MRIs. As he examined her images, he pointed to the wearing away of cartilage in both her shoulders, as well as some neck issues and nerve damage. Confirming Dr. Simon's suspicions, he told Jennifer: *I think you need to see a rheumatologist.*

Dr. Katy M. Setoodeh was pleasant and warm at their first meeting. She held Jennifer's hands as she examined them. "Have you ever seen a rheumatologist before?"* she asked.

"Never," Jennifer said.

"Just from looking at your hands, I can see that you have a rheumatologic disorder."

Jennifer couldn't believe what she was hearing. Her hands had always felt fine.

The doctor pressed different parts of her body, asking, "Does this hurt?" She ordered blood work to check for autoimmune diseases, a bone scan to look for inflammation, and new MRIs of Jennifer's hands and lower back to see if she had joint damage.

At their second meeting, Dr. Setoodeh referred to those images as she

---

*As Dr. Setoodeh attests, many people with unexplained aches and pains don't even know what a rheumatologist does. She's seen patients endure years of joint damage before they even get to the correct realm of rheumatology—when probably all that was needed was for a smart dermatologist to ask, "Do you have joint pain?" or a thoughtful PCP to send the patient to a rheumatologist after discovering that orthopedic consultations were of no help.

counted up the toll: "You have damage to the joints in your hands, wrists, shoulders, neck, lower back, hips, knees, ankles, feet . . ." She went on and on. "I believe you have a severe case of *psoriatic arthritis* characterized by high levels of inflammation, which would explain your pain and exhaustion. I know you've had this pain for a long time. I really wish you had come to me years ago."

Jennifer's psoriasis, an itching, flaky skin condition, had first manifested about seventeen years earlier. There were times when the condition flared up, leaving her with cracked, painful skin, but just on her hands and elbows—and her dermatologist had prescribed medication that helped.

As far as she could recall, no one had ever talked to her about psoriatic arthritis, a chronic autoimmune disorder that causes intense joint pain. Up to 30 percent of psoriasis sufferers develop related arthritis, and most cases present between the ages of thirty and fifty. There is no cure, although a number of drugs introduced in the past decade work remarkably well at controlling the symptoms and restoring joint function—but they can't turn back the clock.

Just looking at the X-rays of Jennifer's hips from three years earlier, it was clear, Dr. Setoodeh said, that she had had the condition back then—and likely long before, given how much damage she now had.

"Many people think that musculoskeletal pains are just part of living life," says psoriatic arthritis expert Dr. Philip Mease, the director of rheumatology research at Swedish Medical Center in Seattle, and a clinical professor at the University of Washington's School of Medicine. "They don't know that there is irreversible damage progressing that could have been halted—and that's a shame when we see people who have years of symptoms, but the dermatologist visit has just been too busy, too short, and too focused on skin issues. It's important to have thoughtful assistant staff in the dermatology office who can say, 'I see you've checked arthritis on the intake questionnaire. Let me bring that to the attention of the physician,' or even just, 'Gee, let me give you this National Psoriasis Foundation brochure, which teaches about the possibility that you may have psoriatic arthritis.' Unfortunately, time is such a precious commodity, and in the medical profession, it's being cut short."

Dr. Setoodeh started Jennifer on a biweekly injection of a biological agent that would relieve her inflammation and pain while also slowing down joint damage. Within weeks she was feeling better. Four months later she reported that her pain level was down by two-thirds. She was back in the office three days a week and working from home, too. Little things that used to hurt so much, like clicking on a computer mouse, no longer bothered her.

"This is a major change of life for me—that's how I feel in my most optimistic mode. But in bleak moments, I know I have all this joint damage that's not going to go away and could have been avoided if I had been diagnosed earlier," Jennifer said. "I think my internist failed me on so many levels. If you look back, on this date I complained about a shoulder hurting, on this date I complained about my wrist. Two years later my hip hurts again. And my knees. Then it's my feet. He sends me to a podiatrist and an orthopedic surgeon and orders X-rays and says, 'Oh, you're fifty. You have arthritis. Time to start taking ibuprofen!' Like it's just another day."

To be fair, when Jennifer initially complained of pain, it was reasonable for her PCP to prescribe ibuprofen and X-rays. And when she continued to complain, he sent her to additional specialists. But when they didn't put the pieces together either, Jennifer got caught in the specialist shuffle: every new doctor she consulted with performed diagnostics in order to determine whether she had a condition that was within his realm of expertise, and if he couldn't diagnose her, he'd prescribe medications to try to relieve her symptoms, and if that didn't work, he'd pass her on to the next specialist, who'd go through the same process. The specialist shuffle can expose patients to unnecessary tests and treatments that cost a lot of money, time, and needless anxiety and stress. For patients like Jennifer, with nonspecific symptoms (fatigue, muscle pain, joint aches, etc.), the shuffle can go on for years with no resolution.

"It's a common situation we run into as rheumatologists, hearing arduous patient journeys," says Dr. Mease, who also consults with Jennifer by telephone. "They go to various doctors first—general practitioners, orthopedists, physical therapists, naturopaths—but the possibility that this is an autoimmune inflammatory disease doesn't come across the radar screens of many in the health care profession. And when you think about the amount of time that is devoted to teaching about these diseases? A medical student is lucky if they get one or two days where they are truly exposed to [them]."

If you have consistent and persistent complaints for which conventional treatments are of no help, it's important to start from the beginning, collect all your records, and work with your PCP to try to find a unifying diagnosis. Having a strong internist who actively coordinates your care is the best defense against the specialist shuffle.

Jennifer began the process of finding a new primary care physician while working with her doctors to carefully monitor her treatment.

"What's really helpful to me is, when I talk to Dr. Setoodeh, if I'm not feeling well, there are ways to manage it," she said. "We can decrease this or increase that, or get off Humira and try something else. To know that there's a way to manage my pain and there's someone who understands it— that knowledge is really important. Most of the time she's saying to me, 'We' should switch to this or 'We' should try this. It's not just 'Sorry, I can't do anything more for you.'"

Months after receiving her diagnosis, Jennifer decided to read through her own medical records. They were a revelation.

Prior to her enrollment in the speak-not-of-thy-aches pain-management program, a number of physicians at the program's hospital had reviewed her health history. One, a dermatologist, had noted in her case file that Jennifer *might* have psoriatic arthritis and even suggested putting her on medication. Jennifer also saw notes from a rheumatologist (even though she didn't recall ever meeting one) who disagreed. That doctor wrote that it was *very unlikely, though possible*, that she was suffering from the nascent stirrings of psoriatic arthritis and that *it should be watched*.

Jennifer was certain that no one ever talked to her about psoriatic arthritis. But who knows? It could have been relayed to her in twenty seconds during a fifteen-minute visit, nearly ten years ago. A simple records request can sometimes become the transformative event in your medical care. The fact that her internist never even inquired about her past records confirms to me that he failed her.

"I don't think I was taken seriously by my internist," Jennifer said. "I asked him at one point, 'Do you think it's anything like rheumatoid arthritis?' He said, 'No, you'd have a lot more swollen joints and pain than you do.' I thought, 'But I *do* have a lot of joint pain.' Recently I said to my psychiatrist, 'Maybe I wasn't clear enough?' She said, 'Stop kicking yourself. You're a patient. Your job is to report pain. That's all you had to do.'"

If only that were true. Far too often patients like Jennifer, who are not getting satisfaction, resist the idea of demanding better care and don't know how to find physicians who will help them reach their objectives. The fact that we are getting less quality time with our doctors only compounds the problem. But there is a solution: We can take the time to find a PCP who's the right fit, then act in a way that consistently gets their attention.

Your primary care physician is one of the most important people in your life. Probably not now, but one day, if you become seriously ill, you are going to need him or her to guide you through rough waters. On a scale of 1 to 10, how is your current relationship with your internist? Do you trust and respect her and feel comfortable telling her secrets that affect your health? Is he someone who, if you were experiencing a variety of symptoms, would have the tenacity to stay engaged until the two of you could wrap a diagnosis around the problem and determine the best treatment plan?

Nurturing that PCP relationship—through mutual trust, respect, and a shared interest in the science behind your care—means forging a bond with someone who will be invested in your well-being for the long haul.

Stop for a minute and ask yourself, *How did I choose my doctor?* Was it based on the recommendation of a friend? I hear this a lot: "I started seeing Dr. Williams because my brother-in-law goes to him and thinks he's great." Really? How do *you* know he's great? Maybe Dr. Williams is "great" because he's nice and doesn't bug your brother-in-law about his bulging waistline or his chewing-tobacco habit or those rising cholesterol numbers. Maybe he's great because he's a Cavaliers fan like your brother-in-law. Not the smartest way to judge a physician.

Remember how you (or your children, or that brainy neighbor kid) chose a college? You studied the best institutions for your major, made personal visits, applied to your top choices, and spoke to teachers and current students before you made a decision. I'm asking you to devote just half as much time and effort to finding the physician who will be the lifelong forensic detective of your health.

Let's say you've had back pain. Months later you get headaches and fatigue. If you don't feel comfortable calling your doctor, you may think, *Oh, I don't want to wait to get an appointment—he's always busy anyway. I'll just pop some aspirin.* You accept the pain. But a good physician who knows you, takes your calls, and has been paying attention will review your collection of symptoms to identify a likely underlying condition: depression. He knows you've suffered it in the past, or that it runs in your family. And he recognizes that depression often manifests as physical pain and fatigue. He'll take it very seriously and work with you on a course of treatment because, according to the latest studies, depression nearly doubles your risk of a stroke. (He'll also be aware that 23 percent of stroke victims suffer from post-traumatic stress disorder within a year of the incident, which would be a vicious cycle in your case.)

Here's another example on the pediatric front. Babies have a higher predisposition to meningitis than adults. Viral meningitis is fairly common—but bacterial meningitis? *That's* a clinical emergency. Hours matter. When your child is sick, if the pediatrician has seen little Jason a bunch of times, he's going to look at the boy and in twenty seconds say to himself, *I've got a whole room of kids with upper-respiratory infections sitting out there, but this one is different. I know this child, and he looks exceptionally sick. His mom is sharp, and she can tell something is really off. We need to get him to an emergency room* right now. It can be the difference between life and death.

Having a close relationship with a good primary care physician means you're not only comfortable going to him when you think something is wrong, you're also giving him the same confidence when he spots something that worries him and he wants to do tests, send you to a specialist, or get you to the hospital *now*. He will be able to say, "You know, this feels important. It's time to do something. I know it's going to disrupt your day, and you're not going to be happy about it. And I might be wrong. But I might be right." You are empowering your doctor to be at the top of his game—in a partnership that won't end when you walk out of his office, or even leave town.

Ben, a forty-two-year-old accountant, was vacationing in Australia when he developed an earache. On the first day of his trip, he had been free-diving down to about thirty-five feet, coming up a few times to catch a breath, hold his nose, and clear his ears.

Later that night he woke up his wife around four a.m. and said, "The smoke alarm is going off."

"What are you talking about?" she asked.

"The smoke alarm—you can't hear that?"

She couldn't hear a thing, which left Ben beyond confused. It turned out that the siren was in his inner left ear.

The next day Ben went to the island physician (a man whom Ben and his wife would later call the "voodoo doctor"). He examined Ben's ear, then pulled out a manual on how to diagnose and treat ear conditions. He flushed Ben's ear very hard with saline solution several times, then clogged it up with cotton balls and told Ben to avoid diving for a few days. *It should be fine now*, he said.

Of course, it wasn't fine. Two days later his left ear felt numb and had no hearing at all. He went back to the doctor, who just shrugged his shoulders.

Worried and distraught, but not trusting his own PCP back home whom he didn't have confidence in, Ben called a friend for advice and was put in touch with a good ear, nose, and throat doctor.

After listening to Ben describe his symptoms over the phone, the ENT said he had a hunch: "The good news is I'm pretty sure I know exactly what's wrong. The bad news? If I'm right, then flushing your ear with saline was the worst thing that doctor could have done."

Ben had an inner ear tear, likely caused by the pressure of diving and then clearing out his ears. The fluid in the inner ear, which aids in hearing, is finite; it doesn't replenish itself. The loss of liquid from the tear—and from the forceful flushing Ben had been subjected to—put him in danger of permanent auditory damage. He needed to be on a heavy-dose steroid regimen immediately to heal the tear fast.

The ENT coordinated with the island doctor to get Ben a prednisone prescription. To minimize the possibility of additional damage to his ear on his flight back, Ben was also coached on what to do during takeoff and landing, a routine that involved chewing gum and using Afrin nose spray. Ben saw the ENT as soon as he returned, and having followed all the instructions to a T, he retained about 95 percent hearing in his left ear.

"I realize now that you have to get to the right specialist, and the *only* way to get to that person is to go through a doctor who really knows you back home," Ben said. "You can't just ask the hotel. People do this all the time: Your kid is sick, you call the concierge, they send you to the nearest doctor. But that doctor has no idea who you are!" More dangerous, you have no idea who the local physician is or if he's any good.

People never think to call their PCP when they are traveling. But whether it's a torn inner ear in Australia, Montezuma's revenge in Mexico, or a sprained ankle in Italy, your doctor has no geographic constraints. If the relationship is there, they will be too, coaching you through it, no matter how far away you are.

"I find that more people get in trouble by not calling me than by calling me," says Dr. Eugene Sayfie, an internist, a cardiologist, an associate professor of medicine, and the medical director of the University of Miami Miller

School of Medicine's Executive Health Program. "I've talked to one patient four times today already."

In Ben's case, there was another reason he didn't call his own PCP. On a gut level, he didn't trust his internist's abilities. "He's nice," Ben said, "but he'd always be getting his books out—like the voodoo doctor—to look up diagnoses and treat me, instead of referring me."

Like Jennifer, Ben had simply stuck with a PCP who was pleasant and well intentioned. A doctor who was good enough—as long as the patient was healthy. It's what many people do, but it's no way to take care of yourself.

"People who aren't in charge of their health tend to wait for someone else to initiate things," Dr. Sayfie says. "I announce to every new patient that I'm a resource for them. I execute a health plan for the future for them. But I tell them that they are the major actor in this relationship and they are in charge of their health."

In 2012 I met Dr. Steven W. Tabak, a Johns Hopkins–trained cardiologist who previously served as the clinical chief of cardiology at Cedars-Sinai. Dr. Tabak had recently started pulling back from invasive cardiology to focus on preventive cardiology.

"When I first went into practice in 1983 . . . balloon angioplasty had just been developed in the late 1970s, and it was really the first time we could intervene on heart disease, short of surgery," Dr. Tabak recalled. "It was an exciting time to be in cardiology, but we were just putting out fires. I was seeing people with acute heart problems, and we were putting in the balloons, treating the heart attacks, when in fact, the treatment for this really should have started thirty years before with better lifestyle, maintaining lean body weight, exercising regularly, avoiding smoking.

"After having done probably ten thousand angiographic procedures, it was hard to get excited about doing the ten thousand and first case," he said. "But more important, I really thought that my role was more productive in preventing patients from getting to that point."

Now Dr. Tabak focuses on *preventing* heart disease.* "I think you have to look at medical care as a partnership, and it obviously involves an active

---

*Many PCPs have become experts on cardiovascular risk reduction because more than 30 percent of the deaths in America are a result of cardiovascular disease. Helping patients to lower the risk—by controlling cholesterol, weight, and stress, and by starting an exercise plan—is one of the greatest benefits a PCP can provide. If you are in danger of heart disease, having a PCP like Dr. Tabak—someone who is also a superb cardiologist—can be really helpful.

role of both the physician and the patient," he said. "As with anything, it really doesn't make sense to wait until you have an acute need to develop a relationship with a primary care physician. You want to have a long-standing relationship in place with a physician who really knows you and who can direct you as you move through the various stages of life and health care."

I would venture that 99 percent of internists begin their careers with the same level of compassion and commitment to patient care that Drs. Say-fie and Tabak demonstrate. But doctors are only human, and their jobs are harder than ever. That's why you need to understand their roles and to help them be their best. Think about your partnership with your PCP on three different levels:

PARTNERING WITH YOUR PRIMARY CARE PHYSICIAN: THE THREE LEVELS OF CARE

1. Ongoing care. This is the level most of us have experienced. Your doctor needs to be someone whom you trust, respect, and like. He or she should work diligently to help you accomplish your wellness goals and objectives. That means being dogged about getting you in for your physical exams, and putting you through, at the appropriate ages and intervals, early-detection and preventive measures such as mammography, colonoscopy, and PSA tests, as well as blood pressure, cholesterol, and dermatological checks. These are the tools they use to help prevent (and catch) disease before it takes hold.

2. Committed attention for a serious illness. The second level kicks in when you have a problem. Whether the pain you are experiencing in your shoulder is orthopedic, neurological, or something else; whether your fatigue is because of dietary, cardiac, pulmonology, psychological, or other issues—your PCP has to consider the possibilities until he determines where your issue lies. He may not get it right the first time, or the second or third time. But that doesn't necessarily mean he is making mistakes. It's a discovery process.

In the best-case scenario, you have a terrific PCP who will proceed efficiently to a preliminary diagnosis, or to a realm of specialty, based on a medical history and a physical—and *then* use blood tests, imaging, and other diagnostic studies for confirmation.

Your PCP's role is to figure out the precise realm of medicine in which your illness exists, then refer you to a specialist in that area who can carry on the detective work and confirm a diagnosis. She should be accessible to your specialist if she has questions; and she or her staff should be monitoring your progress after a serious illness, weighing the need for additional care.

Sometimes the search for an accurate diagnosis is long and arduous, no matter how good the doctor is, and sometimes you'll nail it on the first educated guess. But it's essential not to cut the process short and hurl toward a false diagnosis and unnecessary treatment plan. The further you go down the wrong treatment path, the more difficult it is to turn around and get back to the fundamental cause of your problem.

3. Care that supports the work of an expert. The third tier of your PCP's role comes into play after a specialist has definitively identified your condition. That's when your doctor should work with you to help coordinate your care, referring you to the surgeon or specialist with the narrowest and deepest expertise in the specific problem you have. Sometimes that's the same person who confirmed your diagnosis. But other times—and especially with rare diseases like what Catherine was facing—you may need to dig deeper for a next-level expert, someone who has seen every iteration of your potential illness.

Jennifer, for example, is finally out of the realm of orthopedics (where her internist mistakenly placed her) and into autoimmune disorders. And within that specialty, she has two superior doctors (rheumatologist Dr. Setoodeh, in California, and psoriatic arthritis expert Dr. Mease, in Washington State) who care deeply about her well-being. That's excellence in care. And a top-notch PCP could have gotten her there. If she'd had one, she wouldn't have needed me.

If you don't have a primary care physician at all, it's like driving without a seatbelt. But in the next chapter, I'll give you clear steps to take in order to find the best doctor for you. If you already have a doctor you like and want to build on that relationship, you'll learn some surprisingly effective ways to better engage with him or her, as well as interesting advice from top physicians, including one internist who is truly sorry to have overslept her alarm clock and kept you waiting.

QUICK GUIDE

CHAPTER 1. Why Having the Right Primary Care Physician Will Change Your Life

- Forging a strong partnership with a sharp primary care physician is one of the most important first steps you can take in protecting your health.

- If you have a persistent problem that can't be helped by conventional treatments, start from the beginning, collect all your records, and work with your PCP to try to find a unifying diagnosis. Having a strong internist who actively coordinates your care is the best defense against the specialist shuffle.

- Make the time and effort to find a PCP who will be your lifelong health partner.

- If the relationship is there, your PCP will be there for you, coaching you through treatment, no matter how far away you are. If you have a problem while you're traveling, call your PCP.

- Let the three levels of care—(1) ongoing care, (2) committed attention for a serious illness, and (3) care that supports the work of an expert—guide the way you think about your partnership with your PCP.

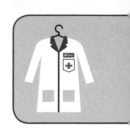

CHAPTER TWO

HOW TO FIND THE BEST PRIMARY CARE PHYSICIAN FOR YOU

. . . or develop a better relationship with the one you have. Plus: advice from doctors on dealing with them

Due for her annual physical, Nicole made an appointment with her primary care physician, who had recently left a group practice to open her own office.

"I had been to her a few times before," Nicole recalled. "She was nice, and I decided to stay with her when she moved."

Nicole was used to waiting twenty to thirty minutes before being called in to see her doctor, so she was pleasantly surprised when she was taken to an exam room in half the time. Then she sat there alone, wearing nothing but a paper gown, for forty-five minutes. "Not a single person checked on me," she said.

Even worse, Nicole could hear the doctor examining a patient in the next room. The walls were so thin and poorly insulated, she was privy to every personal detail. "I realized then," she said, "that they would be able to hear my whole medical history, too."

Frustrated and bewildered after nearly an hour of staring at the ceiling, she finally dressed, marched to the front desk, and informed the receptionist that she would not wait any longer. She was leaving.

Who are you? came the response.

Nicole is a savvy health care consumer. Yet when she shared her story with me, she was perplexed about her own behavior that day. *Why* had she waited so long to be seen? She'd never sit for forty-five minutes at a restaurant table, hoping to be noticed. But when it comes to health care, we accept all manner of poor attention.

Nicole waited because she was sensitive to the fact that doctors today have less time in which to treat more patients. And yet deep down, she knew this scenario was a big red flag. "On some level, I was thinking, 'How can this really be happening?'" she said.

Many patients, when they step into a medical building, leave their values at the door and behave as if they were powerless. Some take on a docile "Yes, doctor, whatever you say" demeanor. Others are in a rush to get in and out; they don't bring their A-game to the conversation, take notes about their doctor's recommendations, or ask pertinent questions.

But Nicole's experience with her PCP was rife with problems that weren't of her making. She hadn't been informed that the doctor was behind schedule; nobody checked on her during her long wait; and given the poor exam room design, she had no expectation of privacy.

"The worst part is, I got an e-mail from the doctor that night—an e-mail, not a phone call—and it was six hours later," Nicole said. "Which to me means her staff didn't think it was important to knock on her office door to say, 'Your patient just walked out.'"

In the doctor's correspondence (written on the fly from her iPhone, as evidenced by the signature line), she apologized, explaining that she'd had to make an unexpected visit to a patient in the hospital. "She blamed it on an emergency," Nicole said, "yet I could hear her in the other room with someone else, and then she just went back to her office. If I'm looking for somebody to be in my corner and really be an advocate for my health, this doctor is clearly not the person."

At least Nicole understands that she is free to hire and fire, so to speak, the PCP of her choice. I recently spoke to a twenty-seven-year-old woman who was unhappy with her seventy-year-old primary care doctor. At her most recent physical, he had chided her for not having married and started a family. As she left that day, reeling over his unwanted comments, he waved good-bye while good-naturedly whispering, *Tick tock, tick tock*—a not-so-subtle implication about her waning reproductive years.

She knew she should find a new physician, not just because of his ignorance and insensitivity but also because getting to his office involved a hundred-mile drive. Yet she had continued seeing him because he was the hometown doctor she'd been with since childhood, and she felt bad about leaving. Plus, the idea of looking for someone new seemed overwhelming to her. "Where do you begin to look?" she said. "And how do you know if they are any good?"

Finding a talented internist can be a daunting task. The standard ways to seek out a specialist just don't exist for PCPs. In many ways, the process is the opposite, as you have to think first about the characteristics in a doctor that are important to you.

As silly as it sounds, among the things people consider—age, training, gender—when choosing a physician, fashion is often an influential factor. According to a 2005 study published in the *American Journal of Medicine*, four hundred men and women were shown photos of physicians in four different styles of dress. Some three-fourths of the study participants said they wanted to see their physician in professional clothing, complete with the white coat. They reported that they'd be more likely to share their problems with a doctor who was dressed this way. Less than 5 percent chose the physician who was dressed casually.

If you don't have a primary care physician, or if you are certain you need to change yours, there's a process to choosing an internist wisely. (And checking out his or her wardrobe may not be the most important part of it.) Just as you would take your time buying a car and test-drive a few models before making an investment, there are steps you should take before selecting the doctor in whom you will invest your health.

Haley, thirty-nine, was happy with the obstetrician-gynecologist who had been overseeing her care for several years, but she had never had a physical exam and was starting to have fears about melanoma, breast cancer, and heart disease—all the conditions that were beginning to crop up in the lives of friends. Plus, as a new mom, she wanted to live long enough to see her daughter's children grow up. She was ready to find a primary care physician and asked me to help her devise a plan of attack.

The three-step plan I gave Haley is the same process I want you to follow, but you should feel free to adapt the goals and questions to fit your needs. I promise that if you do these three things, you will find a doctor who is right for you.

THREE STEPS TO FINDING A GREAT PRIMARY CARE PHYSICIAN

1. Make a list of what's important to you in a PCP.
2. Gather recommendations from people whose opinions you trust.
3. Set up meetings with the doctors at the top of your list to ask questions, collect information, and get a feel for their philosophy, style, and practice.

For Haley, Step 1 was groundbreaking. At first it seemed strange to her to commit to paper what *she* wanted in a doctor and what she *expected* that person to do for her. But then a lightbulb went on. "It was exciting to create a wish list for my health," she said. "Like, all of a sudden I realized, 'Wait, I deserve these things. And there's a doctor out there whose job it is to help me achieve them.'"

Haley's wish list for a PCP started with one who could give her a thorough medical baseline on things like her cholesterol levels, blood pressure, and EKG, and a skin cancer screening, just to see if there was anything brewing she needed to keep an eye on. She also wanted a doctor who was intelligent, up-to-date on the literature, and a good listener. Gender wasn't a concern, but she preferred a physician in her insurance network (she was in a PPO plan through her husband's employer) with visiting privileges at the two hospitals nearest her.

Here's how Haley handled Step 2, gathering recommendations. First she called the doctors she already knew and liked and asked them to make suggestions. And since all doctors *have* doctors, I told her to ask who their internists were.

Haley was nervous about calling her ob-gyn for a PCP recommendation. "What if he says, 'Oh, I can be your primary care physician'?" she asked.

Although that was unlikely, I told her the answer is a very polite "Thank you, but I really want an internist. That's what I'm looking for."

How much or how little you want to divulge when you call your own doctors is up to you. But if you are intimidated by the idea of starting the conversation or are unsure of what to ask, here's what Haley said when she got her ob-gyn's office manager on the phone:

"I'm looking for a really good primary care physician. I've never had one before, and I'm in the process of getting recommendations from people whose opinions I trust. Would Dr. Garcia recommend anyone for me? And also—if he doesn't mind saying—would he tell me who he sees?"

To her surprise, she was given three names on the spot—including the internist her ob-gyn saw—plus reasons why they were good doctors.

Next she called her daughter's pediatrician, who gave her the names of two doctors, including his own. He even called her back later that day to pass along an additional contact, Dr. Philip M. Bretsky, an internist whom he had never met but had heard several patients praising in the last few months.

Haley soon discovered that *Who's your doctor?* isn't a nosy question at all; it's a potent conversation starter. Everybody had something to offer. She quizzed friends and acquaintances about whom they liked and why. If someone said they "really, really" loved their primary care physician, she took special note.

Since Haley wanted a doctor who was in her insurance network, she cross-referenced the names on her list of recommendations with her provider's online database until she narrowed it down to four candidates, including one who was out of network but was so highly recommended, she decided to keep him in the mix.

Before Haley undertook Step 3, setting up the meetings, she checked online with her state's medical licensing board to make sure each doctor was legally licensed to practice in her state (they were) and had no formal disciplinary actions against them (they did not). It's imperative that you do the same before you meet with any potential new physician. (One way to do this is via the directory of state medical and osteopathic boards on the Federation of State Medical Boards' website, at bit.ly/1tXd4a8. From there, click the link to your state's medical licensing body; then from that site, click on the "Look up" or "Verify a license" option, and type in your physician's name.) She also confirmed that the doctors on her list were board certified. As opposed to licensing, which is required to practice medicine, board certification is voluntary; it means that the doctor took extra exams and assessments and participates in the continuing education required for board certification. (A quick check at CertificationMatters.org, a service of the American Board of Medical Specialties, will determine if your doctors are board certified; free registration is required.)

At this point, Haley almost took the easy road and considered skipping the interviews. With a toddler and a busy work schedule, she didn't have a lot of time to consult with physicians, and the first doctor on her list already

HMO VS. PPO: NOT ALL INSURANCE IS CREATED EQUAL

As you begin your search for a primary care physician, you may find that your current insurance plan is putting a serious crimp in your candidate list.

Health maintenance organizations, or HMOs, can be an appealing option, with low to no deductibles and co-pays, but they come with a limited selection of PCPs. And in most HMOs, the PCP serves as a gatekeeper: in order to see a specialist, you must first visit your PCP, and if your illness merits further attention, you'll be referred within the HMO to a doctor who may not be your first choice.

Preferred provider organizations, or PPOs, cost more to join, with higher deductibles and co-payments. In return, you get a wider selection of PCPs to choose from, and you can visit an in-network specialist of your choice (typically without preauthorization), or an out-of-network doctor at a higher cost to you. Obviously, if you're choosing between an HMO and a PPO, you will have more freedom of choice in a PPO.

And yet . . . even within these organizations, there can be great variation. Not every PPO confers carte blanche status. Likewise, there are excellent HMOs—like Kaiser Permanente, the largest and oldest traditional HMO, with most of its patients in the western United States. And a growing number of accountable care organizations provide outstanding preventive services and care for the most common conditions.

The bottom line: Before you commit to *any* insurance plan, carefully review the policy's limitations; consider the size and quality of physicians in the network; find out if it excludes any of the major academic hospitals in your area (that would be a nonstarter for me); and verify with your primary care physician's staff that you are selecting a plan that will allow you to continue to develop this most important relationship.

seemed pretty great: he was a ten-minute drive from her house and came highly recommended by two relatives. Yet deep down she knew this was an incredibly important decision, with long-term consequences. So instead of disrupting her life, she simply slowed the process down and scheduled doctor visits every few weeks, when it was convenient. It took about three months, but in the end her efforts were rewarded.

I encourage you not to skimp on meeting possible doctors. Take your time and explore all your options. Another way to look at it is: If you're spending a fortune remodeling a kitchen, you don't hire the first contractor recommended to you, and you certainly don't hire him without a consult. If you're seeking a nanny, you want to get a sense of her demeanor and ask about her experience and child-rearing philosophy. If you move and would like to find a new place of worship, you'd probably collect several recommendations, get a feel for the congregations at each, and be sure that the teachings and sermons are a fit with your values before committing to a lifelong relationship. Your choice of internist deserves this much thought and care.

Had Haley simply picked the first doctor on her list, sight unseen, as she had been tempted to do, she likely would have received fine care. But she would have soon realized that this person was a family practice physician rather than a board-certified internist. Family practice doctors have broad knowledge about treating everyone from kids to grandparents; internists focus on internal medicine and nonsurgical care for adults. While both are well qualified, the distinction was important to Haley, who wanted an internist. (I generally advise adult clients to select internists as their PCPs, just as children should see pediatricians. But is every internist better than a family practitioner? Of course not! There are some extraordinary family practitioners. The important point is to find someone with whom you have chemistry, and whose skills you trust.)

Furthermore, the doctor's practice was owned by a major local hospital that was not one of Haley's preferred institutions, and the doctor did not have visiting privileges. Hospitals' acquiring successful practices is becoming more common, and it can be a great boon in some ways: record sharing and coordination among caregivers is improved; doctors are on salary rather than a fee-for-service model (which can sometimes contribute to patients getting more treatment than they need). But in Haley's case it meant, as it often does, that her PCP would not be the one who treated her if she landed in the hospital. Instead, she would be seen by a hospitalist, a doctor who cares for patients only while they are in the hospital. (It's advisable to select a PCP who has admitting privileges in your preferred hospital, so that he or she can visit and treat you if needed.) Luckily, Haley pressed on, setting up appointments with the four doctors on her list to learn more about each.

It's important to address the issue of reimbursement here. Insurers usually will not pay for a meet-and-greet. Haley knew that her insurer would cover only one physical exam per year, so she had to be clear when she called to set up appointments that this was not that annual exam—she was simply searching for a new PCP.

In each case, Haley stated her objectives on the phone: "I'm looking for a new internist, and Dr. Smith came very highly recommended. I'm wondering if it's possible to schedule a consult, just to meet with her and ask questions, and see if it's a fit for us both. I'm not interested in a physical exam at this time; I'd just like to sit with her for a few minutes. I'm meeting with a few different doctors before I make a decision."

She also reminded the staff of her situation when she came to the office, to make sure they understood that this was not a physical and should not be coded as such for reimbursement under her insurance plan.

In the end, one doctor billed her insurer for a consultation about Haley's fatigue, which was fair, since they discussed this issue and the doctor made recommendations. Two doctors didn't use her insurance plan at all but simply scheduled her when it was most convenient to them. The fourth doctor, who didn't take insurance, conducted meet-and-greets free of charge, so billing was not an issue.

Although Haley was willing to pay out of pocket for the doctors' time and said as much, no one asked her to. Your experience may be different, depending on your insurance and how the doctors you meet decide to approach your visit. But you'll need to consider ahead of time how much you are willing and able to spend on your PCP search. And you may encounter doctors who can't or won't take the time to meet you, whether it's because they have an overcrowded practice, financial constraints of their own, or a simple lack of interest in the process.

As Haley met with the doctors on her list, she found them all very capable in different ways, but none of them wowed her like Dr. Bretsky, the physician her daughter's pediatrician had recommended.

Dr. Bretsky, an internist in his early forties, was in Haley's insurance network, with visiting privileges at both of her top-choice hospitals. His office was impeccably run, with electronic medical records, appointment reminders via text and automated phone calls, and a friendly and efficient staff, including a talented physician assistant, whom Haley would come to rely on for telephone consults, walk-in appointments, and the treatment of simple ailments.

During their initial thirty-minute meeting in a sunny exam room, Haley asked Dr. Bretsky specific questions about his patient care philosophy.

She learned he was a voracious reader, familiar with the latest evidence on the most prevalent cancers in women her age; he was a big believer in getting second opinions; he preferred to refer patients to the best specialists for their specific conditions, not just to colleagues who practiced at the same hospitals he did; he was sensitive to the way some specialists overtreat; and he talked about sitting with patients after a specialist visit to "bring them back to center" and discuss what the diagnosis means for them. He also described the annual exam process and the additional tests he would recommend for someone of her age and family history.

"He just hit all my wish-list items and was really open and warm, while still being kind of a data geek, interested in sharing the relevant facts and stats concerning my questions," Haley said. She had been through enough interviews by then to feel comfortable listening and evaluating *everything* going on in the doctor's office. And what really clinched it for her was something that happened while she was still in the waiting room.

"Before we even met," she recalled, "I heard him talking to a staffer, asking her to investigate a report on one of his patients. He said, 'I need you to find out more about these labs, because I did not see this patient, and I did not order these tests.' He sounded stern, and everyone really stepped to it, making calls and checking records. I was impressed. To me, it meant that they respected his sense of urgency on the matter and also that he was paying close attention to his patients' care. He wouldn't let things slip through the cracks."

People sometimes ask, *How can I judge whether this is a good doctor?* Don't start from the position that you *can't* judge—that's disabling the intuitive sensors that you use in other parts of your life. Flick that switch to the "on" position, and you'll pick up all kinds of signals. In the interview process, you need to judge these physicians the same way you'd judge the teacher who will school your first grader or the lawyer who is going to write up your will. There may not be a right or wrong answer, but if you pose the same questions to different doctors, you'll hear *different* answers. Collect all the data, and once you've met with everyone on your list, the path will become clear. Your gut will tell you whom to choose, and you will be right.

So what are *you* looking for in a PCP? I would advise against creating a list based on criteria such as educational pedigree (which is more important when it comes to choosing specialists), associations the doctor is affiliated with (any physician can pay to belong to the Association of This and That), or the number of articles published (again, this matters more in evaluating a specialist).

Your list of what's important in a PCP will be personal to your health care needs. But to give you some guidance, here are the five musts that I share with friends and clients, as well as questions to ask during the interview process to learn more about a doctor's practice.

FIVE IMPORTANT TRAITS TO LOOK FOR IN A PRIMARY CARE PHYSICIAN

1. Someone you can have a personal relationship with. If you are worried about a fever, a lump, or chronic fatigue, you want a PCP you'll feel comfortable calling. If you're finding, as you get through the afternoon, that you desperately need one or two or three vodkas—and you know that's not a good thing—you'll want a doctor who will help, not judge. If, at some point, you face important treatment decisions that require a balancing act, you really want a PCP who gets involved in the decision-making process—someone who understands you and whose judgment you respect. To gauge your chemistry with a potential new doctor, ask the following questions, listen carefully, and trust your gut. You'll know by the way she comports herself if she is someone you will like.

"Tell me about yourself."

"I am really empathetic to the fact that it's become more difficult for doctors to spend enough time with their patients. How have you dealt with this challenge in your own practice?"

"I am looking for someone to be a partner in my wellness. What's your philosophy on patient care?"

2. Someone whose practice is organized so that you are seen in a timely fashion and for as long as it takes. This may mean the PCP is supported by a nurse practitioner or physician's assistant. Another consideration: Do you want to see the same doctor every visit? If so, you may want a solo practitioner. But if it's more important that you are able to get an appointment right away, then a group practice is a safer bet.

Keep in mind that a really caring PCP is apt to overbook, never saying no when sick patients call and beg to be seen. A longer wait time can be a small price to pay for a talented PCP who will always squeeze you in. But if you find yourself waiting for ninety minutes, listening to ringing phones that don't get answered, and the receptionist has no idea who you are—you may be waiting for the greatest doctor ever, but this is not the place that's going to be able to handle your case efficiently if you are seriously ill and need special attention.

ASK "What's your availability like?"

"If I become ill during the evenings or weekends, who will I talk to?"

"Do you have a partner who covers for you?"

3. Someone who directs you to the appropriate specialists and makes sure you are seen as soon as necessary. You need a PCP who takes seriously his responsibility for that next step, when your condition is one he is not equipped to handle. Remember the internist who looked at Jennifer's X-rays, diagnosed her with arthritis, and prescribed ibuprofen? He failed to accept that her problem was beyond his ken. When she still complained of pain, he sent her to a foot doctor, then a shoulder surgeon. You want a PCP who doesn't

just dispatch your case to someone else: "Here's the dermatologist I send everybody to. Next!" You want an internist who will continue searching for answers when you have a challenging issue that isn't easily resolved.

"How do you assist your patients with getting timely access to specialists?"

"Can you tell me about your referral network?"

"How do you match your patients to the right experts?"

Did you notice that these are all pretty similar, softball questions? In truth, the questions you ask are not that important. You just want to get the doctor talking about how he makes referrals. And you want to hear an answer that conveys that he regards this as a very important part of his job. For instance, Dr. Bretsky told Haley that his referral decisions really hinge on the patient and the problem. If she was suffering from condition X, there was a guy across town who was doing great work in that arena; for condition Y, he felt that the nearby university hospital had an excellent program that was making strides. And he also considered the patient-doctor personality fit. "Sometimes it happens that I'll send a patient for additional consultation with somebody who I think is good and thorough, but then the patient has a terrible experience, and we need to retool and find a better solution," Dr. Bretsky said. In other words, he focuses on *the patient's needs.*

What do you not want to hear as an answer? *I've got ten doctors I've worked with for twenty years.* Or *I wouldn't worry about referrals; we work with the best doctors in the city.* No, you want an acknowledgment that this is an important task and not an easy thing to do.

4. **Someone who understands the importance of coordinating with specialists.** Internists collaborate with hundreds of other physicians, referring out to rheumatologists, orthopedists, dermatologists, surgeons, and so on. Think of the complexity of interfacing with that

many practitioners. It's no wonder that medical errors, most of them due to human slipups, are so common.

You want to find out how the doctor will coordinate with other physicians. If she says, *Well, I'll get a consultation letter and put it in your file*—wrong answer. Interview more candidates, and see if anybody says anything different. You need to be sure that if you get a diagnostic test done with any outside provider, your PCP will be available to discuss the results with you. Some have a rule: *You hear from us only if there is an abnormal finding.* But the data show that 7 percent of the times in which something is wrong, it *does not* get reported back to the patient. In some practices, the rate is as high as 26 percent.

"When I see a specialist, how do you coordinate with them?"

"What will you do if I get diagnostic testing done? Does someone call me with the results?"

"How will you and I be in dialogue about my illness once I'm being treated by a specialist?"

5. Finally, you want a PCP who is committed to your wellness and health care objectives. You are looking for someone who shares your goals, and will be meticulous about getting you the early-detection and preventive measures you should have—things like mammograms, colonoscopies, PSA tests, blood pressure and cholesterol checks, and dermatological screenings.

If you smoke, you should ask your PCP for help in quitting. I've seen some wonderful doctors nudge and encourage their patients to start smoking-cessation programs or diet and exercise regimens— and get passionately invested in their success. They know that many people just need the importance of this change explained to them, as well as some guidance, in order to get motivated. Of course, not all doctors will feel comfortable being this emphatic about their patients' personal habits. But if that level of input is valuable to you, be sure to let your potential internist know.

"What systems do you have in place to ensure that I'm getting the proper early-detection and prevention tests?"

"How long is a typical physical exam, and what is the process like? Are there any additional tests I would need based on my age, gender, and medical background?"

"I've had a lifelong battle with [weight, tobacco, inactivity—pick your vice]. And there are some years where I'm better than others. My hope is to find a doctor who can help me in that battle."

Notice how that last one isn't even a question. Just listen to the reply, and ask yourself, *Is this a person who will blow the whistle on me when I fall behind?* If this goal is important to you—if it's on your Step 1 list—then you deserve a doctor who really pushes you to win this battle. Listen for a response that is something along the lines of *You know, I think weight is a really important determinant of health, and I appreciate that you mentioned it. One of the things I'm going to want to do with you is get you in here once a year, and if there's more than a ten-pound weight gain in a particular year, we're going to have a serious talk about it.* I'd be very happy with that response or any variation that conveys *I'm with you; I'm your partner on this.* And not *Everybody's weight varies over time, it's not that big a deal.*

When a client asks me for a primary care physician recommendation, I occasionally hear something along the lines of "I want a female doctor who's less than a mile from my house, won't make me wait longer than ten minutes, will spend as much time with me as I need, and is in my insurance network."

That's an assertive patient! But it is also pretty much mission impossible. The unfortunate truth is, if you want or need a PCP who can give you an abundance of quality time at the drop of a hat, then you should expect to pay extra for it. The current health care reimbursement model just doesn't allow internists the luxury of giving you as much attention as they want to. I've heard stories of doctors in group- or hospital-owned practices being financially penalized if they are spending too much time on a single patient.

It's sad but true. And it's why primary care doctors are increasingly moving to direct-pay and concierge medicine models.

A direct-pay model works the old-fashioned way: the patient pays the doctor for services rendered; insurance is not accepted. In a concierge model, the practice collects an annual or monthly fee directly from the patient, which is not reimbursed by insurance. Sometimes that fee is all-inclusive and covers the cost of office visits; often it's an additional charge, like a membership fee. Some concierge practices don't accept any insurance plans; others take both insurance and direct payments from patients. There are many different styles (and quality is not guaranteed—you still have to do your homework!), but the main aim of all these models is greater attention spent on you. That might mean you get same-day appointments, cell phone and e-mail access, and more comprehensive annual exams.

If your problems become so geometrically complex that you need more time and focused reflection from your PCP—and if you can summon the financial resources—then you might want to consider a direct-pay or concierge-style practice. (Just to be clear: When it comes to *specialists*, you can still get some of the best care possible using in-network physicians who practice at major hospitals and academic medical institutions.) It might mean forgoing that annual family vacation, or ditching hopes for a bigger home or apartment, but you have to ask yourself which is worth more to you. If, on the other hand, you can't afford it, or maybe you are in great health and the worst thing that can happen to you is a sprained ankle on a hiking trail, spending the extra money on a private PCP doesn't make much sense.

Let me assure you, no matter where you are on the health spectrum, if you follow the lessons in this book, you will get far better care and outcomes, you will empower your doctor to do more for you, and you will distinguish yourself as a thoughtful and proactive patient. Which sometimes means being aware that it's more difficult nowadays for PCPs to operate as if they had all the time in the world. If you are sensitive to their time constraints and work harder to maximize the time you have together, you and your PCP can forge a wonderful partnership.

Some patients who are getting older face challenging medical issues, or have multiple diseases and must coordinate among several doctors, and may find it difficult to meet their PCPs halfway. Likewise, patients with chronic illnesses or predispositions—such as being highly allergic or having a sup-pressed immune system or an underlying hereditary condition—may desire a PCP who can be more intimately involved in their care. If that's you, and you can afford private care—and I know for most Americans that's a big *if*—then it's a decision that deserves consideration.

One good example comes to mind.

Stephanie, sixty-seven, came to me with a cluster of symptoms: out-of-control blood pressure, gastro-reflux issues, leg cramps, and a gallbladder condition (swelling and infection for which she'd had surgery, but it still wasn't being managed properly). Years earlier she'd had Lyme disease, which was misdiagnosed as a psychological issue. With a family history of heart disease, she feared her aching limbs were a precursor to a heart attack.

Stephanie had been seeing the same PCP for twenty years, and when he announced he was retiring, she found a new one, who was based in her small town. On her third or fourth visit, the doctor asked, *Have I seen you before?*

It was clear that Stephanie was in the throes of a primary care disaster. A friend told her about Dr. Bryan J. Arling, an internist who practices in Washington, D.C.

At their first meeting, an exhausted Stephanie told him straight out: "Listen, I was raised to think doctors were gods, but I've had a lot of bad experiences over the last few years, and none of those doctors listened to me." Dr. Arling responded that he believed patients often know their bodies better than physicians, and he asked her to describe her health history and her goals. He listened for the next hour as she carefully unspooled her medical tale.

In their second hour together, Dr. Arling performed a complete physical exam, explaining each step as he went. In the third hour, his staff came in, drew blood, and did more tests, including a hearing test, something Stephanie had never been given before.

"I had been noticing more and more that I couldn't hear the television," Stephanie said later. "The volume used to be on twenty, but recently my husband walked in and asked why the TV was on so loud. I had it on forty-three! They discovered that I needed a hearing aid."

Things like hearing and eyesight, for most people, erode very gradually over time so we tend to adapt, not realizing how much ground we've lost. A thoughtful physician will do proper testing at the right intervals so that he can improve your situation—whether that entails a hearing aid or blood pressure medication.

Dr. Arling also sent Stephanie to a top cardiologist to explore her heart concerns. Instead of an invasive coronary-angiogram procedure, which her previous doctor had recommended, they altered her diet and exercise, adding vitamins and calcium that successfully alleviated her leg cramps. "I'm taking a low dose of blood pressure medication, and my cholesterol is the lowest it's been since the nineties," she told me. "I'm ecstatic. He's calmed my fears."

Dr. Arling isn't Superman in a white coat, fitting forty hours into a single day. He simply doesn't take any insurance, and Stephanie pays per visit, out of pocket, for his time.

"We always tell new patients that it's going to be between one and two thousand dollars a year," says Dr. Arling, "so they have a framework to build on. We've met all the criteria that are necessary so that Medicare will honor our prescriptions, so that we can get MRIs, we can refer you to specialists, we can hospitalize you. But we don't bill for time on the phone. We don't bill for weekend calls. We bill only for services that happen in our office."

For Stephanie, choosing a PCP who did not take insurance was a very personal decision on her part, based on her dismal history. Her health had suffered to the point where she knew she needed more time and attention than she was getting. She had the financial resources and decided to invest in a physician who could oblige.

But let me reiterate: You don't need to go out of network to find a good PCP (and you certainly don't have to when it comes to specialists). I firmly believe that you can get a higher quality of health care in the United States than any place else even if all you have is an insurance card—but only *if* you assert yourself as a consumer, resolve to make your well-being a priority, and follow the lessons in this book about how to find the best doctors and treatment options.

So what if you like and respect your current doctor but want more from him or her? Start the process the same way you would with literally any other kind of relationship. Be clear about your objectives, and then, in the context of your next appointment, let your doctor know. You could say:

What's important to me is to be able to spend a little more time telling you about my health and my collection of symptoms, as I think we've missed some clues, and I'd be grateful if we could try to solve this together.

Or maybe:

Doctor, I have a new goal that I really need your advice and guidance on. I'm hoping to lessen my dependence on cholesterol medication, and I want to begin a weight-loss and exercise program. Can you help me?

Adjustments are essential throughout life, whether it's with a spouse, a friend, or a work colleague—every relationship changes. Your health care needs will change over time, too. Be courageous enough to share them with a physician you trust. And if you get a negative response? Maybe this is not the right doctor for you. Better to know that now than when you've got a lump in your breast. When you're healthy, that's the time to learn about the strength of your PCP relationship and whether he or she will be there for you when you really need support.

People sometimes say, *I really love my doctor, but should I be looking for someone else? Because he's just not the type to push me to work out more* or *help me to quit smoking* or *call me personally to explain my cholesterol readings.* Just because someone doesn't meet all the criteria on your list doesn't mean they're not a good fit for you. You absolutely have the power to judge whether your doctor is a keeper. Of course, there are a few circumstances in which you can say with certainty that it's time to change PCPs.

THREE SIGNS THAT IT'S TIME TO FIND A NEW PCP

1. You experienced a preventable error under your PCP's care. Some patients endure internist-induced errors that are grounds for changing doctors. The two most common examples I see that rise to this level are (1) a PCP writing a prescription for the wrong drug; (2) a PCP failing to report test results that came back with an abnormal finding. Both of these things can be potentially disastrous to your health. But you owe it to your physician to have a conversation with him about it. Maybe there were missteps by staff, never brought to the PCP's attention, and he may not even know anything bad hap-

pened to you. If, on the other hand, the office seems chaotic, and there's constant employee turnaround—take it as a sign that this medical team isn't capable of looking out for you the way you need.

2. You cannot get timely access to care. When you're feeling *really* bad, you should be able to see your internist or her support staff in a reasonable time frame, say within a day or so. For example, if you are fighting a severe flu and end up driving yourself to urgent care or the ER merely because you couldn't get your own doctor to return your calls, that's not okay. Obviously, for sudden emergencies, you *should* go to the ER for immediate attention. But if you're sneezing, coughing, and have severe gastrointestinal distress, and it takes three days for someone to get back to you—that's a real problem. She may be a great doctor, but she isn't set up to care for you in a timely fashion.

3. Your PCP's communication style is disrespectful and dismissive. There are many reasons why patients don't reach out to their PCPs when they have a problem. Maybe they're reluctant to ask for help, or they're just distrustful of doctors to start. But some patients avoid their PCPs because every interaction ends in a disrespectful dismissal of their complaints and symptoms. This is not good. If a patient has been having piercing headaches, a doctor who isn't really listening might say, *You're probably just under a lot of stress—I see several patients a week with the same problem. Here's a prescription that should help.* This falls under the "Take two aspirin and call me in the morning" trope. In contrast, a thoughtful PCP will listen to your complaints, ask pertinent questions about your symptoms, perform diagnostic tests, and perhaps do more in-depth testing if your status and symptoms merit it. If she doesn't find anything that gives her pause, she may say something more like *Look, these are relatively minor symptoms, and they could mean a lot of different things. But you don't fit the profile for any of these, and I'd like to avoid prescribing anything stronger than ibuprofen if we can. If your headaches continue for more than a week, or if they get worse, I want you to come back in right away, and we can walk through some different tests and scenarios.* That's a caring doctor.

　　If your doctor constantly interrupts you, doesn't let you finish explaining what's wrong, or makes you feel that your own reporting of your health problems is not vital to his viewpoint, then he is disabling the partnership, and this is not a relationship you should continue. You want to feel comfortable talking with your PCP. His office should be a safe haven, a space to be honest and open. And the only way that happens is if the doctor is listening to you carefully, responds respectfully, and explains his view.

In my experience, most physicians—and particularly PCPs—went into the practice of medicine to develop strong emotional bonds with people and help them through health challenges. If you present yourself as someone who wishes to really move forward with a program focused on well-being, reducing risk factors, and identifying disease earlier rather than later, that gives your doctor an opportunity for the kind of satisfaction that attracted her to the medical profession. If you walk in and persuade her that *you* are that patient, I think you're going to get some tremendously concentrated and favorable attention, because she has the *same* need for a satisfying relationship. Patients don't really know that. But doctors do. In fact, in a 2012 survey of more than thirteen thousand American physicians, 80 percent cited "patient relationships" as the most satisfying aspect of their medical practice. The second-most-cited factor, at 70 percent, was "intellectual stimulation." Only 12 percent chose "financial rewards."

A WORD FROM THE DOCTORS: WHAT TO LOOK FOR IN A PCP

For a 180-degree view, I asked some talented physicians for their advice on finding and developing a strong bond with a PCP. Their answers provide valuable insights about what it's like on the other side of the exam table—and they're a reminder of the fact that doctors, like all of us, have biases and foibles. They get frustrated with the increasing time pressure. And they occasionally sleep through their alarm clocks, too.

> "I consider it a personal failure if a longtime patient of mine has a heart attack. The medications and the lifestyle changes I can personally help them make are so good—whether it's exercising more, eating the right diet, or taking a statin drug, an ACE inhibitor, or baby aspirin. It's amazing how much better it can be for patients. . . .
>
> "What's most important for patients is to have an internist who will sit down and spend the time to get to know them, learn what their risk factors are and their family health history, and then come up with a plan. For instance, I would order additional tests for someone whose parents and grandparents had heart attacks or coronary artery disease in their forties and fifties, as compared to those whose relatives are physically active, without coronary artery disease, and living into their eighties and nineties. The same thing with respect to cancer—you have to take a thorough history and make sure patients are properly educated and get preventive screening and immunizations. For example, colonoscopies can prevent colon cancer; immunization against hepatitis B and HPV can prevent liver and cervical cancer."
>
> —Bruce D. Logan, M.D. (New York)

> "Finding a primary care physician, in-network, with ten, fifteen, twenty years' experience? There's just not enough of them anymore. . . . I'm a dean at Harvard Medical School.

I sit on the licensing board that accredits medical schools, and we look at the distribution of the specialties people go into when they graduate. There's been a continual decline over the last twenty years of people going into internal medicine and primary care and an increase in subspecialization. This has a lot to do with the fact that medical students have become disgruntled with the fifteen-minute appointment when meeting a new patient. That's the reality. What I suggest you do is this: All major teaching institutions—like the ones in Boston, Los Angeles, and Chicago—have set up a telephone line, a physician referral network. Call the major teaching center in your area and ask to be referred to a PCP, and they'll set you up with someone who has graduated in the last one to two years. A well-trained young person can be as good as, or sometimes more up to date than, someone with many years of experience. . . . When it comes to communicating with your current doctor? Let the physician know what your concerns are so they have an understanding of what's important to you. Establish up front: 'What do I do if I have a question? And what's the process in your office to get a question answered? If I have a problem with treatment or a side effect or trouble making a decision, who in your office do I talk to?' "

—Anthony V. D'Amico, M.D., Ph.D. (Boston)

"I must tell you, in the thirty years I've been in practice, I can count on one hand the number of times that a patient has wanted to meet first. And I'm happy to do it, just to meet with someone, sit in the office, and see if there's chemistry. I think it's very reasonable. It seems to be much more accepted among pediatricians, when you're selecting one for your child, to sit down and make sure that it's the person that you want. But we don't take that same advice for our own health care, and yet it's a valid thing to do. So much of medicine is the relationship. . . . Here's a red flag: somebody who you really don't feel is listening to you. . . .

"Then there are times when patients aren't forthcoming about a history of smoking, drugs, or alcohol use. And the first time we find out that somebody has been drinking heavily is when they go in for an operation, and they have problems withdrawing after surgery. Openness with your physician is key. This is not legal maneuvering, where you try to hide certain things. Just come in with the mind-set that you're a partner. Come in informed, while also making your information available. Don't rely on your doctor to try and piece together what's happened in the past."

—Steven W. Tabak, M.D., F.A.C.C. (Beverly Hills)

"Sometimes it's good to find a doctor who's about ten years older than you, because they'll have had that much more experience with life situations you'll be going through— whether it's raising children, sending them to college, or having parents die. As doctors, we learn a lot by experiencing these things ourselves and sharing that with patients. . . . Communication skills, I think, are really very important. The patient should have the feeling that if they have a story that they've put together in their own mind, and they want to convey it, the doctor should sit there until there's an absolute silence, and not just a pause. Patients often give us the answers more quickly than would happen if we peppered them with our own questions. And none of us like being interrupted. I think that doctors are smarter if they say less, if they listen more."

—Bryan J. Arling, M.D. (Washington, D.C.)

"When it comes to PCPs, age doesn't matter as much as it does for specialists. For PCPs, you really want someone who's up to date on common things. For example, there are 154 lung diseases. Out of those 154, only eight are common. . . . And 91 percent of everyone with a lung problem who goes to an ER or sees a PCP is suffering from one of those eight diseases. Every organ system is the same way. That's why you really don't need a superstar who has seen everything to be your primary care doctor. What you need is someone who is very willing to refer when he's not sure. In other words, if it doesn't fall into these eight diseases, and he's not sure, he can refer you to quality people—not to his friends but to good-quality doctors. So ask how they pick specialists to refer you to. I would also check to see where that PCP is on staff and make sure it's a good hospital. . . . Another way to tell if it's a good doctor is to find out if he or she is involved in training other doctors. In general, physicians who train others have to keep up better with the latest research."

—Robert R. Simon, M.D., F.A.A.E.M.
(Kalamazoo, Mich.)

"I hear patients say all the time, 'I waited an hour and he didn't spend any time with me.' As a physician, I know how hard that situation can be for patients and for their doctors. Before I went into concierge medicine, I had a busy practice of 2,500 to 3,000 patients. Running on time and giving them my full attention were two of my highest priorities, but there were days that it was near impossible. When a patient is sick or scared, you can't stop your visit after twenty minutes and tell them to come back next week. You have to drop everything and prioritize. And oftentimes that means running late. I'm not saying doctors can't do better. We can and we must. One area where doctors fail miserably is that they don't have enough support staff and/or they don't take time to train their staff to communicate effectively with patients. It's not hard to have someone update patients when the doctor is running late. Most patients just want to know what to expect.

"If a doctor walks in and apologizes for being late, that's a good sign. But even if he or she doesn't, try to extend them the grace that they may or may not deserve. I know that's a lot to ask, especially because you're the one who's already waited forty-five minutes beyond your scheduled appointment, in a cold exam room, naked. . . . There were days when I got stuck in traffic, overslept my alarm, or overbooked my schedule. Those things happen to everyone. But more often than not, I was late because I had to transfer a patient to the ICU after they took a turn for the worse; or a scheduled five-minute call to give a patient test results turned into thirty minutes because we found cancer; or a patient having a routine physical couldn't stop crying because she just lost her husband. I'm never late because I don't care about them. I'm late because I'm caring for someone else. When I walk into a patient's room and the first thing I get from them is their frustration from having to wait, I have to fight shutting down. But when a patient asks, 'Are you okay? It's so good to see you. You must have had a crazy, busy morning,' it's unexpected, and it melts you as a physician that they're extending you grace. It somehow makes everything else we have been dealing with that day a little bit better and allows us to give them our full attention."

—Carrie L. Carter, M.D. (Dallas)

QUICK GUIDE

CHAPTER 2. How to Find the Best Primary Care Physician
for You

- The three steps to finding a great primary care physician are (1) make a list of what's important to you in a PCP, (2) gather recommendations from people whose opinions you trust, and (3) set up exploratory meetings with the doctors at the top of your list.

- Check online with your state's medical licensing body to be sure all the doctors on your list are licensed and have no formal disciplinary actions against them.

- Five important traits to look for in a primary care physician: This is someone who (1) you can have a personal relationship with; (2) has a practice organized so that you are seen in a timely fashion and for as long as it takes; (3) directs you to the appropriate specialists; (4) understands the importance of coordinating with specialists; and (5) is committed to your wellness and health care objectives.

- If your health care problems are complex, and it's important to you to have a PCP who is available at all hours and can spend more attention on your day-to-day needs, those services are available if you decide to devote the financial resources.

- Signs that it's time to find a new PCP are (1) you experienced a preventable error under your PCP's care; (2) you cannot get timely access to care; (3) your PCP's communication style is disrespectful and dismissive.

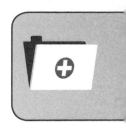

CHAPTER THREE

THREE THINGS YOU CAN DO RIGHT NOW TO BE BETTER PREPARED

Write your family's medical memoir, collect your records, and take inventory

When Amanda, a sophomore in college and a save-the-world kind of kid, gave blood during a Red Cross drive at her school, she received a form letter shortly afterward notifying her that she could not be a donor. Although it was not specific, the letter made a suggestion of hepatitis, a liver disease most commonly contracted from dirty tattoo needles or IV drugs. Amanda had had no experience of either. Her mother, a nurse, knew it had to be something else. She was terrified. Privately, she was thinking, *This could be lymphoma, leukemia, or maybe worse.*

A physician saw Amanda the very next morning. He did tests that ruled out hepatitis, but he agreed that she had some kind of blood anomaly he couldn't figure out. Amanda came home, a week before her Thanksgiving break, and went to see Dr. Michael H. Rosove, a hematologist at UCLA's Jonsson Comprehensive Cancer Center. Dr. Rosove is like a supercomputer when it comes to blood disorders—you can see the disks spinning when he's at work.

During the appointment, Amanda's mother mentioned to Dr. Rosove that when she herself was seven years old, she had had acute anemia—a decrease in red blood cells that left her exhausted. She was so sick, she missed almost a year of school. But when her doctors removed her spleen, because it had become enlarged, she was miraculously cured of anemia. She never had a problem again. Back then, in the late 1950s, the dark ages of medicine, no diagnosis had been forthcoming to explain her illness. But now this very clever woman wondered if there was a link between her condition and her daughter's.

Tests showed that Amanda was also somewhat anemic, even though she had no symptoms. So Dr. Rosove went to work, drawing blood and performing analytics.

"I think I have a theory to explain this," he said. "I think Amanda has hereditary spherocytosis," a condition in which the normally biconcave-shaped red blood cells (imagine a flattened doughnut with no hole) are sphere-shaped (like a ball), making them more fragile and vulnerable to damage as they pass through the spleen. The spleen, located behind the left ribs and above the belly, filters the blood and helps fight infection. When cells prematurely break down inside it, the spleen becomes enlarged and irritated, and the body is deprived of oxygen. In very mild cases, like Amanda's, patients typically don't know anything is wrong because the body compensates by producing more red blood cells. A more severe case—that of Amanda's mother, say—will result in anemia and jaundice. (Although the spleen is a helpful organ, it is not vital; the liver and the lymph nodes will help compensate for functions lost due to a removed spleen.)

The speedy diagnosis was a relief for the family, as no medical treatment (just folic acid supplements) was necessary for Amanda, and her doctors needed only to monitor her periodically in case the day came when she might need a splenectomy. There are many different hematological disorders—and figuring out which one was at play could have been a time-consuming and difficult process. But the family's medical mystery provided the clue Dr. Rosove needed, and a simple blood test confirmed his theory. In fact, they now knew that Amanda's mother also had hereditary spherocytosis—an explanation forty years later!

Amanda's experience underscores the importance of knowing your family health history. Documenting it only takes a few hours, and the results can be both fascinating and priceless. It is the first of three very easy steps you can take right now to better protect yourself and your loved ones. Here they are:

THREE STEPS TO BETTER HEALTH PREPAREDNESS

1. Create a family health history.

2. Collect your medical records.

3. Take inventory.

Everyone knows that the future of high-tech health care is embedded in our genes. Individual genomic mapping is already a reality. And scientists around the world are working furiously to develop new ways to use genetic information to help prevent, detect, and treat a host of diseases. But until the day comes when everyone carries their DNA profile on a flash drive, Step 1, creating a family health history based on the collective memories of your closest relatives, is the best source of information about what may be lying in wait for you.

Dr. Carrie Carter of Dallas, an internist, spends anywhere from thirty minutes to three hours reviewing a patient's history during a first consult. "They probably think I'm just being nice, but really what I'm trying to do is get to know them," Carter says. "When I find out that a patient's mother died when she was fifty-five, I always ask, 'How old were you at the time?' I'm trying to find out the stage of life they were in, what the parent died from, and how that's going to impact them, as well as how they view their health, and what their fears are. . . . I go over their history, but I'm also asking for their life story. It helps so much as I take care of them."

She can spend this kind of time extracting background information from her patients, because she charges an annual retainer. But you can do the same thing by plotting out your ancestral medical history and providing that information to your doctors.

Take the time to be a family medical sleuth. What was great-grandpa's physical and mental condition just before he died of "old age"? Did your aunts, uncles, or cousins suffer from any unusual symptoms? Are there unsolved health mysteries in your family? Has anyone experienced severe—or even fatal—allergic reactions to certain foods, medications, bee stings, and the like? At a minimum, plot the medical problems of parents and siblings—the closer the relation, the more significant the information.

Your doctors can't learn from what they don't know. So write down as much as you remember, then quiz relatives who may have better recollections. Share the information with your extended family, so that they can also reap the benefits.

Step 2 is collecting your medical records and preparing them for distribution to your physicians.

Anytime you privately buy a used automobile, you'll customarily inherit from the previous owner a thick file of repair and maintenance documents, showing everything from the first oil change and tire rotation to serious older-car procedures like transmission work. We're sticklers for keeping auto records—and that's a good thing. But it makes absolutely no sense that a Honda Civic or a Mercedes-Benz has a better paper trail of its "medical history" than you do!

Remember how shocked Jennifer was to discover in her mid-fifties that the practitioners who examined her in her early forties left clues in her records about a possible case of psoriatic arthritis? It *should be watched*, one wrote. Having that file in hand could have saved her years of pain, joint damage, unnecessary treatments, and expense. But she never thought to collect and manage her own records.

There are many possible benefits of having your up-to-date records in one place, including avoiding inaccurate and incomplete diagnostics, harmful drug interactions, and duplicative testing—all things that put you at risk of medical error. At the very least, you're making a tremendous impression on your physicians, who also stand to benefit when you have greater access to and control of your own medical data.

That was what researchers discovered from a 2010 note-sharing experiment. In a yearlong study called OpenNotes, 105 primary care physicians at three U.S. hospitals invited 19,000 of their patients to read their exam notes online (patients logged in to the institution's secure portal) after every doctor visit. The program provided patients with easy access to a detailed account of their visits, including exam notes, lab findings, and the clinician's assessments and instructions, in addition to medications prescribed and follow-up visits scheduled.

Patients who participated said that they understood their medical information better, complied with their prescription schedules as directed, felt more in control and engaged in their own care, and asked their doctors better questions. Physicians reported better trust, transparency, and shared decision making with their patients. At the end of the program, 99 percent of patients and every doctor opted to continue.

In my wallet, I have a plastic USB device the size of a hotel keycard. You can find one online (search for "credit card USB" or "wallet USB") for less than ten dollars. Every clue to my health is right there in digitized form, password-protected. You carry a cell phone, a wallet, and a credit card and consider them necessary equipment—but all these are worthless during a medical emergency.

Some people think they're not allowed to look at their doctor's notes, but under federal privacy laws, it's your legal right. (The one exception is psychotherapy notes.) The Health Insurance Portability and Accountability Act of 1996, or HIPAA, guarantees that:

1. You have a right to receive a copy of your medical records. In most cases, they must be given to you within thirty days. You may have to pay for the cost of copying and mailing them, but state laws limit how much you can be charged. You must be given your records even if you didn't pay for the services you received. And you don't have to give a reason for your request.

2. You can change any wrong information or add to your file if you think something is missing or incomplete. Typically, your file should be updated or amended within sixty days.

3. Your provider must give you notice of how your health information may be shared or used. Patients often receive these notices, as an informed consent letter, at the point when they are establishing care.

State laws govern how long a care provider must hold on to your files, but most doctors retain them for up to ten years or more. (A quick Internet search will pull up helpful FAQs on medical record regulation in your state.) If you are doing this for a spouse, parent, or friend, that person can make you a "personal representative"—someone who is formally authorized to request and collect his or her records. In the appendix and at www.PatientsPlaybook.com is a HIPAA Privacy Authorization form (i.e., medical release form) that the patient can print, sign, and give to you ahead of time. Providers are required by law to comply with the request.

How many years back do you reasonably need to go? The answer depends on your time, patience, and current condition. If you are a relatively healthy person and are beginning this project from scratch, getting files from the last five to ten years should suffice. Here's how you might start:

- Begin with your internist. Call and ask that a copy of your medical files be prepared for pickup or, if you prefer, mailed to you.
- The records you receive from your PCP should include key reports for things like physical exams, lab work, and any tests. They also provide a window into the other physicians you've seen in the last five to ten years, via referrals. Sometimes those doctors' reports will be in this file, too.
- If you don't have a PCP, then just call the offices of the physicians you've visited in the last five to ten years—especially for any surgical procedures or major medical events—and ask for a copy of your records.

If you're doing this for your entire family, and feeling overwhelmed, by all means take your time. You can start with the PCP's office, pick up the phone, and remember the old saw: Mile by mile takes a while, yard by yard is not so hard, but inch by inch is a cinch. Collecting *some* records is better than having none at all.

If you have recently been diagnosed with a condition that your doctors want to monitor, you should collect past records that may provide them with a baseline. With prostate cancer, for instance, if you've had gradually increasing PSA levels, it's important to share any previously recorded levels with your urologist, because the rate of PSA growth over time might determine if you need a biopsy and, if it's positive for cancer, inform your treatment choices. Likewise, for a woman with fibroids in her breasts, sharing past mammography reports helps the doctor interpret your current results. In some cases, you might even save yourself an unnecessary biopsy by providing your doctors with earlier lab reports and images.

If you have a mysterious medical problem, you'll want to dig a little deeper, getting the records for significant and/or abnormal health events from your past that might relate to your present condition. To be clear, you needn't go so far as tracking down your well-baby medical records—*unless* there was something fairly abnormal or significant. But if you're suddenly suffering severe rashes and itchiness . . . remember the time you took a hiking trip in South America and came home with a skin infection? Get the records from that medical consult. If you had a bike accident five years ago that left you unconscious or seeing stars, it might be related to your recent limited vision or terrible headaches. The more closely related a past medical event seems to be to your current condition, the more important it is to collect the records.

For chronic conditions, in addition to procuring potentially relevant records, you can help your doctors zero in on a cause by reconstructing the circumstances of your earliest symptoms. Let's say you're suffering from back pain. Take a minute to write down what happened when you first noticed it: *Was there a bad twist when you were moving furniture? Did you fall on the ice? Wrench your back doing yoga?* Write about what hurt and what helped: *Did it feel better when you iced it or put heat on? What were you prescribed, and did the pain get better or worse? How did it feel to stand, sit, lie down? Did stretching improve your problem? Did exercise?* Your answers will help determine whether this is a structural, muscular, or nerve issue—or something else.

Similarly, chronic autoimmune conditions evolve over time. What seemed many years ago like a stomach disorder, general achiness, or joint pain may have been the first onset of lupus or arthritis. Give your doctor the circumstances, the treatments tried, and your reactions to those therapies. The more facts she gets, the better a detective she'll be.

As you start to collect your files, you may find that your medical history is spread out like a jigsaw puzzle. There are likely to be empty spaces, reflecting moves from one town to the next and other changes through the years. If you can't recall, your PCP should have a record of every referral. Personal appointment calendars may also help fill in the blanks. Past insurance documents, such as explanation of benefits notices, often list who you saw and when.

You'll also begin to see a memoir of your medical self, written in doctors' notes and changing physical exam results over the years. You'll see periods of time where you needed a doctor more frequently, or less so. Don't be surprised if you discover subtle *codes* about yourself in the physician's scribbles. I find them sort of amusing. "Well nourished"? That means: Time to go to the gym.

I like to have my records scanned into an electronic file to keep on my personal USB card and for digital distribution to providers. But some doctors and hospitals aren't ready to accept digital records yet, or they may prefer paper, which is why we also organize all our clients' records in three-ring binders, tab-separated by specialty and physician name.

For example, when we sent a copy of Catherine's binder to Dr. Wechsler, in advance of their phone call, it looked like this:

1. The first three pages were her Medical Summary, which listed:
   - her name and date of birth;
   - known allergies;
   - a few sentences about her condition and health status (and that she was hoping to rule out or confirm a diagnosis of Churg-Strauss);
   - a chronological, bulleted list of notable medical events and changes in her treatment (i.e., *From 1989 to 2001, Catherine took oral prednisone. In 1991 began TAO, Medrol, and an inhaler. Was evaluated in 2001 at [hospital name] and was diagnosed with asthma. A CT scan of her sinuses on February 18, 2012 revealed . . .*).

2. The next section was her Family Health History. This would also be the place to include notes about a first encounter with a chronic problem.

3. Finally, her complete Medical Records. This last section was the largest and included copies from every physician consult during the last two decades, when she had been struggling with the breathing problem. Again, how far back you decide to go will depend on your situation.

About organization: I find it's easier to tab-separate clients' medical records by specialty and doctor name, putting hospital records at the end. Yours, for example, might be organized by tabs that read like this: *Allergy,*

Dr. Smith; Cardiology, Dr. Rothman; Cardiology, Dr. Watson; Dermatology, Dr. Levine; Internal Medicine, Dr. Alsop, etc. The reason is that doctors have different styles for recording your information—and one can get dizzy very quickly looking at medical records in *chronological* order. Separating the files this way enables you and your doctors to easily follow the progression of an illness through each physician and specialty.

However you decide to compile your (and/or your family's) health history, remember to update it. We generally call in records requests for clients quarterly, but you'll only need to ask for a copy of your records (i.e., notes, test results, imaging), as a matter of routine, after every visit.

Now, if you move or need to switch doctors, you have a complete medical story to share with your new physician. If you become sick and are referred to a specialist, you can provide them with years of potential clues that may help solve your problem.

Your records can also speak for you. Carry a digital copy when you travel, especially outside the country. If you are far from home and suddenly find yourself in an ambulance—a situation that is *always* sudden—having your full history with you may become a lifesaver.

But it doesn't take an emergency for this exercise to pay off—not when a majority of medical mistakes are caused by miscommunication and lack of coordination. We see it all the time when we collect clients' records: wildly different documentation, where the drugs and dosages listed by one doctor are different from what's been noted by another doctor. The patient may report to his Monday-appointment doctor that he's on 5 milligrams of a blood thinner, but by his Friday appointment, he thinks it's 10 milligrams. You cannot assume that what's in your medical files is accurate. But by managing your data, reviewing it carefully, and giving physicians the most accurate and up-to-date information, you are taking control and helping to minimize error.

Finally, Step 3: I want you to create an inventory. Make lists for yourself and your family members with the following:

- diagnoses and any major surgeries
- allergies
- any drugs/medications you're taking (including supplements)
- a roster of your physicians

- emergency contacts (who the hospital should call)
- insurance information

In my family, we keep paper copies of this inventory at home and the office, and a digital copy on our USB drives in our wallets. At a minimum, keep your most urgent health information and contact details on a wallet-sized laminated card, because the first thing an emergency response team will do in the case of an unconscious patient is check his or her purse or wallet. (More about this in Chapter 7.)

Some may worry about their health information getting out. But for most people, privacy is less important than giving responders quick access to essential data.

I don't mean to be cavalier about privacy. You are entitled to 100 percent control over who has access to your information. But in my experience, the problem always seems to be on the other side, when privacy protections get in the way of swiftly coordinating patient care. And most physicians and hospitals just aren't very speedy in sharing records with others.

Medical records get collected and moved around all the time for legitimate reasons: a patient applies for life or disability insurance, changes jobs and towns, switches doctors. But when my colleagues and I need to collect a client's records, we have to call numerous times and send repeated e-mails. Sometimes the resistance is because we are a proxy, but often the request is simply a low priority for the person on the other end of the line. Which is why it's a good idea to gather these things now, when you are well and it's not an emergency. Collect the files, review them, and distribute them.

Patients who are afraid to say or do anything that they think might upset or burden their doctors—like asking for a copy of their chart or giving a bulging file to their new physician—should take some comfort in knowing that good caregivers appreciate an informed, intelligent patient who will help them do their job better.

"I love it when patients bring in a big, fat ring-binder of their medical records," says Dr. Gail J. Roboz, a professor of medicine and the director of the Leukemia Program at the Weill Medical College of Cornell University and the NewYork-Presbyterian Hospital in New York City.

Dr. Roboz is a world-renowned specialist. (Writer Nora Ephron and TV host Robin Roberts have been under her care.) And in case one were to believe that only the privileged few can access a doctor of her caliber, she is in-network and cares for people from all walks of life. Dr. Roboz is constantly extracting more information from her patients, especially when it comes to the pills they are taking.

"The new pharmacy-downloading system, where we can see what's being prescribed, is really helpful," she says. "I'll look at it and say to a patient, 'Wait a minute. Who gave you fluconazole?' and I'll hear, '*Oh, yeah*. My gastroenterologist thought I had thrush.' 'Oh? Were you gonna tell me, or is that a secret?'"

Yet Dr. Roboz still makes a point of asking her patients to bring in a ziplock bag of every pill they are on. "I want to see the bottles," Dr. Roboz says. "You discover all kinds of stuff. One doctor prescribed Nexium, the other one prescribed Prilosec, the other one prescribed Protonix. These are all very similar, and the patient's taking *all* of them. It's a window into their other doctor visits. You'd be very surprised. Some of my patients are super-organized, and they'll come in with a whole list of their medications, but I still ask them, 'Are you taking any vitamins?' 'Oh. Yeah. I didn't include the vitamins.' 'Are you taking any herbal supplements?' 'Oh. Do you mean the *gro-bang-go*-whatever that I order from Amazon?' 'Yes.' People assume that all these supplements are benign because they are 'natural.' That is absolutely not the case, especially if you are being treated with multiple medications. There are enormous potential interactions that might be part of cracking the case of a particular side effect."

Doctors may get grumpy or curt with patients who bring in page after page of claims about bogus potions and treatments that they found on the Internet and that don't make much sense for their condition. But when you hand them facts about *you*, you are giving them information to render better judgments, and doctors are glad to have this.

Just by doing the three steps to better health preparedness, you are standing out—in a positive way—from everyone else your doctor sees. You're making his or her job easier. It's a rare doctor who wouldn't appreciate that.

QUICK GUIDE

CHAPTER 3. Three Things You Can Do Right Now to Be Better Prepared

- The three steps to better health preparedness are (1) create a family health history, (2) collect your medical records, and (3) take inventory and keep the most urgent medical information in your wallet.

- The Health Insurance Portability and Accountability Act of 1996, or HIPAA, specifically guarantees your right to: (1) get a copy of your medical records; (2) change or amend your file if you think something is missing or incomplete; (3) be informed of how your health information may be shared or used.

- If you are healthy, gather your records from the doctors you've visited in the past five to ten years. Start with your PCP.

- If you have been diagnosed with a developing disease that needs monitoring, include records that can provide a baseline for your condition.

- If you have a mysterious medical problem, detail significant and/or abnormal medical events from your past, which *might* relate to your present condition.

- If you have a chronic condition, reconstruct the earliest circumstances, treatments tried, and your reactions to therapies—this information will help your doctors zero in on a cause.

- Organize your records in a three-ring binder with: your Medical Summary, Family Health History, and complete records, tab-separated by specialty and physician name.

- If you and your doctors are tech-savvy, scan your records into an electronic file to keep on a personal USB card in your wallet and for digital distribution to providers.

- Ask for a copy of your medical records after every doctor visit and stay current. If you are facing a serious illness, distribute them to each new specialist with whom you consult, to ensure they are getting all the relevant facts about you, and to show them that you are a clinically sophisticated patient.

- Make lists with the following: diagnoses and any major surgeries; allergies; drugs and medications; physicians; emergency contacts; insurance information.

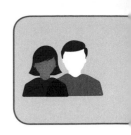

CHAPTER FOUR

DEVELOP A SUPPORT TEAM

*Why you need to recruit an effective health care
quarterback—and how to ask*

Medicine is the only team-performed function in which there is no leader. You could have a brilliant internist, an accomplished oncologist, a savvy nutritionist, and other top-flight practitioners in your stable of health care experts—but nobody is coordinating all that good work.

Imagine having a symphony orchestra composed of the world's most talented musicians but no conductor at the helm. Or a football team without a star quarterback to coordinate the work of ten other players in front of him, bringing out their best. That leadership role is absent in medicine. No one is managing and sharing your medical records, procuring expert opinions about your specific symptoms, and distributing the latest evidence-based science about your illness to the team. Most important, no one is ensuring that all your caregivers are moving in a coordinated way toward the same goal.

"The truth of the matter is that even if you have three or four subspecialists, the onus currently is with the patient to say, 'Hey. Did you know that my neurologist prescribed me this and my cardiologist prescribed that?'" says Dr. Roboz. "Sometimes in an acute situation when somebody is terribly ill, the subspecialists get together to figure things out. But with somebody who is puttering along and doing okay and being treated for several things simultaneously, one doctor has no way of knowing what the others are doing."

This is the way medicine currently works: it's up to *you* to coordinate your care. But it's a rare patient who is able to deftly guide their own case amid the fear and confusion that can arise when you suddenly learn you have a serious problem. You just don't know how you will react.*

"I often suggest to our patients that they need an advocate to help them through the system . . . somebody who drives the process," says Dr. Sheldon Elman, the chairman and CEO of Medisys, Canada's leading provider of preventive medicine and executive health care services. Dr. Elman passionately believes that "You need somebody there to have your back. When nobody's acting on your behalf, nobody is pushing the system to make things happen for you, asking 'When is the next appointment?' 'How can he or she be seen faster?' 'Is this surgery really necessary?' And by having somebody act on your behalf, you become much more proactive."

If you woke up tomorrow to learn you had a potentially fatal disease, who would have your back? Who would lead you through the challenges ahead? It used to be that primary care physicians—who know their patients' health history better than anyone—would play this role, and a small number still do. But the majority simply don't have the time. Which is why you need to think about the people close to you whom you could reliably turn to for help, and ask one or more of them to be your quarterback.

Like most things in life that are worth planning for (college, family, retirement), it's a good idea to think now, *before* you get sick, about who this person could be. As you go through the steps of Intensive Case Management, you'll do so much better if they are at your side.

Sometimes this person's most important job will be helping you to collect and distribute your medical records, schedule exams, pick up medications, and find specialists who can give you expert opinions. If you have a complex or rare condition, she might become your research partner, poring through your records for clues (like the one Jennifer found about her psoriatic arthritis). Maybe she's the one who digs through the medical literature

---

*Here are the three most common dysfunctional responses that I have observed, and that you can avoid by using the lessons in this book: (1) patients become passive and do whatever their doctor orders, without engaging in a meaningful evaluation of the treatment plan; (2) patients are paralyzed with fear and can't make decisions because they need additional information and validation of the plan being proffered—yet they don't know how to obtain it; and (3) patients feel so vulnerable and frustrated with their care that they become prey to con artists and scammers. That last response is not uncommon. Our system has done such a poor job of listening to and actually caring for patients, it's no wonder that so many reject it altogether and embrace the harmful overtures of snake oil salesmen.

to find the right experts to call (as we did with Catherine and her diagnosis of Churg-Strauss) or the latest drugs and clinical trials that could be helpful therapies for you. Other times she'll accompany you on doctor visits, posing questions you may not be thinking of.

In most families, there's a lot of sharing of the role of a quarterback (i.e., your best friend goes with you to chemo appointments, but your spouse does the research, appointment making, and general heavy lifting). It's important to always have someone in the lead role, but this position may be fluid and evolve over the course of your illness.

I recently heard from a physician who had just finished a consult in which there were fourteen people in the room: the patient, her husband, six kids, and their spouses. For initial visits, when you're getting news for the first time, it's great to bring a support team. Because when patients come alone, they frequently forget or misunderstand what the doctor is saying.

Studies show that when a family member or friend participates in visits, we feel better about our care, we can discuss difficult topics, and we have a greater understanding of our physician's advice. This is especially true, according to researchers at Johns Hopkins, when the patient is elderly: having a companion in the room made both the patient *and* the doctor more task-focused and productive. What's more, patients were less likely to passively accept information from their physicians, and doctors got a fuller understanding of the patient's problem because companions contributed information the patient failed to mention.

Under HIPAA, as long as you do not object, your doctor may discuss your health information with you in front of others. In some cases, she may signal that she plans to discuss delicate information (such as past surgeries, disease history that may be relevant to your problem, or genetic proclivities that may affect your family) and give you an opportunity to ask your companion to leave the room. Or she may use her professional judgment to determine that you do not object. It's up to you to let your doctor know if there are matters that are too private to discuss in front of your advocate, but keep in mind that this is someone whom you have decided to trust with your most personal medical details. It will be hard for her to do research and help you make the right decisions if she is missing important pieces of your case history.

When a spouse plays the team leader role, it's a good idea to gently remind him or her that the assignment goes far beyond simply being a loving and supportive husband or wife. For a little guidance, here are the four ways they can aspire to support you during your illness:

1. Emotionally
2. Logistically
3. Clinically
4. Intellectually

Having played this role many times in my life, I find you can usually provide at least two kinds of support. The challenge is to give all four.

I was on the phone the other day with a client who recently had surgery for an aortic dissection, a tear in the large blood vessel that branches off the heart. "Gavin," I said. "I've been thinking about you. How are you doing?" (*Emotional support.*)

"You'll probably be in the hospital three or four more days, so you and your daughter need to think about what kind of care you're going to need once you go home. Do you have a home health aide lined up? Can your daughter set things up so you won't have to walk up and down the stairs for a few days? Is there someone who can help with meals for the next week?" (*Logistical support.*)

"In the meantime, here's some more information for you: the most serious complications typically occur immediately after surgery. But since yours went well, there's less likelihood of a major complication. Also, remember that healing is not entirely linear. People often think that each hour and each day should be better than the last, but that's not always the case. You're going to have up days and down days. It's all normal." (*Clinical information that no one had given him yet.*)

"How are you feeling in this moment? . . . A little spacey and useless? Well, you're an alpha male—let it go. The doctor said your surgery went extremely well. You don't need to be doing anything else except getting better. That's where you are in this process right now." (*Intellectual support.*)

I spend a lot of time thinking about the qualities that make *outstanding* health care quarterbacks. In the best of all possible worlds, that person is a nearby physician, nurse practitioner, or friend with broad clinical expertise, who can read and interpret medical reports and mine the research on the patient's specific illness. They are organized and can manage medical records, appointments, and prescriptions. They can go to appointments with the patient, listening carefully with their radars attuned, bringing a gentle sensitivity or a take-charge, think-outside-the-box approach, depending on what's needed.

And yet I realize that most people just don't have a superhero like this in their lives! And that's totally okay. Because you will still benefit remarkably by having friends and family members standing by, doing what they can for you if you become very sick. Try to ensure that the one you turn to most possesses a few key qualities. Your trusted point person should be:

1. Someone you trust. A lot of your outcome will depend on how well he plays this role. You're going to feel vulnerable a lot of the time, and you need to be comfortable around your helper even in your most unguarded moments.

2. Someone who is a good communicator. A lot of the breakdowns in medicine are due to poor communication. Your helper should be the kind of person who knows how to make friends with the front-office staff. She can explain your latest aches and pains and pursue answers for you when you are feeling too sick to speak for yourself. And she does it without yelling at staff or harassing physicians.

3. Someone who can commit for the duration of your illness. You don't know how long that's going to be, but during this time you will become pretty dependent on this person, and you don't want your spirits to suffer from continual changes in leadership.

It's important, especially for elderly patients, that the quarterback lives close by and can handle on-the-ground coordination. However, there are plenty of opportunities for siblings who live far away to do research, schedule appointments, and lend support. If it's not feasible for one person to take on this role, having two or more can be a great solution. Try to select people who have strengths that match your needs as a patient. One way to think of it: it's kind of like a job, and a really great partner for this job is someone who possesses (a) **methodical organization**; (b) **adeptness at research and data** collection; and (c) **emotional savvy.** If you want to divvy up the job among two or three different people, as parents do among children, be sure they have one or more of these skill sets.

Look around you. Who is the detail-oriented person in your life? The vibrant team leader who keeps everything running smoothly and on time? That's your **organization person.** The one who will help you to update your medical records, schedule appointments, manage prescriptions, and take notes at doctor meetings.

Now, who is the investigator? The computer-savvy resourceful friend who's great at research and networking? That's your **research and data person.** (Oftentimes she may be your organization person, too.) They'll help you set up Google alerts and engage with disease-specific philanthropies, to keep you abreast of the latest developments about your condition and the specialists who have the deepest expertise. You might even lean on them during decision-making processes, when it's time to weigh the pros and cons of various therapies.

Now think about the person you turn to when you need to talk. We all have people in our lives who intuitively sense when we're feeling down. That's your **emotional support person,** someone you can trust to pick you up when your reservoirs are exhausted.

Relationships change over time. The best man at your wedding may be a distant acquaintance ten years later, and the godmother to your child may move far away someday. But if you are at a place where you are ready to ask someone to be your quarterback—either now or in the future—how you begin the conversation depends on the relationship. It often helps to start with a shared experience. Everyone has a friend or relative who's dealt with a serious health problem. Your opener might sound a little like this:

> *I wanted to talk to you about something that's very serious and that I've given a lot of thought to. You're the one person I want to have this conversation with because of my respect for you, and my trust in you. [Or if you are asking two or more: You and Patty are the only people I'm having this conversation with.] I saw how difficult it was for Joe when he was sick. We all tried to be helpful in our own ways,*

but as I reflect on that time, I wonder if we could have provided better, more efficient guidance. At some point in time, I might be in Joe's shoes, and I wanted to talk to you, to see if I could rely on you to support me through it.

If you're stumped for a meaningful *shared* medical experience, there are other ways to get the conversation started. Here are a few:

I was so impressed with all that you did for your aunt when she was diagnosed with lymphoma. I had to help my father get through a pretty tough illness, and I've seen how hard it is to try to manage these things by yourself. So I wanted to ask you: If the day ever comes that I get a serious diagnosis and need someone to help me, would you be there for me?

You know, when my older brother got very ill, it was devastating to our family because we all wanted to help him and we tried to provide him support. But I'm not sure we were as organized as we could have been. I worry sometimes that if the day comes when I get sick, I don't think there's anybody in my family who I'd trust to guide me through some tough decisions. I wanted to talk to you about being my quarterback, taking an active role in helping me through it, if I'm ever in need of help.

George was such a hardworking guy who planned ahead for every problem life dropped in his lap. But when he got sick, everything went south so fast. It made me think: I'm healthy now, but what if I get sick? I've got a lawyer, and life insurance, and a financial planner, and a plumber on speed dial. But who's going to be there to help me through something really serious, like cancer? I would sleep much better knowing that I've got one of my most trusted friends at my side if that day comes.

So what does this all mean for the person you're asking? Even though it's a theoretical scenario you're proposing, it's important to be specific about the role they will play in keeping you safe. Here's one way to explain the concept:

I've been doing some reading, and I know now that when it comes to the management of complicated medical issues, there's three or four really important things that need to get done: I may ask you to help me collect my medical records, come with me to doctor appointments, or do research with me on my condition. I'll need help finding experts, maybe getting second or third opinions if there were a variety of treatment options to choose from. We saw what happened when Mary found a lump in her breast. There were so many decisions she needed to make, but she was exhausted. You've always been so organized and detail-oriented; it would be a relief to know that I had your brain on this. The other thing is, I'm pretty strong, but I don't want to have to tough out a serious illness alone. If I ever got really sick, I know I'd get through it more successfully if I had you by my side.

If you find yourself suddenly caught unprepared by a serious diagnosis, your language will be more specific, more urgent, and more like this:

As you know, I've got this condition. I need to do a lot of research on it. I have to find experts to consult with. I've got a half-dozen treatment options to consider. And I'm basically going to have to dive headfirst into the health care system. I really need someone to help me logistically with collecting my records, making appointments, coordinating among my doctors, and getting things ready at home for my recovery.

Describe the tasks this person is good at and could potentially help you with. If you are asking for help from several people, let them know what you need from each of them:

I'm going to have my brother come with me to appointments, and he's very organized and disciplined, but we just aren't as close as you and I are, so it would mean a lot to me if I could count on you for emotional support. You really helped me get through that terrible period in my life a few years ago. Can I count on you again, to just check in on me once a week? To be a sounding board. Maybe remind me of why I need to keep battling this thing?

You're the most wonderfully compulsive research person I know. Our freshman year—you lived in the library. I don't know anybody who is as good as you on digging up data. I need your brain on this thing. I'm going to have to make some tough decisions, but I don't have enough evidence yet about my different options, and I want to talk to the real experts on this condition before I commit to a treatment plan. Would you help me by digging into the research?

Be clear about how important this job is. Give the other person an opportunity to ask questions. Let them take some time to think about it:

This is one of the most difficult challenges I've ever confronted. You are the person I trust most to keep me steady and help me through it. Can you help me to navigate this thing? It's a big responsibility, and I certainly understand if you can't do it, but let's talk about it.

People always say, "How can I ask anyone to do that? I'm uncomfortable with the idea of dragging my cousin to my medical appointments or having him make calls for me." But you probably *have* asked a friend or family member to serve as the guardian of your children should you die. Letting someone help you to navigate the health care system is a similar bestowing of trust. It feels hard at first, but as this person partners with you, supporting you in your journey, your experience will be easier, and your outcomes will be better. And the bond between you will deepen.

I realize that this is a step some people really want to skip. But stay with me, because I *know* you can do it. I believe with all my heart and experience that if you follow the lessons in this book, the health rewards will be enormous. Pick your team leader carefully, and share what you've learned here with that person. And as you begin to proactively take charge of your care, your doctors will feel even more empowered to give you *their* very best, too.

QUICK GUIDE

CHAPTER 4. Develop a Support Team

- Think about the people close to you whom you could reliably turn to for help. When the time is right, ask one or more of them to be your quarterback.

- The four ways he or she can support you during your illness are emotionally, logistically, clinically, and intellectually.

- This person should be someone you trust, who is a good communicator, and can commit for the duration of your illness.

- A really great quarterback possesses (1) methodical organization; (2) adeptness at research and data collection; and (3) emotional savvy. So, if you want to break this job up among two or three different people, just be sure they have one or more of these skill sets.

- Begin the conversation around a shared medical experience; be specific about the role you're hoping they can play; describe the skills they are good at and the tasks they could potentially help you with; be clear about how important this job is; and give them time to ask questions and think about it further.

PART II

➤ *Experts and Emergencies*

When a potential health crisis looms, how to get to the
bottom of the problem and the top tier of medical care.
Plus: how to handle yourself in an emergency (room).

OVERTREATMENT CAN BE AS DANGEROUS AS UNDERTREATMENT

How to find the right level, no matter your condition

O ne morning in April 2010, I got a surprising call from a friend. "Jim is dying," he said. "We have to help him *now*." I play the role of quarterback for clients all the time, but this was different—Jim and his wife were dear friends. In fact, the last time I'd seen him, he looked great, the picture of robust health. How could he be dying?

His harrowing journey began in November 2009, while riding the stationary bike at the gym near his home in northern California. As Jim, sixty-five, progressed to higher-resistance levels, he felt his chest tightening and his lungs laboring. Assuming the worst, he called his cardiologist, who ordered a nuclear stress test and an EKG.

Mindful of the fact that his mother's side of the family suffered from heart trouble, Jim had kept his cholesterol down over the years with statins, a healthy diet, and plenty of exercise. So when his test results came back normal, he figured, *Okay—maybe I'm just not in as good shape as I used to be?* His doctor also didn't seem concerned but mentioned that if Jim's symptoms persisted, they could do a coronary angiogram, a procedure that would enable them to get a real-time visual on his arteries to see if there were any obstructions. Jim kept that option in his back pocket.

Over the next few months, he worked out frequently but saw little improvement in his conditioning. Then one day he heard from a friend who had recently suffered a heart attack, falling to one knee while his grand-daughter was in his arms. In the hospital, the man had another massive attack and almost died. The news weighed heavily on Jim—he and his friend had grown up in the same town and been fraternity brothers in college.

Two months later, while coming home from a business trip, Jim was carrying suitcases up the steps to his front door when he suddenly felt weak and went down on one knee. The coincidence seemed uncanny. Now he was distressed. He called his cardiologist and was dismayed to discover the doctor was out of town. By chance, Jim's interior decorator had just raved about her cardiologist, who practiced at their local hospital. Jim picked up the phone to call, figuring he'd have to wait to get an appointment. But the receptionist said she could get him in for an angiogram the *very next day*. Jim took it. In his rush to judgment, he didn't consider that it was a really bad sign that he was scheduled for an angiogram before his new cardiologist had ever met or examined him.

When it comes to his work as an engineer, Jim is a methodical problem solver who carefully considers all aspects of a project. He's not normally a superstitious guy, but when he got sick, he stopped thinking rationally: As he dropped to the steps that day, he pictured his college buddy. *A sign that his heart was in trouble!* When his decorator gushed about her cardiologist, Jim thought to himself, *Synchronicity!* And when he was able to get an immediate appointment? *More evidence that the stars are in alignment.* So often, when we face important medical decisions, we abandon our ability to reason, fact-find, and judge, and we start to follow paths that actually might be wrong for us.

When you are experiencing a medical issue that's not life-threatening but is causing you real concern, it's important to stay steady. Your first call really should be to your internist—the person with whom you've placed deep trust in your health. Your PCP should help you figure out what your problem is and whether you need to consult a specialist. Whether the pain you are experiencing is orthopedic, neurological, cardiovascular, or something else, give your internist the opportunity to sequence through the possibilities and then refer you to a specialist in that realm, before resorting to invasive pro-cedures that might be harmful.

Jim's wife Sandra drove him to the hospital the next morning for his angiogram. The procedure typically begins by inserting a very thin catheter into an artery in the leg or arm and guiding it through blood vessels to the heart. A contrast dye is injected through the catheter, and a special type of X-ray machine allows doctors to see the patient's real-time arterial blood flow. If there's serious blockage, patients may opt for angioplasty, in which the doctor inserts a stent—a small mesh tube that looks like a Chinese finger trap—to keep the artery open. The whole process can be done while the patient is conscious and able to watch what's happening on a TV screen, but that wasn't offered in Jim's case. He was in his gown and being prepped for surgery when his new cardiologist arrived and delivered a nonchalant recitation of his approach: "I've done hundreds of these; 70 percent of the time everything is fine. If, by chance, I find any serious blockages, I'll put in a stent; you'll wake up in a few hours, and we'll discuss the results."

To Jim and Sandra, he seemed cavalier, but he had come so highly recommended that they romanticized his behavior: He was "a smart cowboy."

Minutes before going under general anesthesia, Jim was handed a consent form giving the doctor permission to stent him if necessary. Not working with his PCP was his first mistake; signing that consent form, Jim would later admit, was his second.

When Jim woke up, Sandra was holding his hand and smiling at him. The doctor was not smiling. He announced that he'd had to put in two stents and pointed to an X-ray: "clogged arteries, here and here." Jim, slightly dazed, just nodded. It was hard for him to see the blockages. The hospital would keep him overnight for monitoring, the doctor said. He'd see him in a week for follow-up; and then again in six months, because a third stent might be necessary. Jim's statin dosage was quadrupled, and he was put on new drugs, including blood thinners (to prevent the stents from creating clots) and blood pressure medication.

At his one-week follow-up, Jim told the cardiologist that he hadn't gotten better at all. In fact, he felt like he couldn't get enough oxygen in his lungs. He described it by recalling the time he'd tried to play tennis in a smoggy city—now when he took a breath, he felt the same tightness and burning.

The doctor closed Jim's file and said, "Well, it's not your heart; I did my job."

In other words, hearts were his specialty, and Jim's heart looked fine, so his work was done.

Jim called his primary care physician next. Thinking his problem might be viral, the internist referred him to an ENT, who didn't see anything in

Jim's ears, nose, or throat but prescribed antibiotics just in case. After ten days, Jim felt well enough to go to his first cardiac rehab appointment. It had been a month since his stent surgery.

At rehab, he was hooked up to a heart-lung monitoring machine and put on a stationary bike. After five minutes, a nurse stopped him. His blood-oxygen saturation level—the concentration of oxygen in his blood—was dangerously low. Normal is about 98 or 99. Below 95 means there's a problem, and your organs are not getting the oxygen they need to properly function. Jim's was at 82. The nurse immediately scheduled him for a CT scan in the pulmonology department.

"See this 'broken glass' here?" the pulmonologist said, pointing to an X-ray of Jim's lungs. The dense, whitish material at the bottom of his lungs looked like tiny, shattered glass fragments, and it represented serious scarring and inflammation.

Jim had lung disease.

He could see his problem clearly now: his damaged lung tissue couldn't deliver oxygen to his bloodstream. The pain in his chest had had *nothing* to do with his heart. (In fact, independent cardiologists who later reviewed Jim's angiograms determined that the stents he received were completely unnecessary.)

But there was a new problem. The pulmonologist couldn't give Jim a true diagnosis until they biopsied his lung tissue. But he couldn't possibly do a biopsy, because Jim just had heart surgery and was on blood thinners.

To get him well enough for a biopsy, Jim needed to be injected daily, for ten days, with a drug that would temporarily wean him off the blood thinners. But it would be a dangerous balancing act: taking him off anticoagulants increased his chance of his stents becoming clogged and potentially causing fatal blood clots.

He left the pulmonologist's office on a Thursday. By Friday morning, he couldn't breathe on his own. That afternoon a portable oxygen generator was delivered to the couple's home, and Jim spent the rest of his recovery wearing the face mask and hose that pumped precious oxygen into his diseased lungs. As the days passed, and he waited for the blood thinners to leave his system, his lungs grew weaker. "I'm not sure I'm going to make it through ten days," he told Sandra. She soldiered on, trying to stay upbeat as she watched over him.

On the tenth day, Jim went back to the hospital for his biopsy. The pulmonologist had explained previously that there were two ways to collect the lung tissue: a bronchoscopy procedure, entering through Jim's nose or mouth; or a video-assisted thoracoscopic surgery (VATS), which required an incision through the chest wall. The pulmonologist recommended the bronchoscopy. Since this was the doctor who had identified Jim's real problem, the grateful couple was happy to let him do whichever procedure he preferred, no questions asked.

After his biopsy surgery, Jim went back on the blood thinners for his stents, remained on the oxygen for his stricken lungs, and waited for a diagnosis. Three days later he got terrible news: they didn't get enough tissue.

Specialists will sometimes steer a patient toward the procedure they feel most comfortable with—and that makes sense for them. But it doesn't necessarily mean it's the right course for you, the patient. Jim's bronchoscopy likely had been unsuccessful because the damaged tissues that needed to be examined were in the *lower* part of his lungs—a more difficult place to reach. Sandra and Jim hadn't thought to get a second opinion, and most people don't when they are feeling vulnerable. But rushing into surgery again only set him back further. Now he would have to do it all a second time: stop the blood thinners for ten days, get another biopsy, and wait for the diagnosis that he desperately needed in order to start the *right* treatment.

Privately, Sandra was terrified that Jim really might not make it through ten more days. He looked sallow and ashen. She could see him physically aging.

That's when I got the call from our mutual friend. The last time I'd visited Jim, about six months earlier, he'd seemed strong and energetic. To see him now, wasting away and hunched over like an old man, was heartbreaking. Time was short, and his failing body couldn't tolerate any more mistakes.

We decided pretty quickly that Jim needed the VATS procedure this time. And no more small-town hospitals—he would have to go to a major medical institution and be treated by physicians who had deep expertise in cardiology and pulmonology, doctors who would work like a team as they considered the complexity of Jim's situation.

I gave Jim and Sandra two options. If you want to stay in northern California, I told them, you're going to the UC San Francisco Medical Center, where you'll be wonderfully looked after. Or come to Los Angeles, where you'll get excellent doctors at Cedars-Sinai, and I can coordinate your care—no more unnecessary surgeries at your local hospital. Thankfully, they chose L.A. and allowed me to be their quarterback.

For the next few weeks, Jim was bedbound, tethered by a thin lifeline to the whirring oxygen machine and measuring his days in worsening results from breathing tests. His lung function (how much air he could get in and out of his lungs) was about 30 percent.

Two days before his second biopsy surgery, Jim went to see an internist who was double-boarded in pulmonary medicine and critical care (just the kind of expert you want on your team if you have lung disease). In the middle of the exam, Jim's heart rate suddenly plummeted to 38 beats per minute. The doctor was alarmed but remained calm and immediately sent him to Cedars-Sinai cardiology, where he was monitored for the next twenty-four hours.

The heart and lungs are intricately connected, and it's impossible to tinker with one without affecting the other. Jim's stents were having a severe effect on his respiratory condition. The night before surgery he stabilized. It was only later that the doctor told him, "You know, Jim, you almost died that day."

At Cedars-Sinai he was operated on by Dr. Robert McKenna, Jr., the medical director of the hospital's Thoracic Surgery and Trauma Program, and co–medical director of the Women's Guild Lung Institute. Dr. McKenna met with Jim and Sandra well in advance of the surgery. He explained the VATS process, step by step, and what to expect along the way. He asked if they had any questions. There was nothing cavalier about his bedside manner, and they knew now that this was a good thing.

This time, enough lung tissue was procured for a diagnosis, and the doctors were quickly able to rule out cancer and a host of other life-threatening diseases. According to Dr. McKenna, Jim had something called hypersensitivity pneumonitis: a systemic inflammatory disorder in which his lungs had become extremely sensitive to typical allergens—dust, mold, pollen, and the like. As part of his treatment, he was immediately put on a large daily dose of prednisone, 60 milligrams. He felt better within days. Three weeks after the biopsy he was able to breathe without his oxygen machine.

Jim also saw a hypersensitivity pneumonitis specialist who told him that half the time the exact trigger for the disease is unknown, but it's typically caused by organic, environmental factors. "Do you have birds?" the specialist asked. "Do you live near hay? Do you have a hot tub?" Jim's life involved none of these factors, and he was determined to get to the root of his problem, so he hired inspectors to test his and Sandra's home.

Three men in white hazmat suits spent a day crawling under the floorboards, swabbing the attic, digging in carpets, and collecting samples that they sealed in plastic tubes. A week later the couple received a room-by-room report: spores had been found in the ceiling of the living room, where there had been a slow water leak. The shady side of the house was redolent with mold. And one of Jim and Sandra's favorite features, a British black walnut tree near the steps where Jim had first gone down, also tested positive for allergens. Jim and Sandra embarked on a major remodeling project to rid their home of mold and mildew and create better-ventilated spaces throughout.

About a year later Jim's lungs were functioning at about 65 percent, which may be the best they will ever be, considering how much damage was done while he waited for an accurate diagnosis. He was back to working out on the stationary bike. He was also down to 5 milligrams of prednisone a day, though he will probably need to take it for the rest of his life, along with the blood thinners and statins.

Jim came to see that his own fear and bias had led him to turn off his keen instincts and move rashly to a cardiologist on autopilot. "When we were younger," he said, "our health problems tended to be one-dimensional: stitches, a broken arm, chicken pox. These were easy things for the medical profession to tackle. The doctors were heroes because they could solve stuff. And the system worked, so you develop the confidence that it always will. But as you get older, your problems aren't so one-dimensional anymore. They get fairly complicated for the doctors. To me now, every specialist is someone who has a compartmentalized view of my health. I accept the fact that that's the case, which means I have to manage them.

"Still," he continued, "I wish that the cardiologist that day would have stopped to think, 'Wait a minute—this guy just had a clean echocardiogram in November, and his angiogram shows *some* blockage but not the kind that would cause his symptoms. His heart is not the issue. He may need a stent someday, but that's not what the problem is today.' The reality is that *I* was biased, and I walked straight into cardiology land. The doctor wasn't thinking, 'This might be pulmonary'—he does hearts and a lot of stents. You give a carpenter a hammer, he's going to see every problem as a nail."

If Jim had waited and not scheduled angiography, he and his PCP would have found their way to a pulmonologist, and he would have had a true diagnosis in a few weeks. Instead, he raced toward a treatment he did not need and spent seventy-seven days in bed hooked up to an oxygen machine. Unfortunately, his case is not unique.

According to a 2013 special report in the *Journal of the American Medical Association*, the United States spends $2.7 trillion a year on heath care. About 30 percent of that—roughly $750 billion a year—is wasted on unnecessary treatments, tests, and procedures, according to the Institute of Medicine.

Heart catheterizations with stents are done at the rate of about half a million a year. But that number has been on the decline since 2007, when researchers found that the procedure didn't prevent heart attacks any better than drugs, exercise, and diet in patients with stable angina—predictable chest pains that occur during overexertion and are not due to severe heart disease. In a true coronary emergency, stents can absolutely save lives. But for everyone else? A 2011 *JAMA* report found that only half of 144,000 non-emergency heart catheterizations they studied were appropriate (38 percent were "uncertain" and 12 percent were "inappropriate").

What factors lead to overtreatment? Sometimes it stems from overdiagnosis, in which practitioners want to "catch" and "cure" conditions early, even when those discoveries are unlikely to progress into full-blown disease: for example, finding a tumor and recommending surgery, chemotherapy, radiation, and other therapies, when a wait-and-watch approach might be more appropriate. (This is especially harmful when the patient is elderly and won't live long enough for the disease to develop.)

Other times a clinician who trains for years to develop the skills and expertise to perform a complex, lifesaving technique may be overly invested in it. Imagine how emotional and difficult it is to be a doctor, with lives at stake every day. You really *need* to believe in what you do. But that sincere commitment sometimes translates into patients getting the wrong remedy.

Remember Jim's pulmonologist, who had more experience (and success) with bronchoscopies, even though, in Jim's case, a VATS procedure was more appropriate? We all tend to favor things that have worked well for us and avoid those that have not.

Another piece of the overtreatment puzzle is the practice of defensive medicine, ordering unnecessary treatments and tests to guard against liability in malpractice suits. Many physicians have the perception that they will be safer from liability claims if they prescribe *more* interventions.

Then there's the role *we* play, as patients. When we are sick,* we like to be diagnosed and treated on the spot. We also count on being able to run, wrestle with our grandkids, or play golf much longer than our parents did, and we want the latest high-tech treatments to keep us mobile. When we're not given fast fixes, we are disappointed. But if we consistently expect physicians to intervene, we are conditioning them to prescribe drugs needlessly, order useless invasive tests, and do potentially dangerous surgeries.

To help doctors and patients better communicate about treatment decisions, the American Board of Internal Medicine collaborated with a half-million physicians from the major specialty societies (American Academy of Pediatrics, American College of Surgeons, American Society of Clinical Oncology, etc.) to create questions patients should ask about certain types of tests, medicines, and procedures that may be unnecessary. These "Choosing Wisely" lists (at www.choosingwisely.org) cover such wide-ranging topics as ways to ease heartburn without drugs, the treatment of blocked leg arteries, and why you may not need bone density tests, allergy tests, CT scans, and other therapies for certain ailments. These recommendations don't cover everything—they focus on the most egregiously overused interventions—and they aren't a substitute for medical advice. But they're a worthwhile read on the current best-practices thinking from the leading medical organizations.

There's another pretty awful, but avoidable, factor that can contribute to overtreatment: financial incentives. Jim's story offers just a glimpse into

---

*Here's a simple example. When you show up at your primary care physician's office with a bad cold, you *expect* her to give you something to make you feel better. If she sends you home with a recommendation to rest, drink more fluids, and take an over-the-counter decongestant, you're dissatisfied. Far too many physicians prescribe antibiotics that are ineffective and potentially counterproductive at defeating colds and flu (which are caused by viruses, not by *bacteria*), simply to keep their patients happy.

what has become a nationwide controversy, that is: Are patients being over-stented? Stents are a huge moneymaker, billed at an average of $30,000 apiece, and Medicare has spent tens of billions on them in the last decade. When hospitals invest millions of dollars on catheter labs and state-of-the-art technologies, they naturally want to see a return on their investments. Sometimes the incentive becomes so powerful it veers to full-on fraud. In 2009, the year Jim got sick, a series of Justice Department investigations were slowly made public, revealing lawsuits chiefly filed by whistle-blower nurses and physicians horrified by what they had seen: doctors getting kick-backs from hospitals for cath-lab referrals; cardiologists giving patients the "full metal jacket" treatment—inserting as many as twenty to thirty stents—when they didn't need even one; and untrained surgeons regularly tearing open patients' arteries yet being allowed to continue to practice because they were cath-lab cash cows.

Which is not to say that all doctors and hospitals are greedy. It's just recognizing that we are all fallible. Doctors struggle, as we do, with personal pressures, anxieties about professional growth, and fears about meeting the needs of our families. People sometimes think that having the initials *M.D.* after one's name makes a person superhuman, immune to the same forces that motivate others. That's asking too much. Everyone responds to incentives. When you walk into a car dealership, you know that the salesperson is rewarded for selling you the top-of-the-line model, with lots of fancy extras. As a result, your guard is up. When it's time to take the car in for repairs, you're mindful that you'll be charged on a piecework basis and are wary of getting things fixed that are not broken. The vast majority of physicians and hospitals are also paid per procedure: the more they do, the more they make.

In fact, the procedures you receive when you get sick can have *more* to do with your zip code—and the medical approach of the hospitals in your area—than with your actual illness. There's no better data I've been able to find on this issue than the Dartmouth Atlas of Health Care, a series of reports from the Dartmouth Institute for Health Policy and Clinical Practice, which captures the rates of use of different medical procedures within hospital referral regions and then compares those rates from city to city. (Curious about your region? At www.dartmouthatlas.org you can slice and dice the statistics by zip code, surgical topic, key health care issue, and more.)

For instance, a 2012 report that studied elective surgical procedures among Medicare recipients found that patients in Casper, Wyoming, were seven times more likely to undergo back surgery than patients in Honolulu, Hawaii; meanwhile, women over sixty-five in Grand Forks, North Dakota, were seven times more likely to have a mastectomy for early-stage breast cancer than women in San Francisco, California.

When the researchers looked at elective stenting procedures (like Jim's), at the high end was the city of Elyria, Ohio, where doctors performed 19.8 per 1,000 patients; at the low end was (again) Honolulu, with just 2.6. (Although it would be lovely to assume that Hawaii's continual skewing to the left of the bell curve is the result of island physicians who are acutely sensitive to overtreatment, it's more likely a consequence of the doctor shortage in Hawaii: not enough orthopedic surgeons means fewer knee replacements. In other words, the data are helpful but have to be viewed in context.)

Jim, it turns out, resided in the region that held the record for greatest variation. Depending on what hospital you went to in his area in 2010, doctors performed anywhere from 4.2 to 18.1 stenting procedures per 1,000 patients. (The national average was 7.6.) Jim unwittingly went to the hospital that hit the 18.1 mark. Geography is destiny for lots of things, but medical care should not be one of them.

Jim's story illustrates an important lesson that anyone can follow: Unless you are in a life-threatening, emergency situation, do not start invasive treatment until you reach an evidence-based diagnosis. To get to that place, partner first with your PCP to dig into your problem and get to the right realm of medicine. Then see specialists who can confirm or rule out the disease in question. After you reach a diagnosis you feel very confident about, insist on having informed discussions with experts in your specific illness about the pros and cons of different approaches.

When you're lying on a gurney in a hospital gown, getting prepped for surgery, it takes an enormous amount of courage to *not* sign the consent form being handed to you. Your illness warrants careful examination. So take the time you need to be certain you have the right diagnosis, and the right doctor, before that happens.

"When my friends go for angiography now, I say, 'Do *not* sign that paper,'" Jim said. "Tell the surgeon, 'Unless I'm ninety percent blocked and at huge risk, you wake me up and we talk about it before you put that stent in.' And if he refuses to continue? I tell you what, I'd be fine with that, because I don't want him operating on me."

Jim learned how to advocate for himself after suffering through many missteps. Richard's story, on the other hand, shows how good care can be when you take the time to get it right.

In 2012 Richard got an upsetting phone call from his elderly mother, Sally, who lived in Dallas. Her hip had been bothering her recently, so her internist referred her to a top orthopedist. After one visit, and an MRI, the orthopedist told her that she needed to get her fifteen-year-old artificial hip replaced immediately.

That just didn't sound right to Richard, but on the phone from New York he wondered if perhaps his mother had gotten confused about the doctor's orders.

"Mom, are you sure?" he asked.

Actually, Sally wasn't sure. She had leaned for guidance on her physician husband until his death two years earlier. But now that she was on her own—and at eighty-seven had a short-term memory that wasn't what it used to be—thankfully, Sally was in the habit of bringing a friend along on medical visits. That companion was with her as she spoke to her son.

"When we went to see that doctor," Sally turned to ask her friend, "do I remember correctly that he told me I needed to have surgery?"

"Not only did he tell you that you needed a new hip," the pal confirmed, "he went ahead and scheduled a date for you."

Richard was worried now. His mom was not making this up. In fact, she had been told by the orthopedist that if he didn't operate on her quickly, she would be bedridden for the rest of her years.

His worry quickly shifted to skepticism: *Why had there been no talk about conservative options? Why the rush to operate, when her life wasn't in danger?*

Trusting his gut, he said: "Mom, hold on. I think we need to get another opinion."

Sally's first hip replacement surgery had been excruciating for her. Recovery was painful, and she hated doing the rehab therapy. But her husband had been there to help and to push her to do her exercises. Richard didn't think she would survive a second operation. After he discussed the matter with his brothers, the family summoned the courage to put the brakes on this fast-moving train.

"My father raised me with a couple of values toward medicine," Richard said, when we spoke about his mother's case. "One is, there's no such thing as minor surgery. Minor surgery is when it's on *you*. Major surgery is when it's on *me*.

"The other value he gave me," he continued, "is that medicine is still an art—it's not a science. When every doctor gets the same outcome for every procedure, then medicine will be a science. Until then, choosing the right surgeon is critical."

My own father taught me that you never ask the barber if you need a haircut—so I got what he was saying. We would need first to determine whether Sally really needed this *major* surgery. If she did, then we had to be sure she was seeing the right surgeon.

We began—just as you would at the beginning of your own serious diagnosis—by collecting her entire health history and sending her recent MRIs to several hip experts for a second round of opinions. They didn't find what her Dallas doctor saw, so we approached him in a very diplomatic, respectful way and shared the differing perspectives to get his take. He was reasonable. He agreed that perhaps it wasn't so urgent. But we weren't sure a new hip was necessary at all.

About 332,000 hip replacements are done in the United States annually. (Knees are replaced at more than twice the rate.) According to a 2013 *New York Times* investigative report, nearly all the artificial knees and hips used in this country are made by five companies that have been able to maintain a death grip on prices. An artificial hip like the one that Sally's doctor wanted to implant probably costs about $350 to manufacture, but the final hospital bill could range from $11,000 to $126,000. Sally was on Medicare, so she wouldn't be writing the check. And hospitals know that.

I wondered if geography was a factor in Sally's case. Probably not. According to the Dartmouth Atlas, Dallas doctors performed 3.2 hip replacements per 1,000 Medicare recipients that year, just under the national average of 3.9.

Sally's doctor seemed like a reasonable person, not driven by monetary incentives. It's more likely he was just being a hip expert, responding to what he saw on an MRI: "This socket looks a little worse for wear. Let's fix it." Instead, he needed to step back and look at the totality of the human being in front of him.

It took about two months to get all of Sally's records, but it was worth the wait, because within them was the clue we had been hoping for. Many years earlier Sally had had an unsuccessful cornea transplant and lost the vision in her right eye. Afterward Richard had implored his parents to go to the Jules Stein Eye Institute in Los Angeles, so that his mother could get a thorough exam with experts.

"We have good news and bad news," the institute's doctors had told Sally. The bad news was that she was not going to get vision back in her right eye. The good news? "Your blindness was caused by a surgical mishap—so you don't have to worry about losing vision in your left eye based on what happened in your right eye."

How's that for good news? Sally didn't complain, though. She simply adjusted to her compromised sight.

When we found Sally a new orthopedist, Dr. Michael H. Huo, a professor of orthopedic surgery at the University of Texas Southwestern Medical Center, we sent him her full medical history, including the eye surgery reports. Dr. Huo had a hunch after reviewing her file. And when he spoke with her during their exam, he saw her problem instantly. He told her, "Sally, from now on, I want you to pick up your right foot and point it in the direction of the person you're conversing with."

What had happened was this: Ever since her botched cornea transplant, whenever someone was standing to her right, Sally would lean over so she could see the person through her good left eye. This action, repeated over and over throughout the years, was putting stress on the joint where her right hipbone connected to her femur. Once she made the small adjustment, her hip pain went away. It was that simple.

She was thrilled, of course, as were her children. "There are very few doctors who really understand how the whole system works," Richard said. "You're either a brain surgeon or a heart surgeon, or you take care of the eyes, feet, skin—but nobody really knows how the whole body works together. I don't want to suggest that her first doctor was trying to take advantage of a situation. I just think his training led him to the conclusion that, whatever he saw in that MRI, the best way to fix it was surgically. A doctor with a more holistic approach might look at it and say, 'You know, let's see if physical therapy can solve the problem.'"

Richard had the competence to recognize that his mother's condition was probably not an emergency. But he also had the courage to question her surgeon's treatment plan and cancel the scheduled operation, even though he was a well-known and respected orthopedist. He understood that having the world's greatest doctor does not always mean you get to sit back and let him or her call the shots.

Orthopedic surgeons and cardiologists are consistently the highest-earning doctors, according to physician compensation surveys. As in most professions, the best-paid "stars" often receive the most respect and deference—and less scrutiny than their peers. All of which allows the occasional cowboy in their midst to get away with appalling errors. The problem is compounded when Medicare is paying the bill and elderly patients blindly follow the doctor's orders.

But there's another level of dysfunction that we, as patients, are guilty of, and it's equally frightening. Because we're not paying our doctors directly out of our own pockets, the financial insulation makes us lose sight of the *responsibility* we have to assume control of our own care. Further, we don't recognize that the real currency we are tendering in this transaction is our well-being—a currency that is extremely fragile. What you are putting on the line when you relinquish responsibility for your medical decisions is your capacity to walk, to breathe, to function.

So what can you do? It comes back to competence and courage: the competence to do your research and ask the right questions, and the courage to get expert opinions and say no to bad proposals. If you can summon these two traits when you're in the market for a new cell phone plan, a gym membership, or a home loan, then I know you can do it when you are talking to practitioners in white lab coats.

"It used to be, whatever a doctor said, the patient did. Now, there's a lot more back-and-forth, and honestly I prefer that," says Dr. Michael Davidson, an expert in heart disease prevention and a clinical professor of medicine and director of preventive cardiology at the University of Chicago's School of Medicine. "I prefer a patient who's really going to dive into the issues, understand them well, and work with me on making the right decisions."

In fact, one thing Dr. Davidson always asks his patients when he sees them is "What things can we stop or take away?"

If your physician doesn't take the same approach, it's totally fine (even courageous!) to ask: *Is this procedure necessary? Do I really need to be on these drugs? Can we lessen my dosage?*

"Look, if there was one thing that I thought was a hundred percent the right way to go, I would try to push that. But in most cases there's multiple options to consider," Dr. Davidson says. "Hearing what the patient has to say, trying to find out their options and hurdles . . . helping the patient to come up with their own solutions . . . makes the ultimate success of the therapy a lot more possible. And when the patient acknowledges it's the right path for them, it's more likely that they're going to adhere to and be successful in the plan."

Good medicine is a collaborative effort, and good doctors *want* you to be courageous and competent in your dealings with them. Here are some ways to get there.

HOW TO BE MORE COMPETENT

- Immerse yourself in the literature on your proposed diagnosis, and do online research on the physicians recommending your surgery or treatment.
- Talk to friends and family members who may have been through similar experiences.
- Get expert opinions from specialists on your condition.
- Study the websites of the major medical institutions in your state and find out if they have specialists and departments solely devoted to your illness. If you like what you see, call for a consultation.
- Look up your region in the Dartmouth Atlas of Health Care to see if the treatment your practitioner is recommending has been cited as being prescribed more or less often than the national average.
- Review the "Choosing Wisely" lists to find out if the treatment your doctor is proposing meets standard-practice recommendations.

HOW TO BE MORE COURAGEOUS

- Engage in a dialogue with your doctor:

"Why is this surgery/drug/test necessary?"

"What are the risks/side effects of this procedure?"

"How long is the recovery period, and what will it involve?"

"How many times have you done this surgery/used this protocol, and have you had any complications?"

"What will happen if we don't do it?"

"Are there nonsurgical/less aggressive options we can try first? How do they compare to my surgical/more aggressive options?"

- Tell your doctor you'd like to get an independent second opinion, and ask for a copy of your medical records.
- Send your records in advance of your new consultation, and call the front office to make sure the doctor has read them before your appointment.
- If you get differing advice, consider getting a third opinion.

In the next chapter, I'm going to show you how to do smarter online research, as well as the best ways to find and interview the right specialists for your problem. As you gain more practice in savvy health care consumption, your medical instincts will become more finely tuned. And like Richard, you'll attain a healthy dose of skepticism when someone tries to sell you or your loved ones something they don't need. Always be as cautious of overtreatment as you are of undertreatment. In medicine, as in many things, sometimes less is more.

QUICK GUIDE

CHAPTER 5. Overtreatment Can Be as Dangerous as Undertreatment

- When you are experiencing a medical issue that's not life-threatening, your first call should be to your PCP.

- Be aware of the factors that lead to overtreatment. Recognize the role you may be playing in the problem when you self-diagnose, fail to ask questions, don't get expert opinions, and demand fast fixes from your doctors.

- Unless you are in a life-threatening, emergency situation, do not start treatment until you reach an evidence-based diagnosis.

- Be more competent and courageous in your interactions with your providers, using the suggestions on pages 104 and 105.

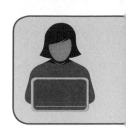

CHAPTER SIX

HOW TO FIND AND INTERVIEW THE MEDICAL EXPERTS YOU NEED

Don't just Google it—here are smarter ways to get the right specialists.

Rachel had always enjoyed perfect hearing, but at thirty-eight she started to notice diminished function in her left ear. "It felt like my ear was plugged," she recalls. "My ob-gyn told me that because I'd recently had a baby, I was experiencing a normal hormonal surge, and my membranes were swollen. So I didn't think much about it. But then I had a second and third child, and it got worse."

In her late forties, Rachel saw an ear, nose, and throat doctor who diagnosed her with something called otosclerosis, an abnormal bony growth in her middle ear. In Rachel's case, it was preventing her ear bones from vibrating as sounds passed through, a crucial part of auditory function. Surgery would cure her, but since she was a busy mom, and her condition wasn't life-threatening, she decided to wait.

Fast-forward to age fifty-one. Rachel was now down to about 15 percent hearing in her left ear, which was affecting her life in so many negative ways. Imagine missing almost half of what people say to you. She was unable to decipher what teachers were announcing at her children's school functions. She had to watch TV with headphones to avoid annoying her family with the high volume. Her kids were constantly yelling "Mom! Mom!" to get her attention. And she had specific trouble with low-pitched tones, which meant that men who spoke in a bass voice appeared to be mouthing their words.

(The opposite could be said of the kids' Saturday-morning cartoon programs, which sounded like screeching to her.) Rachel's husband had to sit strategically to her right in order to avoid scream-pitch conversations. They could forget about talking when he was driving them anywhere. "You *really* need to get that fixed," he kept saying.

Rachel knew he was right. It was time. So she began meeting with potential surgeons (the doctor who first diagnosed her was not a surgeon), starting with a woman who practiced at a center that specialized in ear disorders. To her surprise, this doctor told Rachel that her problem was *not* otosclerosis but a neurological condition for which there was no cure. A hearing aid would help, she said. Rachel bought one that she could try risk-free for thirty days. It was of no help whatsoever, so she returned it.

Undaunted, she made an appointment with a new surgeon (if you're keeping count, doctor number three) who agreed with doctor number one: "This is most definitely otosclerosis." Since doctors two and three worked at the same institution, she asked them to explain their difference of opinion. Each insisted that the other was not only wrong but also pretty stupid. Rachel was bewildered by their behavior. She asked if they would be willing to meet to discuss her case. They refused. Rachel wisely decided this was not the right place for her surgery.

She next saw an ENT at a large teaching hospital. He confirmed her original—and ultimately correct—diagnosis of otosclerosis and recommended the same surgery that the first and third doctors had, which involved removing either all (a stapedectomy) or part (a stapedotomy) of her stapes bone and inserting a prosthetic.

The stapes, a tiny horseshoe-shaped structure, is the smallest bone in the body (about one-tenth of an inch). It's tiny even in someone who's six foot four, so you can imagine how little it was in Rachel, who barely topped five-two in her high heels.

The doctor described the procedure and gave her a pamphlet to take home. She'd lost count of how many times she'd been handed the same old *What You Need to Know About Your Stapes Surgery* leaflet. Every time she looked at it, one figure gnawed at her: the surgery would completely restore hearing if it went well, but in about 1 out of 100 cases, hearing becomes even worse.

Those odds might sound okay. But Rachel wasn't willing to trade the poor hearing in her left ear for total deafness or grim possible side effects like tinnitus, a continual, high-pitched ringing. She also wondered why every doctor was telling her about the same procedure that had been around for decades. *Doctors don't even have to crack open ribs to do heart surgeries anymore*, she thought. *So why are they still going in manually with their big fingers to take out the tiniest bone in the body? What are the cutting-edge options? How come no one's talking about lasers?*

She didn't have full confidence in any of the doctors she met. So she turned to the resource that everyone uses when facing an important medical decision. "I'm going to go on the Internet and find out for myself who's the best," she announced to her husband one summer day. She started by typing the phrase "best ear surgeon in the world" into Google—and discovered that virtually every ENT with a website claims that title. She got more specific, trying "laser ear surgery" and "stapes surgery + best." This led her to many more advertisements for ear surgeons, as well as a slew of random clinical articles and an endless supply of blog postings about other people's surgeries. She read countless horror stories of painful recoveries and disastrous outcomes. Unfortunately, none of it brought her any nearer to finding the right surgeon.

So she took a stab in the dark. "What do you think of this guy?" she asked her husband. "He claims he's the best, *and* he does laser surgery."

"I don't know about this, Rachel," he said. "His office is in a shopping center in Minnesota."

Rachel was waist-deep in what I call the tragic treasure trove. Type "stapes surgery" into Google, and you get about 50,000 returns for a procedure that's pretty uncommon. Where does one begin? If you really want to be overwhelmed, try looking up common conditions like "skin cancer" (about 1.4 million hits on Google and counting), "heart disease" (4.9 million), or "breast cancer" (11.2 million).

If you focus only on the sites of respected institutions and medical journals, you'll still be faced with a mountain of data. More than sixty thousand medical articles are published every month (twice as many as a decade ago), offering a body of literature containing deeper understandings of the causes of disease than ever before, faster ways to get a correct diagnosis, and the latest teachings on the best treatments. The treasure trove is overflowing with invaluable information. The tragic part is that doctors do not have the time or resources to mine it in order to help their patients get the best care.

When you retain a lawyer to figure out a problem, she's paid to do research. Her firm has junior staff who study evolving issues and keep the firm on its toes. Doctors don't have this luxury, and they don't get paid to read. There is no insurance reimbursement code for studying up on a patient's condition. As a result, many physicians don't do it. It takes years, even decades, for better surgical techniques, medical procedures, and drug treatments to become the norm because not everyone is in the know.

"It's true that a lot of doctors are not up to date on the literature," notes Dallas internist Dr. Carter. "In my primary care practice, I'll see a new patient come in, and they are on the same blood pressure medication they started in 1978. But here's the reality: Some of those drugs are tried and true. They are still the gold standard, and if they are working for you, it may make sense to stay with them. But for other patients who come in, and their blood pressure isn't that well controlled, I know we can do better. We have drugs now that can control blood pressure *and* protect your kidneys against the effects of diabetes if you also have that. But when your doctor's not reading, they may miss things and potentially impact your overall health."

If, like Rachel, you decide to immerse yourself in the literature—which I would encourage you to do, because you cannot assume your doctors will—there's a better way to do it than poring over anecdotal blogs. Throughout this book, I'm going to share smarter ways to do research. Here's a quick look at how we did it in Rachel's case.

First, I asked for her top three medical questions. Rachel wanted to know:

- Should I do a stapedectomy or a stapedotomy?
- Who's the best surgeon for the job? (In other words, who's done the procedure thousands of times and won't leave me deaf?)
- Is anyone using lasers, and is this the right option for me?

Your research questions will vary depending on your condition, but I suggest writing them down so they can serve as a compass, keeping you on course if you start to get overwhelmed by the sheer amount of information. As you learn more about your condition, your questions will become more refined, and you'll bring them with you to consultations with specialists. If you need a little help getting started, the Agency for Healthcare Research and Quality has a thoughtful "Question Builder" application (www.ahrq.gov/apps/qb/) that allows you to create and prioritize a list of important things to ask your doctor, based on the nature of your visit.

With Rachel's questions in hand, we were able to begin our online research. Where *you* start depends on where you are in the process:

1. I have symptoms, and I want to learn more about the underlying cause.
2. I have been given a diagnosis, or I may have this condition, and I want to learn more about it.
3. I am trying to find experts who can consult with me on my illness.

If you're at the beginning of your journey (numbers one and two) and just need basic information, it's fine to start with Google, but as your search becomes more sophisticated, you'll get more reliable data by turning to the stalwart institutions, like the National Institutes of Health (NIH), the Mayo Clinic, and WebMD.

When you are ready to dig deeper into your condition, and find out who the most research-invested specialists are (number three), as Rachel was, I guarantee that you will get better information if you search PubMed (www .pubmed.gov), a database of medical articles maintained by the U.S. National Library of Medicine at the NIH.

At PubMed you can read the abstracts (and in some cases the entire article) for free. You may find, at first, that the content is dense and difficult to understand. But if you stick with it, you will come to learn the language and landscape of your illness—and that will keep you firmly in the role of decision maker. Having even a small understanding of what the latest studies say about your condition will make your doctors take notice—especially if it's *their* research.

"More often than not, when you see a patient whose condition is relevant to your research, you're relaying information to them that you've already published," says Dr. George Wilding, an oncologist, cancer researcher, and former director of the Carbone Cancer Center at the University of Wisconsin in Madison. "If a patient actually looked up the stuff and read it? I'd think that's great. It's good for patients and their families to know as much as possible about their disease and treatment options."

When we search online, we typically begin with broad search terms that become more precise as we learn the terminology. But the more specific you can be, the better your results. For instance, when I type "ear surgery" into PubMed (with quotation marks, to tell the search engine I want this exact phrase), about 1,600 articles pop up. Oops. Let's try "stapes surgery." That gives me 3,200 articles. Still too broad, but a good sense of the breadth of literature. (You may be wondering why there were more results for "stapes surgery" than "ear surgery." Here, the keywords of these papers are adhering to the medical nomenclature. As you begin to understand your condition better, you'll also start describing it the way physicians and researchers do: with precision.) How about "stapes surgery" + laser. Bingo! Now I've got nearly 300 of the most recent articles about one of Rachel's specific questions, written by international surgeons and researchers who are passionate about this treatment.

Because many of the papers are off-topic for Rachel's case (i.e., "The Role of Imaging in the Diagnosis and Management of Otosclerosis"), I can ignore a lot of them. To get more granular, click on the filters located at the top left-hand side of the window (to search, for example, for clinical trials, or only English results). For instance, if I click on "Review," the algorithm will find studies that summarize the literature on laser stapes surgery. You can also type the word "review" next to your search terms in the main PubMed search engine box, like so: "stapes surgery" + review. Once you become adept, try an advanced search to direct the engine to show only the articles that contain your key words in the title and/or abstract fields. (In the PubMed Advanced Search Builder window, scroll down and select "Title" or "Title/Abstract," type in your search term, then click "Search.") This will help you find papers most focused on your problem. Helpful features, located in the margins of your results, show you papers with related citations, free-to-read articles on your topic, and more filters to help manage your search.

When we go online, we tend to circle. As new terms pop up and the same phrases catch your eye, they spur more discoveries, then more inquiries. After reading dozens of abstracts on stapes surgery, I go back to the beginning to get more granular, typing in the phrase "stapedectomy versus stapedotomy." That pulls up 35 results—a nice short list of the most recent studies that speak to Rachel's narrow question: *Which procedure is right for me?*

But here's the exciting part: After a few hours of researching, I see the same authors' names cropping up.* With PubMed, you can click on a byline (the first name cited is the lead author, typically the most involved researcher) and get a list of every article written by that person. (If there are multiple authors with the same name, PubMed lists all of them, so double-check middle initials to be sure you've got the right person.) You can add these names to your list of potential experts to call on. (In Rachel's case, not all of them would be surgeons, of course. But they might be excellent resources, people who could refer her to great surgeons for her condition.)

An additional online resource that we frequently use to supplement PubMed research is Expertscape.com, a site that helps patients track down the most-published specialists on a topic. Enter your condition into Expertscape, click on "Show Experts," and a broad list of names comes up. If you click next on your country, region, city, or desired medical institution, a smaller list shows the most-published clinicians who match your request criteria. Click on these names to see their article titles and abstracts.

It's important to remember that the number and depth of papers a doctor has published can be a good indicator of how devoted he or she is to a specific condition. But that doesn't always mean this doctor is going to be the best specialist for you. You still need to pick up the phone, ask questions, and gather data. View these sites as valuable starting points in your research.

Another fast, reliable way to find a specialist is to study the websites of the top medical institutions in the biggest city near you. Go to the department that fits your need (whether it's endocrinology, dermatology, pediatric allergies, etc.), and pull up the bios of the staff members to identify practitioners whose education, training, and research areas match your concerns. You can also find expert physicians by studying the names on the medical/scientific advisory boards of the nonprofit philanthropies and disease-specific foundations that focus on your illness. Go deeper by typing these names into PubMed to review any published works. You will have done more to learn about them than 99 percent of their patients do.

I ultimately gave Rachel the names of three surgeons with whom I wanted her to consult by phone: a physician in France, whom she ultimately

---

*It's important to keep in mind that just because someone's name is on a paper, it doesn't mean that person played an active role in the study. You have to look at the names of the people who are leading the study (or clinical trial). In general, the lead author, the first name listed, is the person who led the research and preparation of the article.

decided against because she had excellent options in the United States; Dr. William Lippy, in Warren, Ohio, who had performed more than seventeen thousand stapedectomies and invented many of the tools and techniques of the procedure; and Dr. Herbert Silverstein, the president and founder of the Silverstein Institute and Ear Research Foundation in Sarasota, Florida, who had also pioneered techniques and tools in the area of stapedotomy (he had more than two hundred articles in PubMed), lowering the risk of hearing loss from 1 in 100 cases to about 1 in 400.

After speaking to all three, Rachel chose Dr. Silverstein. The clincher for her was that he wanted to perform a partial stapes removal, leaving part of the bone behind—and he would do it using a laser.

But any of these doctors could easily have been *the* one: Rachel was in the No-Mistake Zone. By that I mean:

- She had a true, evidence-based diagnosis.
- She was convinced that now was the right time for treatment— as opposed to waiting and watching.
- She had explored her treatment options and consulted with experts who were focused on her condition.
- She clearly understood her treatment plan and all that it entailed.

A few weeks later Rachel flew to Sarasota for her early-morning operation. It took about an hour, and there were no complications. A surgical success. Because she wouldn't be able to fly for a week, she had invited a girlfriend to tag along and keep her company. Rachel had pored over terrifying blog posts about postsurgery nausea, vomiting, dizziness, and blackouts— she was prepared for the apocalypse.

"I'm going to get in bed now," she told her pal when they got back to the hotel room. "I'm probably going to be throwing up soon, crawling to the bathroom, it's going to get ugly."

"Okay," her friend said. "I'll just stay here on the couch and watch you."

Rachel carefully put on her pajamas, got in bed, and waited. An hour passed.

"It's going to hit me any minute," Rachel said.

"Do you mind if I put the news on?" her friend replied.

Another hour passed.

"I'm sure it's coming—just hang in there."

"Of course. Just let me know," said her dutiful pal. By three in the afternoon, she asked: "Rachel, are you sure you don't want a cocktail while we're waiting?"

Rachel decided to get dressed and, if she didn't collapse first, maybe take a walk around the grounds holding her friend's arm. She discovered she had the strength not only to walk but also to go shopping and have a cocktail before dinner.

After twelve years of near deafness, it took a while for Rachel to get used to the enhanced volume. Sounds seemed so loud, they almost hurt. "It's amazing to get something back that I never thought I could," she said.

It's likely that Rachel would have gotten a fine result with any of the skilled surgeons she had met on her own. But because we took the time to properly research her treatment options and interview physicians, she had an *excellent* outcome and recovery.

Rachel wanted a cutting-edge procedure with a master surgeon, and she was willing to fly anywhere to get it. May we all be lucky enough to have the same time and resources. But the extra expenses she incurred in order to restore her hearing—and ensure she wouldn't go deaf—were not as high as one might think. She had to pay out of pocket for her travel expenses and phone consultations. The rest was covered by her insurance.

I understand that many people find it difficult to travel for care or pay for any additional costs beyond what insurance covers. But when faced with a technically demanding procedure or rare disease, at the least, you should get to the closest large hospital, which is more likely to have volume and expertise in your specific condition.

Most Americans live within one hundred miles of a major metropolitan city. Almost every large city has an academic medical center or distinguished hospital that is in-network, with specialists and surgeons who take Medicare and most kinds of insurance. When you live in a small town and find yourself with a serious condition, if you are well enough to travel, you owe it to yourself to get to a prominent hospital—at least for a second opinion. Because if something goes wrong (and you have to consider that it might), the quality of care and resources at a small, community hospital are just not optimal.

"I see a lot of mistakes," says Dr. Robert Udelsman, an expert in endocrine oncology and surgery and the chair of the department of surgery (and surgeon-in-chief) at Yale–New Haven Hospital in Connecticut. In fact, 20 percent of Dr. Udelsman's practice is revision surgery—meaning he fixes other doctors' mistakes. He's like the surgeon's surgeon, the cleanup guy who knows everybody else's operation notes, their handiwork, their sutures. But what I wanted to know, what I asked Dr. Udelsman, was what kinds of mistakes he sees *patients* make.

"Sometimes they treat surgery like it's a commodity," he said. "They run and get the quickest guy, because it's convenient, because they want this problem to go away before the holiday."

Slow down a little bit and find the right person, Dr. Udelsman says, especially if you're having an elective procedure: "Don't go to your local hospital when, fifteen miles farther, you can get the world-class expert. For something as precious as your health, when bad, irreversible things can happen, I would be sure to go where my odds are improved. Shop a little bit. When you buy a house, you probably look at fifteen or twenty houses before you pick one. Nobody buys the first house they see. Picking a hospital for an operation is probably just as important as that."

Harvard researchers wanted to find out if patients who underwent certain risky operations had better results when they were done at "high-complexity" hospitals—institutes that offer a wider range of services and technologies (such as an adult catheter lab, oncology care, hemodialysis, PET scanners)—than at typical rural hospitals. So they studied the outcomes of patients who had one of five common, high-risk surgical procedures: above-the-knee amputation, abdominal aortic aneurysm repair, coronary artery bypass graft, colon resection, and small bowel resection. As you might imagine, patients who had their procedures done at the *lowest*-complexity hospitals had a 27 percent higher risk of death than those who went to high-complexity hospitals—which, in addition to having more resources, also tend to be large, nonprofit institutions with academic teaching programs.

Think you can't afford the bigger, city hospitals? Here's a trick of the trade that most people don't realize: In most cases, it doesn't cost you more to get better care. Think about the major purchases we make. In virtually every sector of the economy except for health care, there's a pretty tight relationship between price and quality. Nobody would argue that flying coach is better than first class or that the super-deluxe ocean-view suite at a hotel will cost the same as the parking-lot-facing single. But in medicine? Price and quality aren't demonstrably related. If your health insurance plan is accepted at both your small local hospital and at the nearest major academic center, why wouldn't you go to the one with more technology and experienced practitioners?

As Tom Gordon, CEO of Cedars-Sinai Medical Network, recently put it to me, "Look, if you're an HMO patient or a PPO patient, you're treated exactly the same way here. If you're an HMO patient or a PPO patient and you need to be hospitalized, you get to go to Cedars-Sinai; and if you need brain surgery, you get to see Keith Black"—a world-renowned neurosurgeon—"so it doesn't much matter here."

A few years ago, when Walmart was looking to lower its health insurance costs, executives discovered that a small number of workers with complicated health care problems were being treated locally and getting the wrong diagnoses, wasteful interventions, and error-prone care. Walmart found it could actually save money by sending employees who needed certain pricey surgeries (i.e., knee and hip replacements, organ transplants, spine surgery) to bigger, better-equipped institutions with proven track records, and pay for 100 percent of the care and costs (i.e., travel, lodging, and living expenses for the patient and a caregiver). Walmart negotiated flat fees with a handful of "centers of excellence" and initiated a travel medicine program for its full-time employees, allowing them to have their heart surgeries at the Mayo Clinic in Rochester, Minnesota, or hip replacements at Virginia Mason Medical Center in Seattle.

Home improvement chain Lowe's has a similar plan in place, whereby employees and their dependents enrolled in the company's medical plan can have cardiac surgery at the Cleveland Clinic, in Ohio, and Lowe's picks up medical costs, travel, hotel, and food expenses for the patient and a caregiver. Beverage and snack food giant PepsiCo has an alliance with Johns Hopkins in Baltimore to provide heart procedures and complex joint-replacement surgeries at no extra cost to employees. These money-conscious corporations aren't just getting deals on surgery for millions of employees, they're getting lower complication rates, fewer repeat procedures, and better long-term outcomes.

The point is: When you have a complicated illness, if you are well enough to travel, it's worthwhile to consult with a major institution, at least for an expert opinion.

"It's not true for *everything* in medicine that the places or the individuals who do more of something are necessarily better," notes New York hematologist Dr. Roboz. "Nonetheless, I think it's fair to find out from your surgeon, 'Have you done this before?' and 'How many times? Once or a gazillion?' and 'If you've done it once, are you going to do this procedure with somebody who's done it a gazillion times?'

"The other thing to think about—and this is important—you have to imagine that everything will go wrong," Dr. Roboz continued. "If you're having a baby and everything goes right, then the taxi driver can deliver, and it's fine. But you always have to think *What if everything goes wrong?* Your surgeon might be phenomenal, but if you're in a small community hospital, what's the intensive care unit like? If the doctor is telling you that this surgery is 'high-risk' or 'complicated,' those are buzz words that might make you think about going to a bigger teaching hospital."

Some pregnant women pick their ob-gyn based on the peacefulness and comfort of the maternity ward where the physician delivers, but Dr. Roboz picked her ob-gyn by who did the best C-section—just in case she needed one. "It turns out—I ended up needing two," she says. "I picked the guy who does an eight-minute, perfect C-section with a really good scar. I don't give a banana about the curtains. I don't care if they hold my hand. I don't need a best friend. So again, it's a useful principle to ask, 'What could go wrong?,' 'How's my doctor?,' and 'How's my hospital if it does go wrong?'"

For Rachel, learning how to interview her doctors was one of the most important things she gleaned from our work together. "It just never occurred to me that you can send a list of questions to physicians and then set up a conference call to ask them about their procedures and track records," she said. "It was really eye-opening."

Not every doctor will welcome your inquiry with open arms, but in my experience most of the good ones do. And it *never* hurts to ask. Make friends with the doctor's administrative assistant and be honest:

> *I realize that Dr. McDaniels is very busy and in great demand, but I've read all of his articles, and I'd really like him to do my surgery. I'd just like to ask him a few questions first. Could we set up a time to meet? Any time that works for him.*

I've also found that if you hit a wall, having your internist—or even a friend or family member—call for you works wonders. I do this for people all the time, by just saying:

My friend needs to have this surgery. I know Dr. Smith is the best. I realize her schedule is stacked, but my friend can drop everything in a moment's notice. Can we get him in for a consultation? If you get a cancellation, just call me and we'll make it happen.

Rachel discovered that doctors treated her very differently when she interviewed them, because she was approaching her surgery with a significant level of knowledge. She felt more respected and *remembered* as a patient.

"They've got five hundred patients. It's like a college application—how will you stand out so they treat you better?" she said. "I didn't do surgical interviews with my previous physicians—I just walked in and was like every other patient they had. I think it made Dr. Silverstein feel important—as silly as that sounds. But if someone says to you, 'I'd like *you* to perform my surgery, but let's do a call first, because I have a lot of questions for you,' I think you'd respect that person more because they are taking charge of their own situation."

And when you've made your choice, it doesn't hurt to ask that your doctor be the one holding the knife the day of your procedure. That conversation goes something like this:

Dr. Howard, I've got the highest respect for your practice and your accomplishments. This is a complicated and sensitive surgery. I frankly have concerns about it. I've met with several physicians, but I knew after meeting and speaking with you that you are the only one I want doing my surgery. I realize that we're in a teaching facility, and you have fellows you need to train. What I'd like is to make sure that you're the person who actually does the surgery on me. Would that be okay with you?

If this is really difficult for you, you could ask your trusted primary care physician to make the request. I've known a few cases in which the surgeon not only agrees but also invites the PCP to scrub in and watch. It can be extremely comforting for a patient to know that his or her internist will be in the operating room.

Debbie, a college-aged woman with a thick, wavy black mane, noticed one morning that her hair was noticeably thinning. Soon she was losing a brushful every morning. Her father, Michael, had reason to be worried. He and his wife had previously lost an infant child to cancer. As a parent, he was imagining the worst.

Debbie's PCP did blood tests and allergy panels. He asked her to keep a log of her diet. But he just couldn't come up with an answer. All Debbie kept hearing was: *There's nothing wrong. You're probably under a lot of stress.*

Michael wasn't satisfied. On a hunch, he researched all of Debbie's prescriptions, which included Loestrin birth control pills and Topamax migraine medicine. Pretty easily he discovered that alopecia, or hair loss, is a potential side effect for both Topamax and Loestrin. (A simple Google search can churn up plenty of reliable information on prescription drugs. The NIH's Drug Information Portal has detailed technical information, and Drugs.com has full package inserts, a drug interactions checker, and a pill identifier.)

Normally, one might pop the champagne corks and call it a day. But because of the family's history, Michael wanted to make absolutely sure. So he found a hair-loss expert at a nearby teaching hospital. Debbie didn't necessarily need *the* best in the country—any alopecia expert should have been skilled enough to do a simple follicle test under a microscope. Which is exactly what this one did, determining that Debbie's hair loss was indeed a side effect of medication. There are lots of treatments for migraines, and many other forms of birth control, so she stopped taking both drugs. Her hair grew back, and everyone had peace of mind.

Fifty years ago, if your car broke down, you could take it to the gas station for repairs. It didn't matter what type of car you had; they were all similar enough that any mechanic could figure it out. But today there's so much technology in an automobile, you might get the best results by taking it to a repair shop that specializes in your make, where they have the diagnostics, the training, and the experience to fix it. The same is true with health care. Which is why you needn't risk your well-being by putting it in the hands of someone for whom your condition is a novelty. There are many different kinds of breast cancers, brain tumors, ear disorders, reasons for hair loss—and many experts are trained in the very specific types of diseases and procedures you may need.

When it comes to solving unique or rare health problems, you sometimes have to stop and ask yourself, *Am I going deep enough? Have I found a practitioner who spends all her time thinking about my condition?* Debbie's internist hadn't sent her to a hair-loss expert because PCPs often don't take it as their responsibility to get patients to the specialist with the greatest and narrowest expertise in exactly their condition.

I saw someone the other day whose ten-year-old nephew's epilepsy was being managed—not very successfully—by a primary care physician. "Why don't his parents take him to an epileptologist?" I asked. The PCP had never suggested it, and it hadn't occurred to the family that anyone like that existed. But for almost every profession and condition, there's an expert. If your PCP doesn't recommend one, you should ask for his help and do some legwork yourself.

We found Catherine's expert, Dr. Wechsler, much the same way we found Rachel's ear surgeon: while reviewing her condition on PubMed. But seeking out disease organizations was another important expert-seeking step we took—one you should take as well. Dr. Wechsler was one of several capable doctors listed on the Churg-Strauss Syndrome Association's medical advisory board, and his published work on the disease was prolific. We sent a brief, professional e-mail to his university address, asking if he would be willing to review a new potential case. He was delighted to hear from us— this was his life's work, after all.

Look at the medical advisory boards of the organizations devoted to your illness, and cross-reference the names with PubMed to see who has made this condition a research priority. Are any of these doctors located near you? Might they be seeing patients or be open to a phone consultation? When you reach out to your chosen experts, remember that a little flattery goes a long way. First, introduce yourself:

I have just been diagnosed with . . . or *I am struggling with . . .*

Then let the doctor know you've done your homework:

I've been doing extensive research on this topic, and your name keeps coming up again and again. I really appreciate the work you are doing. I learned so much from your paper on [name of your condition].

And get to the point quickly:

I'm looking for some guidance, and I would so appreciate the opportunity to talk with you. Any input you might have would be helpful to me.

Do you ever do distance consultations or medical record reviews?

And remember, if you ask for these things, let the doctor know that you respect his time and expertise:

My insurance company has told me that they are willing to pay for . . .

I know you are very busy, and I am happy to pay out of pocket for your time.

Even if this doctor turns out to be unavailable, you can ask for a local reference:

Thank you so much for your reply. If your schedule opens up, I'd love to speak with you. Until then, is there a doctor in [your state] whom you would recommend? If you've noticed other physicians who are doing good work in this area, I'd be grateful for a reference.

While it's true that doctors can be competitive, the ones at the top of their game really do want to help and will often guide you to colleagues who are *also* really good.

Here's something I do all the time: Call the chairman of surgery or medicine at any one of the best teaching institutions to ask for a referral. Dr. Udelsman, of Yale–New Haven, gets calls like this about twice a week.

"I got one this morning," he said to me recently. "Maybe it's a colleague, someone I can't remember from medical school. I don't even know who most of these people are, but they say, 'Rob, can you help me out? I've got my uncle, my aunt, my daughter . . .' I do a quick e-mail, I figure out who the right person is, and I try to refer them on. If they ask me for a name in another city, I probably can get at least a contact, and say, 'I don't know, but I have a good friend at so-and-so hospital, and I bet they could help solve this problem.' So yes, call the chair of surgery, the chief medical officer for the hospital, the chair of medicine if it's a medicine-related thing. I think they're all valuable resources, and depending on their schedules and their interest levels, they may be helpful."

Another fantastic resource, should you have a connection you can use, is the nonsurgical staff at a hospital. If you want to know who is the institution's best gastrointestinal surgeon, ask the gastroenterologists, anesthesiologists, or operating room nurses. They know who's a maestro and who's one stitch short of a disaster. They can't advise you on when and how to operate, but they know the stars and the flops in their midst. Next best is to reach out to a hospital nurse, administrative person, or anyone else who can inquire on your behalf.

It's also important to keep in mind, as you are doing your specialist search, that there are many different ways to slice an apple. The important thing is to have that gut feeling that you are in the No-Mistake Zone.

I speak from experience. About a decade ago I developed bunions in both feet, a condition in which the big toe angles drastically toward the other toes, causing an abnormal protuberance at the base of the joint. I couldn't run anymore. It hurt to walk. I had to get it taken care of, but I was scared to death. Bunion surgery is not very complex, but it has to be done with great precision because the recovery period after a bunionectomy can be long and arduous, and the pain *truly* excruciating—a 10 on a scale of 1 to 10.

I started by asking my PCP for a recommendation, and he referred me to a podiatrist at a major teaching hospital. Our meeting went well. He walked me through the traditional surgery process, just as I'd heard about. I thanked him for his time. You can probably see where this is going. My goal (which probably sounded like sheer folly to people who know from bunion surgery) was to find a doctor who could do this procedure pain-free (or at least with minimal pain).

My problem wasn't time sensitive, so I decided to do more research. I asked friends for recommendations, looked up the orthopedic staff at the best local hospitals, and cross-referenced names on PubMed. I checked in with medical colleagues to ask if they'd heard of anyone who was blazing trails in the field. I interviewed a lot of physicians, my list of questions in hand—but like Rachel, I wasn't really comfortable with any of them, so I waited.

Then one day (about two years later) I noticed that one of my friends was wearing a walking boot. He had just had bunion surgery, and he raved about his surgeon: "My guy is the best in the world. He's absolutely wonderful. I felt no pain at all."

I'd *never* heard that before. No pain? I was very skeptical when I made an appointment to meet Dr. Marc Selner. When I arrived for my consultation, I noticed that his office was next door to a gas station and across the street from a pizza joint. The waiting room furniture, to be polite, was nothing fancy; the X-ray machine looked ancient. I was ready to walk out. But instead, I stayed and talked to him.

He gave me quite a surprise. Dr. Selner said that his father, brother, and daughter were all podiatrists. (Can you imagine the conversations at that dinner table?) He explained in great detail exactly how he performs a very special, pain-free bunion surgery, in which he cuts out a chevron-shaped piece of the bone, then uses a single, hollowed-out screw to tighten the two pieces together, which results in significantly less pain because the bones aren't moving as they heal—they're fixed together.

I was still skeptical, though, and asked for references. He provided me with a multipage list of patients who had given consent to discuss their cases. I thought, *Either the guy's a total fraud and has a call center in India, or this is really interesting.* I phoned about thirty-five of them. Because of privacy laws, it's rare for a doctor to have such a list, but I always ask if there are patients who would be willing to discuss their experience, and there's no reason why you shouldn't do the same. Here's what I said when I phoned people on Dr. Selner's list:

> *Hi, my name is Leslie Michelson. We've never met, but I'm calling at the suggestion of Dr. Selner. I'm considering bunion surgery, and he said that you might be willing to discuss your experience?*

All of them were happy to talk to me. So I got right to it, asking:

Was your surgery unilateral or bilateral? What was your recovery like? What was the pain level like? How long ago did you have it done? How are you feeling now? Have you had any issues?

The response was unanimous: they were satisfied with their results and had felt little to no postsurgery pain.

And that was my result too. My surgery with Dr. Selner was a success. Afterward, I felt fine and needed no pain medication at all.

If I had simply Googled Dr. Selner or researched him on PubMed, I wouldn't have found anything very persuasive. But after having a conversation with him, I *was* persuaded—by the logic of his technique, his focused commitment to my specific condition, the volume of surgeries he'd performed, and his patient references.

The questions you bring to a specialist during your interviewing phase will be unique to your condition and your personal goals. But here are my four must-asks:

FOUR QUESTIONS FOR A SPECIALIST

"What portion of your time as a [cardiologist/orthopedist/ENT, etc.] do you spend on this specific type of condition/illness/procedure?"

"How long has this been a specialty for you?"

"Have you done research and published on it?"

"Doctor, you told me you spend about 70 percent of your time on this procedure. I'm sure there's an enormous amount of research and literature on the topic. What do you do to stay on top of the rapidly advancing science?"

This last question requires you simply to listen, then check with your gut. Does the response satisfy you that he or she has figured out how to stay abreast of developments in the field?

First-rate physicians will give all sorts of answers to this question: *I sub-scribe to these journals. Twice a year I go to these conferences. I have a research team that helps me gather the latest information.* But while the responses may vary, they are given without hesitation. If this specialty—whether it be a specific disease, surgical procedure, or treatment regimen—is a very important part of a practitioner's life, his or her answer will come spontaneously, and your instinct will give you a strong signal. Listen to it.

If you are interviewing a surgeon, then you need to broach the track-record question. While there's no foolproof predictor for surgical "expertise," one commonly used measure is volume—the more procedures a surgeon has performed, the more likely *you* will have a successful outcome. You needn't be rude or pushy, just ask, during an appropriate time in the consultation, *How many of these surgeries have you done?*

I have to applaud Rachel, who showed tremendous courage during our phone consults with ear surgeons. Her main goal was to lower her risk of hearing loss. So she asked each of them, *Has anyone gone deaf on your watch? How many? What happened? How old were they?*

You can pose similar questions about your own condition. Do not—I repeat—*do not* be alarmed if a doctor tells you he's had complications. A physician who claims perfection either hasn't done enough procedures or hasn't paid sufficient attention to his outcomes. The surgeons Rachel interviewed didn't have perfect track records, but what mattered to her was getting straight, honest answers.

Keep in mind that some physicians and medical institutions tend to treat patients who have more complex and advanced diseases. Which means their statistical outcomes may not be as glowing as those who primarily care for patients with less challenging cases. That shouldn't be held against them.

I always appreciate a physician who provides specific information about the likelihood of success, the nature and frequency of complications, and what to except in terms of recovery. That is the information you need to make an informed decision and, after a surgery or treatment, to determine if your recovery is on track.

Anytime you hear a beating-around-the-bush response—*Oh, these things happen,* or *Well, you never really know why it doesn't work*—that's a red flag. Maybe the doctor is reluctant to admit error or to learn from mistakes.

I've been in situations where we had to ask very awkward things. Sometimes, because we'd already met the physician, we'd ring the person in charge of his office to inquire, very politely:

This doctor is a little older, and we just need to know, is he still sharp? How many of these procedures has he done? Is he still doing at least three a week? Has he had any bad outcomes? How does he handle them?

People feel anxious about challenging their physicians, so I recognize that some of these questions will make you uncomfortable. But if you were interviewing a nanny, for instance, it would seem perfectly reasonable to say, "Has a child ever been seriously injured on your watch?" And if the response was, "Oh, I can't recall, probably not," or "Yes, but you know how kids are, always getting into trouble," that probably wouldn't inspire confidence that this is the person to care for your baby.

Sometimes after patients have gone through a careful vetting process and consulted with several well-qualified specialists, they get cold feet and are unable to make a choice. To me, this is like watching a homecoming queen who can't decide whether she wants to go to prom with the team captain or the class president. That's when I have to remind them that they are already in the No-Mistake Zone: You've done your homework, you've interviewed some outstanding doctors, and you've even rejected one or two. Your list has been narrowed down to a few very good choices. Any of these doctors could do the job. So let your instincts take over and you won't go wrong.

A WORD FROM THE DOCTORS: HOW TO COLD-CALL A PHYSICIAN

Patients are reluctant to question doctors or ask for help, for fear of provoking a negative reaction. But doctors are just like us—they want to please and satisfy. They make mistakes, but they try to do their best. Instead of being intimidated by the white coat, engage doctors as partners in your care. I asked a handful of extremely talented physicians if there were good and bad ways for patients to reach out to them. Their answers may surprise you.

"If your doctor can initiate the call, that works a little bit better. But if the patient's going to reach out directly, then they should get the phone number of the specialist's assistant and say, 'I understand that the doctor has a good level of experience with this problem. What's the best way for me to have an opportunity to avail myself of his expertise? Can I speak with him on the phone? What method would be easiest for him?' . . . Some doctors are a pain in the butt, but most of them are gentlemen and ladies. Some will call the patient right back: 'Tell me about your case. I'll arrange for you to come up, whatever's convenient for you.' They're human beings like that. That's why you want to ask, 'What is the best way for you to help me?' As a doctor, I'd appreciate that very much. To pound your fists and scream and holler, that doesn't do any good whatsoever."
—Eugene J. Sayfie, M.D., F.A.C.C., F.A.C.P. (Miami)

"Most doctors, when they are the ones confronting a personal medical issue, don't hesitate to call an expert locally or even nationally. I get calls from all around the country: 'I'm the chief of medicine at so and so, and my wife may have Churg-Strauss Syndrome. Can you help me out? Can you talk me through it?' Someone I don't even know. And I'm happy to do it. My mission is to help people. That's how I practice. I make

my contact information public. Not everyone is like that, I think, because people want to protect themselves, and they don't want to be inundated. There are a lot of pressures—time, money—that prevent most physicians from doing the right thing. When I get a personal e-mail from someone—'Can you help me,' 'Help my mother'—I respond promptly because I want to help them and do what's right."
　　—Michael E. Wechsler, M.D., M.M.S.c. (Denver)

"For me personally, e-mail first is always best, followed by phone calls, which are harder to get through to me. I've had situations arise where the patient has seen one or two rheumatologists [elsewhere], and they learn I'm a specialist in this because they've seen my publications. They e-mail me and they say, 'Look, we'll pay you to just have a phone conversation. Give us some guidance here. We're very concerned.' I like that. Recently, [a father in Italy] was worried about his daughter's health, and her physicians were not doing a very good job. We had a preliminary conversation on the phone, and then they ended up coming to Seattle, making a family vacation of it. I set them up with a really good rheumatologist in Rome, but they still check in. We got her on the right therapeutic path . . . and she's doing beautifully. That was a good example of using the Internet to find out who is knowledgeable, and then making contact. . . .

　　"I'll be honest, if the patient e-mails with a certain sense of entitlement that I will e-mail them back with advice, sight unseen, without really knowing carefully their history or presentation, or if they expect free advice, that's irritating. If I receive an e-mail from a patient who describes that they've seen twenty different physicians, including one or two rheumatologists who I recognize as being really good in their evaluation of things—it's very awkward. You find yourself going, 'Uh-oh, I don't want to get involved here. This may be a big sinkhole.'"
　　—Philip Mease, M.D., F.A.C.R., F.A.C.P. (Seattle)

"In order to give somebody the right kind of advice, you need information. Occasionally, the patient is self-diagnosing, and saying, 'I want to see an orthopedic surgeon for my leg pain,' but it's really vascular, not orthopedic. As a doctor, you have to take into context: Who is asking for what, and what advice did they get before they called you? A patient who says: 'I have these symptoms, I went to this hospital, I saw this physician, I was diagnosed with this condition, but I'm not sure, and I'd like to get a second opinion'—that makes a world of difference than somebody coming out of left field who's had no professional input at all, but their nail aesthetician says they have liver disease. Referring a patient without having the right information does that patient, and my colleagues, a disservice. Let's say someone says, 'I really need a good gastroenterologist for my abdominal pain.' So we make a referral to a GI specialist. The patient walks in, and after five minutes, the gastroenterologist realizes this is not a GI problem at all—it's cardiac. We look like idiots for taking up this guy's time and creating a scenario with expectations on both sides. . . . You're not making the proper referral, and you lose credibility. And the next time you call the gastroenterologist, they won't necessarily bend over backward to see a patient urgently."

—Sheldon Elman, M.D. (Montreal, Canada)

"I've gotten [cold calls] for years and years. Especially when I was the director of the Carbone Cancer Center, I would get calls and e-mails from different directions and all days of the week. If they lived in an area I was familiar with, I'd raise specific doctors' names. Or I would send a note to someone I knew at another institution, asking for who they would recommend within a certain specialty, and then get back to the patient: 'This is what I've inquired, and this is what I've been told.' If someone reaches out to me, looking for help, it's my business to help. Some people are more aggressive, though. I think all physicians have had experiences where someone they don't know approaches them, starts pouring out personal information and asking for advice—while you're at a family wedding or sitting on a long flight. It's easier if you get an e-mail. It gives you time to ponder, send a note to a colleague, get some preliminary information about an expert in this procedure or that disease so you can send an informative response to the patient. . . .

"How would I do it myself if I weren't a physician? I'd probably start on the computer, looking for the main institutions in my city, starting with university health systems or National Cancer Institute–designated cancer centers, if it's cancer related, and try to narrow it down to the point where I can send someone an e-mail. That's part of being a doctor these days: people can get to you in a lot of different ways. I hope that most, if not all, of my colleagues would respond to such queries. You don't have to know the person. You're here to serve people and help them. It's part of what we do."

—George Wilding, M.D. (Madison, Wis.)

SMARTER RESEARCH ONLINE AND OFF: WHERE TO FIND THE EXPERTS AND INFORMATION YOU NEED

STATE MEDICAL LICENSING BOARDS

www.fsmb.org/directory_smb.html

- To find out if a physician is licensed to practice in your state, and whether there are any criminal, license, or malpractice judgments against the doctor.

AMERICAN BOARD OF MEDICAL SPECIALTIES

www.certificationmatters.org/is-your-doctor-board-certified /search-now.aspx

- To see if this physician is board certified in his or her specialty and if certification is up to date.

PUBMED/MEDLINE

www.pubmed.gov

- To read peer-reviewed published articles on a specific topic, and to study the articles of a specific expert.

EXPERTSCAPE

expertscape.com

- To search for the most-published experts on a specific condition.

GOOGLE SCHOLAR

scholar.google.com

- To read published works that have been cited by other authors. Google Scholar lists articles in the order of most citations, so this can be a good way to find so-called classic papers on a subject.

CLINICALTRIALS.GOV

www.clinicaltrials.gov

- To find clinical trials for a specific drug or disease, as well as the names of trial investigators.

DRUGS@FDA

www.accessdata.fda.gov/scripts/cder/drugsatfda/

- To find information on drugs approved by the FDA, including background approval documents and research data.

DRUG INFORMATION PORTAL

druginfo.nlm.nih.gov

- To find information on drugs and dietary supplements.

PILL IDENTIFIER

www.drugs.com/pill_identification.html

- To find images of brand and generic prescription drugs, which can be especially helpful when pills get separated from their bottles.

QUESTION BUILDER

www.ahrq.gov/apps/qb/

- A simple app that helps you create, prioritize, and print a list of questions to bring to a medical visit.

CHOOSING WISELY

www.choosingwisely.org

- Sometimes the type of care a patient wants, or is recommended, may be unnecessary or even harmful. This site, an initiative of the American Board of Internal Medicine Foundation, provides talking points and information for patients and their physicians on the most overused tests and procedures.

TO FIND RELEVANT INFORMATION ON SPECIFIC CONDITIONS, I LIKE AND RELY HEAVILY ON:

- Mayo Clinic (www.mayoclinic.com/health-information/) For basic, well-vetted information about myriad conditions and their symptoms, causes, treatments, and prognoses.
- National Institutes of Health (health.nih.gov) As the nation's medical research agency (housing twenty-seven different institutes and centers),

➤

the NIH has a lot to offer for clinicians and patients, from practical advice on how to communicate better with your doctors to in-depth clinical trial databases and the latest scientific discoveries.

- MedlinePlus (www.nlm.nih.gov/medlineplus/) For authoritative information on research, drugs, and treatments for more than nine hundred different medical conditions, this NIH website provides lay-friendly materials, videos, and educational resources.
- UpToDate (www.uptodate.com/home/uptodate-benefits-patients) This site provides original peer-reviewed articles on countless medical topics, with practical recommendations for diagnoses and treatments. Because it is so in-depth and constantly updated, it is often a starting point for the research projects my company tackles. Patients can access articles for free, but there is a subscription fee to obtain the more detailed, physician-level content.
- Major academic institutions that have centers of excellence devoted to a specific disease.
- Disease-research foundations that meet one or more of the following criteria:
  - Has a medical/scientific advisory board
  - Provides research grants
  - Receives educational grants to produce independent scientific and medical information (i.e., from pharmaceutical companies, governmental agencies, and other foundations)

TO FIND SPECIALISTS:

- Visit the websites of the major medical institutions near you to research the bios and medical interest areas of the specialists on staff in the departments that fit your condition.
- Seek out physicians listed on medical/scientific advisory boards of disease-specific foundations.
- Research names of physicians on editorial boards of specialty-specific associations.
- Contact the investigators leading the clinical trials that relate to your condition, or reach out to the lead author of published clinical trials.
- Get in touch with the authors of review articles found on PubMed,

Expertscape, and/or editorials in the *New England Journal of Medicine* or *JAMA*.

- Attend conferences held by foundations related to your condition, and make connections with the presenting doctors and medical staff.
- Ask for recommendations from the nonsurgical staff at respected teaching hospitals and major medical institutions.

QUICK GUIDE

CHAPTER 6. How to Find and Interview the Medical
Experts You Need

- Start your research by making a list of questions; use this list to keep yourself on course if you start to get overwhelmed. Refine your questions as you become more competent and conversant in the language of your illness. Bring your questions to consultations with specialists.

- When you are facing a technically demanding procedure or rare disease, a large, distinguished hospital is more likely to have volume and expertise in your specific condition than a small community hospital.

- Major academic hospitals and so-called centers of excellence take Medicare and most types of insurance. If it doesn't cost you more to go to a larger, better-resourced hospital, you may as well go there.

- When interviewing specialists, approach the process with a significant level of knowledge; let them know how important the surgery is to you and how impressed you are with their body of work; ask about their volume and track records; then listen with your gut.

- For every disease, there are experts. Never risk your well-being by putting it in the hands of someone for whom your condition is a novelty.

- When reaching out to a doctor for advice from afar: introduce yourself and explain your problem; let him know you've done homework on your condition and his expertise; state your needs clearly; and let him know how much you appreciate his time. If he is unable to help, ask if he can make a referral to someone else who can.

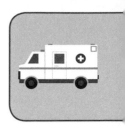

CHAPTER SEVEN

EMERGENCY ROOM 101

The four most common mistakes made in the first twenty-four hours of a medical emergency

Tracey, a forty-year-old bookstore clerk, regained consciousness one Monday morning to find herself sprawled across the threshold of her shower stall. The water was off, but she was wet. She remembered feeling dizzy as she showered. *I must have turned off the water seconds before fainting,* she thought. She suddenly realized that she couldn't feel her arms or legs.

Alone and scared, Tracey managed to get to the phone to call her sister Jane. By then, her limbs were prickly, as if they'd fallen asleep.

"I just passed out," she told her sister. "My arms really hurt, and I think I may have fallen on them."

Jane asked her if she thought it was serious.

"I think I'm okay. I'm just really frightened."

The sisters shared the same internist, across town, and Jane suggested Tracey ring the doctor to make an appointment, offering to drive her there after traffic died down. When Tracey called, the office was closed, but an operator said she could try the drop-in clinic later that morning.

At eleven a.m., with Jane at her side, Tracey was finally able to tell her PCP what had happened. She described fainting in the shower, hitting her head, waking up temporarily paralyzed, and feeling pain in her arms.

"You need to go to the emergency room right away," the physician said, explaining to Tracey that she needed imaging and tests that couldn't be done in the office.

Tracey and her sister drove to the nearest ER, at a hospital in a suburb of Chicago.

After Tracey was seen, two details about her captured the staff's attention: This was the third time she'd fainted in the last year; and her family had a history of heart attacks. She was sent to the hospital's cardiology unit and given a full workup. All the while, she complained about her arms and upper body. Her paper ID bracelet felt like a ring of red ants, and the sleeves of her gown burned against her skin. She was given painkillers and scheduled for an X-ray the next day.

When she called her father to let him know what had happened, he said, "Tracey, it sounds like you may have hurt your neck or your spine." But she didn't mention her father's hunch to the medical staff, thinking, *Wouldn't they have asked me about my neck or spine if my symptoms had warranted it?*

The next afternoon, as Tracey returned to her hospital room after a walk around the floor with Jane, a young neurosurgeon was waiting. "Why are you walking around?" he asked her, chiding, "You're lucky you're not paralyzed."

The doctor showed Tracey her X-rays and explained that she had Central Cord Syndrome: an acute cervical spinal cord injury. He ordered MRIs and a neck brace and told her that he needed to operate immediately. Surgery was scheduled for the next day.

When Tracey recalled this moment, many years later, this was the point in the story when she said, "I was in complete shock. My family took over."

If you get sick, it's important to know your limitations, because it's challenging for even a healthy person to successfully navigate their way through turbulent waters. The first misstep Tracey made, when she woke up in the shower that morning, was that she didn't call 911.

"I actually felt very badly about it right after," her sister Jane told me. "I live about forty minutes from Tracey. When she called, it was rush hour, and we are on opposite sides of the city. So I told her I would come get her and take her to the doctor after traffic died down, but we really should have called 911."

It's a situation anyone might face, and it brings us to the first of the four most common mistakes that people make in the first twenty-four hours of a medical emergency.

1. TOO CLOSE TO CALL

In those first few minutes, it can be difficult to decide: Go to the ER or to an urgent care clinic? Dial 911 or wait it out? Car or ambulance? To get the best advice on this common issue, I turned to an emergency medicine guru.

Dr. Robert Simon (the physician who first helped Jennifer with her psoriatic arthritis mystery) is the founder and chairman of the global relief nonprofit International Medical Corps and the author of six textbooks on emergency medicine. He has trained hundreds of ER doctors, and developed many of the surgical techniques being used today in emergency departments.

"As with anything," he says, "it requires a serious judgment call. You have to consider a patient's age, their health history, and the mechanism and seriousness of their injury."

For example, if a robust twenty-year-old falls down and bruises his chest, but he has only mild discomfort and tenderness, no serious injuries, no prolonged pain or tingling in his extremities (like what Tracey experienced), and no shortness of breath, then going to see his internist or urgent care (also referred to as a walk-in clinic) is probably fine. But when an eighty-year-old takes the same spill, her chest wall is more delicate; she likely has osteoporosis and may have broken a rib or punctured a lung—that requires ER care.

"Shortness of breath, vomiting, severe abdominal pain, or any pain that increases instead of decreases over time—those are danger signs," Dr. Simon says. "Look at the patient, think about his or her age and medical history, and ask yourself: 'Does he seem sicker than normal?'" For example, a young man with a cough or cold and shortness of breath is probably fine to go to urgent care or his PCP. But a sixty-five-year-old with chest pain and shortness of breath? Call 911. If she's got a neurological condition, like multiple sclerosis, and she's suddenly having difficulty swallowing: call 911. An unusually severe headache with intense vomiting? Call 911. Spinal injury? 911.

"Asthma is another one for the ER, because it's extremely unpredictable, and it's a killer," Dr. Simon says. "If it's a minor asthma attack that responds nicely to an inhaler, but they're just not getting complete relief, you could safely take them by car to the emergency room. Otherwise, call 911—fast. I will never forget the tragic case of a woman in her thirties, who had two kids and a husband with severe asthma. He was having an attack, so she got him in the car and raced to the hospital, running lights and weaving through traffic as he got worse and worse. By the time she arrived to the ER, he was dead. Asthma is a really dangerous disease. You must be careful."

At the opposite end of the spectrum: If a patient has a relatively minor injury to the arms or legs—and none of the danger signs mentioned above are present—urgent care is usually fine. But if the broken limb looks deformed, rotated, or blue—or if it's a femoral or thigh bone fracture in an older person and they can't bear weight and/or get up—in both of these cases, call an ambulance. "Whenever an elderly person falls and can't get up due to pain in the thigh or hip, assume it is a broken femoral head or neck until proven otherwise," Dr. Simon says. "In fact, the X-ray may even be negative since there is osteoporosis, but a CT scan will show the fracture.

"For trauma to the head or torso, I would lean going to an ER," he advises. "But for a simple cut or minor sprain? I would go to urgent care. You can't always be sure of the skill level of the doctors, but these centers tend to be less expensive and faster." How to assess your local facility? One way is to ask which hospital it's associated with. (Every urgent care clinic must be affiliated with an ER.) Those that are connected to the larger, higher-volume hospitals are generally going to be staffed by more qualified and experienced practitioners."

And don't forget to bring your PCP into the loop. If you've got a non-emergency health problem like a cut, sprain, or bruise, and you're not sure if you should go to your PCP, urgent care, or ER, just call your internist and ask. Medical advice is always advised.

Sometimes, when an injury isn't life-threatening, people struggle with whether to drive the patient to the ER or call for an ambulance. Although you should always err on the side of caution, there may be circumstances, as Dr. Simon points out, when an ambulance isn't optimal.

"I've seen ambulances delayed in rush hour traffic on the way to a patient and it takes them thirty extra minutes to pick up someone with a broken arm, when that person could have easily been driven one-way, by a friend, much faster," he says. Meaning: If it's simply a broken arm, and the patient is breathing fine, his pulse is normal, his complexion is clear (not cold or clammy), and there's no chest pain, taking him to the nearby ER yourself, in some cases, might be faster than waiting for an ambulance that has to make a round trip in heavy gridlock. But again, age and past medical history are essential factors to consider. In serious situations, ambulance technicians can stabilize the patient, start an IV, perform lifesaving techniques, provide pain relief, and alert the ER to be ready to admit.

One other point Dr. Simon impresses upon patients whenever he can is this: Learn more about how your local ambulance company functions. This is especially important if you live in a rural area.

"I live in a rural area, so I can give you an example," he says. "One time there was a kid who jumped into the lake headfirst, hit his head on a tree stump, broke his neck, and was drowning. Somebody dived in after him, brought him out, and started CPR. Another person called 911. I wasn't there—I was at home. But here's what I saw: an ambulance driving back and forth on the road, with its sirens on, trying to figure out where to go. It was a volunteer service, and they were lost. The point is, contact your ambulance company and say, 'I'm a resident and you cover my area. I want to learn more about your service.'"

Specifically, Dr. Simon says, you want to know if it's paid or volunteer. And does it function 24/7 from a central location, like a fire station or a medical facility? (Sometimes, with a volunteer service, if a 911 call comes in during a low-volume shift, the volunteers may be coming from their own homes, which could add precious minutes to response times.) And how is the training? Ideally, you want a paid staff that's EMT-trained, stationed in a central location 24/7, and not on call. On-call ambulances can take a lot longer to get to you, and you may be better off taking the patient to the ER yourself.

Another piece of information that might be helpful to ask about, Dr. Simon adds, is whether the ambulance is based at the hospital or the fire department. Because if the crew is working in the ER, as extra hands, they will have far more emergency medical experience under their belts than if they are based solely at a fire department.

"If you live in a rural area, and you find yourself in an emergency situation where the service isn't optimal, but you have little choice and you *need* them to come to you," Dr. Simon continues, "then when you call 911, direct the operator to stay on the call. Say, 'Here's how you find my house . . .' and 'I need you to stay on the line with me until they get here.'" As he points out, if you call from a landline, your location can be easily traced. However, if you are calling from a cell phone—as in the case of the drowning victim—then it's much more difficult to find you, and you must keep the operator on the line until help arrives.

A peculiar situation can arise when you live in a major metropolitan city where there are several hospitals to choose from. Suppose you tore your Achilles tendon running in the park, and your injury isn't life-threatening, but you need an ambulance, and your preferred hospital is not the nearest one.

In a case like this—when you are not at serious medical risk—it doesn't hurt to ask the driver to take you to your first-choice hospital. Explain that all your records are there, and it's where your internist has visiting privileges. If they're wavering, ask to contact their supervisor about your request. "In the bigger cities they will usually do it if it is as close as the nearest facility, or they may charge extra for going a few extra miles," Dr. Simon says. "But if they perceive any threat to your life, they won't do it."

You can also call your local service ahead of time (in large cities, your call might be to the fire department, which commonly handles ambulance services) to ask about their policy and how they'd handle such a request.

In an emergency, after 911, your next call should be to your primary care physician. It's very difficult to break through the triage-style shuffling of patients that happens in emergency rooms every day, particularly on weekend evenings and holidays. Your PCP is in a position to give the treating physicians the full context of your health history and provide an extra level of coordination and involvement.

Based on Tracey's imaging, it appeared that her fall in the shower had herniated the disc between vertebrae C4 and C5, the neck area. The injured disc was protruding toward her spine, causing bruising and swelling of the cord, instability, and a weakening from her neck down. All of which explained the pain in her arms. The spinal cord is about eighteen inches long from the base of the brain to the pelvis, and the higher up the injury, the greater potential danger for quadriplegia (what actor Christopher Reeve suffered after his fall off a horse).

Tracey's surgeon was recommending an anterior cervical discectomy and fusion, or ACDF, in which he would make an incision through her throat, remove the offending disc, and then fuse together the vertebrae above and below the disc with a bone graft. ACDF, like any spine surgery, is a highly technical procedure; you have to be in good hands. And while her doctor was skilled and thoughtful, he was, as they learned, just two years out of residency training. This is the moment when anyone in a similar position should say to him- or herself: *This is a very complicated surgery. This guy has been practicing medicine for two years. No criticism of him, but let him get a little more experienced, and then we'll talk about it.*

Could he have done the surgery? Yes, and it likely would have gone just fine. But when the risk involves never again being able to walk, then your job as a patient is to make sure the surgeon has performed this surgery hundreds, if not thousands, of times. Tracey's parents asked the head of neurosurgery if he would do the procedure instead. But he refused to reassign the case. That's a common and understandable response: it might signal a lack of respect if the head of your department takes over your case. But this code of etiquette can run counter to the patient's needs.

When it became clear that the hospital was not going to budge, the family got Dr. Simon to weigh in. He believed that Tracey was at risk of paralysis *only* if she suffered another fall, another fainting spell. But as long as she remained stable, she wouldn't need surgery *right now*. This meant they had a small window of time to collect her records and ask for an expert opinion from a new neurosurgeon. The family already had one in mind.

Dr. Richard G. Fessler, a well-known pioneer of minimally invasive spine surgery, practiced at Northwestern University. The family had two questions for him: *Does Tracey need this surgery? And, if so, is it an emergency?*

What happened next is no surprise. As soon as they expressed their desire to get a second opinion and a possible transfer to Northwestern, the family was treated terribly by the hospital. Tracey was left in the cardiac unit, even though her problem was neurological; the neurology nurses and doctors stopped coming to see her; and her neck brace was bothering her and didn't feel properly placed, but no one would fix it.

Even more maddening, when Jane went to the nursing station to ask for a copy of her sister's records in order to get an *emergency* second opinion, she was told it would take weeks to get them—yet Tracey had walked into the ER just thirty hours earlier. Jane asked to speak to a supervisor. She was told that, because it was after-hours, there was no one there who could help her—she'd have to come back in the morning.

Jane was already mentally and physically exhausted, and now she felt as if she were being stonewalled by people who should have been helping her.

You can imagine the panic and helplessness she felt. The clock was ticking, and she had to have those records. She went home frustrated and angry. It was eleven p.m. What could she do now?

If you find yourself in a similar situation, don't give up. You can still get help—you just need to aim higher and use the communication tips that Dr. Simon gave Jane and her husband that night. Here's what he taught the couple about who to ask for, and what words to use:

When it's after-hours and the hospital CEO (i.e., the boss) is off duty, **there's always a senior administrator in charge.** Very large facilities **also have junior administrators** or what might be referred to as **first on call.** Dr. Simon told Jane's husband (who had taken over at this point) to call the hospital operator and **ask for the administrator on call.**

"You've got to be pretty firm when you reach that person," he said. "You've got to say, 'My sister needs a second opinion. This is a serious matter. It's really not something that can wait until the morning. I simply need all her records collected. I know that staff is short in the evenings, but I'm not getting any cooperation, and I desperately need your help. Can you find someone who can copy her records for us?'"

Dr. Simon suggested following up this request with a reminder: "I know we will be getting a patient satisfaction survey about our experience"—these surveys are critical to the hospital, and many institutions change their procedures based upon responses—"and I really *want* to be able to complete that survey positively. I understand how hard everyone's job is, and that the staff is doing all they can, but we need to get a second opinion *urgently*, and I really need your help here."

"If you still can't get any satisfaction," Dr. Simon said, "then call the operator back and say, 'I want to speak with **the senior administrator on call.**'"

Over the next two hours, amid a flurry of calls, they were able to track down an administrator who empathized with their case. By two a.m. the records were being assembled. They were delivered to Dr. Fessler hours before Tracey's scheduled surgery.

Dr. Fessler agreed that Tracey needed surgery. But as long as her condition wasn't deteriorating, they could transfer her to Northwestern, keeping her stable, and he would operate as soon as the swelling had gone down.

The next night, after more hard-fought administrative sign-offs, Tracey was transferred to Northwestern's neurosurgery unit. She immediately felt more at ease. The staff explained her condition in detail, conducted additional tests, fixed the position of her neck brace, and put her paper ID bracelet on her ankle (instead of her arm) so she'd be more comfortable. Dr. Fessler personally performed her surgery, which was a success.

Tracey later figured out that the fainting spells she suffered from that year were due to low blood pressure, caused by her sleeping pills. She switched medication and hasn't suffered from a fall since. Unfortunately she did suffer permanent nerve damage, and parts of her arms will probably always be sensitive to touch, but she'll feel nothing like the burning pain she was dealing with at first.

"My biggest frustration with the emergency room was, I hit my head, I had a bruise. You'd think that someone would have thought to look at the possibility of a head or neck injury," Tracey said in reflection. "But because of my family's history, everyone was thinking 'Heart, heart, heart.' I don't think I made it clear enough that I was having serious symptoms in my arms."

Even very smart people like Tracey, when they are in the ER, become paralyzed by the frenetic pace, the suffering around them, and the fact that they are not familiar with the medical jargon. Tracey discovered that she wasn't even in the right unit because the ER hadn't paid attention to her arm pain and her head and neck trauma. And when her diagnosis and treatment was presented to her, she reacted the way any of us might if we got earth-shattering news from a person in authority: she gratefully agreed to whatever the doctor said. Tracey had never spent a night in a hospital before, and it wasn't in her nature to advocate for herself; that felt like making a fuss. As a result, she suppressed her keen capacity to judge. Which brings us to number 2:

2. A FAILURE TO COMMUNICATE

If poor communication is one of the biggest factors leading to medical error, then your job as a patient is clear: full disclosure. Good physicians often say that patients know their bodies best, so share your knowledge with your doctors.

This is crucial in an ER setting, where care providers are often residents who may not have the luxury of time or depth of experience to provide patients with the kind of attention needed. Likewise, patients underplay and underreport their symptoms and history, assuming that doctors will simply ask for more information if it's needed.

In a study out of the University of Pennsylvania, researchers tape-recorded ninety-three encounters between emergency room residents and patients and analyzed the communication patterns. They discovered that only 8 percent of the residents indicated to patients that they were trainees; the average amount of time patients were able to explain their problems before being interrupted was twelve seconds; discharge instructions lasted a little over a minute (only 16 percent of patients were asked if they had any questions); and not once was a patient asked if he or she had understood the information given. The evidence is pretty clear: We have a responsibility to ask questions and provide information, even if we are being interrupted.

Give the staff your full range of symptoms and medical history. Be clear and detailed about what you think your problem is. Be assertive about your needs. And if for some reason you cannot, that's when the inventory you created after reading Chapter 3 will have to speak for you. This may become especially important for elderly parents. Think of the peace of mind you'll have if a crisis arises and you're not there, but all the crucial information a responder needs is readily available on a laminated card in their wallet.

Just assume, for safety's sake, that you are going to be unable to communicate in the ER—maybe you had a stroke or became delirious—and you have to have this information on you. Attach it to your driver's license, because police, ambulance, and ER staff will always look there first if you are unconscious. Unfortunately, most people don't keep this information in their purse or wallet. In the rare instances when ER staff do find it, the patient is typically a doctor.

EMERGENCY MEDICAL INFORMATION CHECKLIST. KEEP THESE DETAILS ATTACHED TO YOUR DRIVER'S LICENSE OR IDENTIFICATION CARD.

- Any allergies you have
- Any medications you are on, including dosages. This is essential, because some have serious side effects, and the physicians must know what you are taking and how much. This also includes medical marijuana, as well as any vitamins and supplements.
- Any diseases or serious diagnoses you have or have had. Provid-

ing information about your diseases is key and will help lead physicians to the most likely cause of your problem. Failing to disclose even a small issue like eczema could cause doctors to miss a potential autoimmune disorder.

- A baseline EKG. Ask your PCP for a copy of your "12-lead EKG," Dr. Simon recommends. This report, he says, can be very worthwhile for emergency physicians to have, because your ER EKG can be compared to your baseline, allowing them to confirm or rule out any abnormalities.
- Pertinent family health history (heart attacks, strokes, etc.)
- The name and phone number of your PCP
- An emergency contact person. Who do you want the hospital to call?

And while you don't necessarily need insurance details in an emergency (all ERs are mandated to care for you regardless of insurance), it might be helpful to have your card on hand.

Here's another communication error that surprised me when I first heard about it: An increasing number of women are dying of undiagnosed heart attacks simply because they don't perceive their symptoms as serious and aren't describing them to emergency responders in a way that gets attention.

Dr. C. Noel Bairey Merz, director of the Barbra Streisand Women's Heart Center at Cedars-Sinai, specializes in the myriad ways women experience heart attacks differently than men do. At least three times a week, Dr. Bairey Merz has to remind her patients to tell medical responders the universal declaration that will get their attention: "Always say 'I have *chest pain!*'"

"I saw a patient last week in follow-up, who I hadn't seen in a couple years," Dr. Bairey Merz said. "She had been to the emergency room again. She said, 'I'm so frustrated with my local ER. When I go in, they don't do anything.' I asked her, 'What do you say?' She said, 'I tell them I'm not feeling well.' I said, 'No, no, no—you have to say: *I have chest pain.*' The patient said, 'But it's *not really* chest pain. I just don't feel well.' I told her again, 'You *must say:* I'm having chest pain.' And if they don't give you an EKG and do the blood test, demand it."

Heart disease is the number one killer of women. In fact, one in three will die of heart disease and stroke. But one-third of all women (and 10 percent of men) do not experience heart attacks the way they've seen it on TV: falling to their knees and clutching at their shirt buttons as if their chest is about to explode. While men are more likely to experience pain in their chest and left arm—and they communicate that to a doctor—women tend to have more general aches accompanied by cold sweats, shortness of breath, and other symptoms that they underplay. They say to themselves, *I'm just feeling a little dizzy, a heavy pressure.* More often they think they're having troublesome heartburn or hot flashes. They don't consider that this might be a heart attack.

Every woman needs to be aware of the symptoms of a heart attack, which, according to the American Heart Association, include:

- Uncomfortable pressure, squeezing, fullness, or pain in the center of your chest that lasts more than a few minutes, or goes away and comes back
- Pain or discomfort in one or both arms, the back, neck, jaw, or stomach
- Shortness of breath, with or without chest discomfort
- Other signs such as breaking out in a cold sweat, nausea, or light-headedness

Sometimes a sudden and inexplicable dizzy spell can be a danger sign if it's coupled with an increased (or markedly *decreased*) pulse rate, a slow heartbeat, or other cardiac symptoms such as clammy, pale skin. The point is, use your best judgment, and call 911 if you are unsure. If you think it's nothing, but you already suffer from high cholesterol, high blood pressure, diabetes, or a family history of heart disease, it's better to be safe and call 911.

3. OOPS! I'M AT THE WRONG PLACE.

Tracey had no way of knowing, when she walked into that first hospital, that she was going to have to move to a different institution. Luckily, it worked out for her. But I have seen too many cases where patients got stuck in challenging situations that could have been avoided with a little research. There's a crucial reason why you want to learn more about your local ERs ahead of time, when you are well. And it's something no one realizes until they've experienced it: When you enter the ER, once you are admitted it's extremely difficult to get transferred to a hospital that's better suited to care for you. Here's why:

- You have to prove to your insurance company that what you need is not available at Hospital A, or it will refuse to cover the expenses, which include a transfer to Hospital B (you *have* to be moved by ambulance), duplicate testing, and extra care costs.
- Nobody at Hospital A wants to let you go because they don't want to risk moving you if you are not stable enough; they have real fears about being sued over poor quality of care; and frankly, you are a revenue source. They don't want to see dollars walking out the door.
- The receiving Hospital B is also going to be very cautious about taking you. They're scratching their heads and wondering, *Why is the patient leaving Hospital A? This one's going to be trouble. It might be a botched case, and we know that those are always much more difficult.*

When clients ask me to help with a hospital-to-hospital transfer, I tell them that it's one of the hardest things we do. It requires literally dozens of phone calls and two to three days of work coordinating among the hospitals, the carrier, and the medical transport. Everyone has to sign off. And if they don't, and you decide to leave under what's called Against Medical Advice, or AMA, your insurance company may threaten to not pay any costs at the new facility, or any claims related to your illness.

Here's how to avoid all that: Now, while you are healthy, research the facilities of your local emergency rooms, so that if the time comes when you need one, you will already have made an informed decision about which is best for your needs. Now, let me be perfectly clear: If you're having a heart attack, stroke, or other life-threatening event, you don't have time to research which local hospital has a state-of-the-art cath lab. Call 911, and the ambulance will take you to the nearest ER. Studies show that your chances of surviving a coronary event are best when doctors can do angioplasty and open your blocked blood vessels within an hour and a half—the golden ninety minutes—from when chest pain starts.

Okay, so what are your emergency room research criteria?

"First, you want to pick an ER that has trained *and* boarded emergency physicians—not just those who have been grandfathered in," Dr. Simon says, explaining that before emergency medicine became a specialty, most doctors who practiced in the ER had only a year of general training. Ideally, you want to be seen by physicians who have more than just an M.D. in their title. They should also have an F.A.A.E.M. (Fellow of the American Academy of Emergency Medicine) or F.A.C.E.P. (Fellow of the College of Emergency Physicians) affiliation.

How do you find out? Most hospitals' websites provide enough information by which to judge their emergency department, but some don't. You can always call the hospital's medical staff office—not the main switchboard but the department where the CEO and other administrators work—and ask for the names of the chairman of emergency medicine and the ER attending physicians. A quick check online with the American Board of Medical Specialties will reveal whether they specialize in emergency medicine.

You also want to be at an ER that sees enough patients a year to have experienced all the different ways things can go wrong. "ERs that have less than twenty thousand visits annually, in general, won't have enough experience with difficult cases, which they need in order to become good at them," says Dr. Simon. "For example, a small ER may only see a few asthmatic patients a year. They treat them and send them home. An ER that has cared for tens of thousands of asthmatics will know how dire it is, they'll have patients who have died, and the physicians will be much more attuned to and careful about sending a patient home too early." Asthma is just one scenario. The same can be said of other potential time bombs, such as abdominal pain that ends up being an aneurysm; a headache with vomiting that's due to a ruptured aneurysm; or even back pain that is so severe it ends up being an aortic dissection. You want to ensure you're at an ER that has seen it all.

Again, ask the medical office; they should be able to tell you the number of emergency room patient visits per year. If they can't, take that into consideration too. (*U.S. News & World Report*'s annual Best Hospitals rankings also provides this data free online for some five thousand hospitals.)

Another important consideration is whether the hospital is designated as a trauma center, a place with the manpower and technology to handle the worst types of physical injuries from car crashes, high falls, gunshot wounds, and more. The American College of Surgeons (ACOS) has designations for a trauma center's ability to deliver optimal care, with Level I being the highest (meaning it's the local community's place for major emergencies) and

Level V the lowest. You can find your state's trauma centers at www.facs.org /trauma/verified.html.

At a minimum, find out where your PCP has admitting privileges. Because if you end up in a facility where your doctor has no affiliation, she is not allowed to visit you, can't get access to your chart, and can't prescribe. The attending physicians may not even take your PCP's calls. You will be stuck fighting for yourself.

If you have infants or small children, then you really must do research and select your ER *carefully*, ahead of time. And ask your pediatrician for a recommendation.

Angela, a highly competent forty-three-year-old caterer, learned this the hard way when her newborn son became ill. Little Adam arrived strong and healthy on a Saturday morning in a maternity ward that was first class. All the nurses and doctors who walked into her room washed their hands at a sink by the door, introduced themselves, wore ID badges, explained in detail what they had come to do, and asked for verbal approval from Angela before administering medications, conducting routine tests, or even just touching her baby. Angela felt safe and cared for.

When she and her husband took Adam home, however, it soon became clear that something was wrong. The baby cried inconsolably, spit up his food, turned a pale shade of yellow, and wasn't soiling his diapers. Angela feared jaundice. On Monday morning, she brought two-day-old Adam to the emergency room of the same hospital where she had delivered.

"I gave birth there, so it just made sense to go back to the people who had brought Adam into this world," Angela said. "It turns out lots and lots of people do the exact same thing." Lots and lots of well-meaning parents also didn't know—and weren't told after their perfect delivery—that this hospital did *not* have a dedicated pediatric ER.

The difference in care infants receive at a pediatric ER is extraordinary, as Angela soon discovered. She was eager to share her story, she said, because she wanted to keep other parents from making the same mistake.

Adam's exam that morning started out well enough. The attending physician was very gentle. But he seemed uncomfortable. "He told us that he wanted to run some tests first, but he was inclined to believe that we were right, that it was jaundice," Angela recalled. If the tests confirmed jaundice, he said, then Adam would have to be transferred to another hospital (let's call it Hospital B), a few miles away. As he got up to leave, the doctor said he would order an IV of fluids for Adam, who appeared dehydrated, and would also consult with the head nurse of the maternity ward because they weren't used to seeing babies.

"We're not used to seeing babies"? That doesn't sound right, Angela thought to herself.

She asked the doctor if he could also ask one of the maternity ward nurses to put the IV in Adam. He agreed that was a good idea. Angela's husband sneaked her a look that said, *Why didn't he suggest it first then?*

An ER nurse arrived a few minutes later to inform Adam's parents that the maternity ward was completely swamped, so she would be doing the IV. "She said to me, 'Look, I'm going to be honest with you,'" Angela recalled, "'I see a baby maybe once every six months, and never one this small, but we're going to do our best.'" Three additional nurses had to come in to help pin Adam still, stick the IV into a vein in his hand, and tape it down. It took a torturous twenty minutes. Angela fought back tears.

Adam mewed in pain again as another nurse punctured the heel of his tiny foot to fill three vials of blood. Sometime later a man walked in and told Angela, "I'm so sorry, they made a mistake with the test and we need to take more blood."

"Really?" Angela said. She was upset, but the guy was so apologetic, she thought to herself, *Okay, mistakes happen, let's get through this.*

Something in Angela, a mother's instincts, had been pinging at her nervous system again and again, making her feel uneasy. But she pushed it down. And who can blame her? She had just given birth. She was exhausted. She couldn't tell if her feelings of alarm were real or an overreaction. But we have to keep listening to those protective prompts *even* when we are in the presence of genuinely well-meaning doctors.

Angela watched the nurse fumble with plastic containers and heel pricks, filling a vial with blood and setting it on the top of a filing cabinet, since there was no counter space. Another nurse came in asking for something, and he gestured toward an empty chair, doing a double-take as he said out loud, "Wait, where did I put that?" Angela looked around and noticed discarded medical wrappers on the dirty floors.

A half hour later the nurse came back and said, again, *I'm so sorry.* Two of the tests were in process, but one had to be redone because he didn't get enough blood—the vial had been about a drop short.

Angela knew something was really wrong. She started shaking. "Can we please get it right this time!" she said through tears. She hated feeling like she was being dramatic. *They have to do what they have to do*, she told herself. But Adam's heels were already covered in marks.

In the meantime, the attending physician confirmed that Adam had jaundice, and they'd need to transfer him to Hospital B. While they waited for the ambulance to be ordered, the doctor said, "Let's begin phototherapy, get a head start on treatment." Angela liked the sound of that.

The busy maternity ward couldn't spare any biliblankets (light-emitting vests that help reduce a jaundiced infant's bilirubin levels), so they sent down an old-model phototherapy machine instead: a plastic box with a blue-light lamp affixed to the top and rubberized holes for reaching in to the baby. Angela watched as three nurses pulled at the contraption's cords, trying to figure out how to start it up.

One even asked Angela if she could see where the power button was located.

"Is it that one?" she said, pointing, and trying to be helpful but beating back the voice in her head screaming, *This isn't right!*

Her husband was in the hallway, unable to hear but watching the nurses' body language. When he saw one of them smirk, putting her hands up in the air with a shrug, he lost his cool and went into the room.

"Do you need some help?" he barked with exasperation.

"We're not really sure how to get it working," a nurse responded.

"Well, can you get someone else who knows what they're doing?" he said. "Or do you want me to kick the tires for you?"

"Honey," Angela tried to calm him, "that's not going to help. They're doing their best."

Then one of the nurses got caught on Adam's IV line.

"Oh my God," Angela said. "You just knocked it out!"

The nurse reached over and shoved the needle back into Adam's hand, obviously hoping that no one would see.

The baby screamed.

One of the head nurses walked in to see what the commotion was about.

"She just knocked out his IV," Angela said.

"No," the junior nurse said, "I put it back in. Look, it's fine."

But it wasn't fine. They would need to start a new IV.

The head nurse apologized to Angela, who had lost count of how many times she had heard the words *I'm so sorry*.

At that point, someone who looked like a social worker walked in and asked Angela's husband if everything was okay.

"No!" he yelled, startling everyone. "It's not okay. And nobody in here seems to know what they're doing. I understand that people make mistakes, but everybody has made their mistake for the day on my child!"

The room was quiet.

"I want you to get someone who knows what they're doing to take care of his IV and to figure out how to work this machine. This is an infant you are dealing with—and I've *had it* with him being the guinea pig."

Although I don't normally advocate screaming or pointing fingers to get what you need, in poor little baby Adam's case, I'd say his dad was well within his rights to raise hell.

Minutes later the head nurse of the maternity ward marched in with three assistants, put in Adam's new IV in about ten seconds, set up the phototherapy machine, and said she would personally call Hospital B to make sure Adam was well taken care of.

At about five p.m., Angela and Adam arrived at the pediatric emergency department of Hospital B. Angela was immediately approached by a doctor who had reviewed Adam's lab work from the first ER.

"Your son has a blood-bacterial infection," the doctor said. In infants, Angela learned, this is a very serious diagnosis that can go from bad to worse very quickly. They would need to give him a spinal tap in order to deliver the proper treatment. Tears streamed down Angela's face. But then the doctor said something that gave her hope: "The odd thing is, he's not exhibiting any other signs of an infection. I heard about how chaotic it was for you today, so part of me wonders if perhaps the blood sample was contaminated."

Thank goodness this new doctor had the intellectual curiosity to pause and think before ordering painful treatments on Adam. Angela's mind raced back to the dirty exam room and the nurse's confusion as he placed vials here and there. She urged the new doctor to take (yet another) blood sample. "Please," she said. "Let's do the test again."

The doctor agreed and said they'd monitor Adam carefully while waiting for the results. One last thing, she added: This was a teaching hospital, so there would be residents checking on the baby, but if Angela needed anything, the head nurse could reach one of the attending doctors.

By the time Adam was admitted to Hospital B, he was almost three days old. Mother and child had had virtually no sleep since his birth. Every hour, someone would come into the room to take the baby's vitals, administer drugs, and ask questions. Attending doctors who popped in were trailed by a group of residents, and Angela dutifully retold Adam's medical story each time. At some point in the middle of the night, she passed out, delirious from a lack of rest.

Around four a.m. her son began screaming, a different cry from the usual, and it barely roused her. She could make out that someone else was in the room. He spoke to Angela briefly, but she couldn't make out the words. He left. Adam continued to rage, but no one came back to tend to him. Angela felt incapable of rising.

When she woke up, Adam was in her arms, but she couldn't recall having gone to him. Hours later a resident came in to ask Adam's weight.

"You know what?" she said calmly but firmly. "I know that this is a teaching hospital, and I'm happy to answer your questions, but you obviously haven't read his chart. So go read it. Then we'll talk." The resident apologized and backed out of the room.

A little rest had reawakened Angela's instincts. She was also thinking like a savvy health care consumer now, and she couldn't help but compare this experience to the standards of her own profession. Over the years, she had interviewed candidates for positions at her company. When someone walked in without having done any homework on her business, it was a sure sign that they weren't fit to work there. She couldn't understand why no one would take three minutes to read her son's chart.

Later that day a woman in scrubs rolled a cart of glass vials and solutions into Adam's room and announced that she needed to do a blood test.

"What test?" Angela demanded. "Because he already had one, and I don't want to do it again if we don't have to."

"Really?" the nurse said, confused. She held up a small, sealed container filled with yellow liquid and asked, "Did it look like this one? Is this the test they gave him?"

Angela was furious.

"Are you *kidding* me? I've had two and a half hours of sleep in four days.

I'm not a nurse. You're holding an ambiguous vial in my face, and you want me to identify what was given to him? No. Go read his chart. Go ask the head nurse. I have no idea what blood test he had."

Angela called her husband in tears. She felt that Adam's life was in her hands, that she had to be on guard 24/7 to protect her child from the people who were supposed to be helping him. She smartly recognized her own limitations in this situation and had gathered the courage to ask for help. From then on, her husband made sure that someone—he, another family member, or a trusted friend—was at Angela's side to help her coordinate Adam's care.

By the end of the day, she finally got some good news. A doctor sat with her and told her that Adam didn't have a blood-bacterial infection. The test at Hospital A had indeed been contaminated. The baby was responding well to his jaundice treatment and could go home very soon. The physician was sorry for the ordeal she had been through.

"He told me that one of the number one problems at big hospitals like this, with so many staff, is miscommunication," she recalled. "He said, 'I'm so glad that your son is well now. If anything, you've learned in all this that you really do have to advocate for your own health, and you should always have someone else with you to listen and make sure things are being communicated properly.'"

His words are a reminder that doctors are only human, working as best they can in an imperfect system. They *need* us to be partners in the management of our own care.

Angela also learned that day that Hospital B frequently received infants from hospitals that did not have a pediatric ER and were not equipped to care for babies. He suggested she go see the ombudsman or patient advocate at the first hospital to make a formal complaint.

A few weeks later Angela had that very meeting. The woman who greeted her was warm and welcoming and asked her to start from the beginning. As Angela narrated each unbelievable detail of her story, play by play, the ombudsman's face turned dark. At one point, she laughed out loud when Angela described her husband asking the nurses if he should "kick the tires" of the phototherapy machine. She apologized and said, "This sounds like a bad movie. I don't understand how things could have gotten any worse, but they did."

Angela learned for the first time that day that even though the hospital had an excellent maternity ward, its ER wasn't prepared to treat infants. *Why didn't anyone say anything?* she wanted to know. The ombudsman explained that hospitals are prohibited from sending patients away, or even inferring a refusal to treat, because of federal law meant to protect mentally ill and homeless people from being denied care.

Angela thought of what the attending physician had said to her: *We're not used to seeing babies.* Maybe he was trying to signal to her that she was in the wrong place? It wasn't until Adam's jaundice was confirmed that he was able to recommend transfer to another facility—one with a pediatric ER, equipped to handle babies. Angela understood now that the entire outrageous fiasco could have been avoided if she had simply driven her son straight to Hospital B—or any hospital with a pediatric ER.

Angela will never make mistake number 3 again (being at the wrong ER). But equally valuable for her was learning how to assert herself in an emergency. Which leads us to number 4:

4. FORGETTING WHO'S IN CHARGE. (HINT: IT'S YOU.)

When you're not getting satisfaction from the ER staff or the admitting hospital's nurses and physicians, it can be very difficult to figure out how to ask the necessary questions and get the appropriate people to help you. You have to keep asking yourself, *Is this right?*

"I don't know why I didn't just leave," Angela says now about those first few hours in the wrong ER with her son. "When the doctor examined Adam, I kept thinking, *He looks like he's never held a baby before.*" She deferred to the doctor, telling herself, *I'm going to be open-minded and withhold judgment.* But if that doctor had been interviewing for the role of babysitter, even just for one night? You better believe she would have sent him packing.

At Hospital B, she learned that it was up to her to coordinate her son's care. She started demanding that they read his chart, asked staff to explain their actions before they proceeded, and complained to the head nurse when something was done improperly.

If you become a patient in a teaching hospital, you have to do the same. And find out who you are dealing with. If a clinician doesn't introduce himself, ask, *Are you a resident or the attending physician?* Chances are you will have numerous students coming to your bedside throughout your stay, and that's fine, but if you are dealing with a complex issue—more than a flu or a sprain—be sure to ask to be examined by the attending physician.

In Tracey's case, her family would have been happy for the head of surgery to do her procedure, but he refused, and they weren't interested in other surgeons at the hospital. While it might be a considerable challenge, asking for a change of doctors is worth the effort if you are really dissatisfied with yours. In my experience, it's hard to switch, but depending on the hospital's policy, you can sometimes get a different doctor if you are flexible about the reassignment.

"You don't have to be aggressive about it," Dr. Simon says. "Here's how you do it. Go to the medical staff office and say, 'I want to talk to the medical director'—in a smaller hospital, they might be called the president of the medical staff. Say to this person, 'I'm really unsatisfied. All I want to do is switch to a different neurosurgeon'—or whatever the specialty—'and I need you to recommend one.'"

Be firm but polite. Above all, you don't want to be the kind of patient who introduces himself by yelling at staff and threatening lawsuits. Comport yourself like a confident health care consumer.

"At the end of the day, they have to be a profitable business," Angela said. "And if people are having bad experiences and word gets around, their business suffers."

One last suggestion: Before you leave the ER or hospital, get a copy of your records, including lab reports and imaging. In fact, the best time to request imaging is when you're with the technician, getting your X-rays and MRIs done. Sometimes it's easier to get an extra CD on the spot than to try to procure one later. (We've even had clients, during a consult, take out their cell phones and snap beautiful, clear images of the screen if it wasn't possible to get a quick copy.) Keep all your records in your personal medical file. They hold potential clues for future physicians.

And remember that a visit to the emergency department isn't meant to be a substitute for primary care. For better or worse, the ER's main concern is to rule out or treat life-threatening issues. Which means that if you've been seen and released, and a day or two later you're still feeling lousy, work with your internist to find a specialist who can help you figure out the cause of your problem. In the off chance that you and your doctors discover a much more serious condition, take a breath, stay strong, and make sure your support team of family and friends are there to help you navigate the rough waters ahead.

QUICK GUIDE

CHAPTER 7. Emergency Room 101

- In an emergency, it can be difficult to decide: ER or urgent care? Dial 911 or wait it out? Car or ambulance? In every case, consider (1) the patient's age, (2) health history, (3) the mechanism and seriousness of the injury, and (4) the capabilities of your local ambulance service.

- Call 911 when there are signs of a more acute medical condition, such as shortness of breath, severe vomiting, or abdominal pain, or any pain that increases instead of decreases over time, especially if the patient's age, health, and medical history are a reason for concern.

- Asthma is an extremely unpredictable killer. Call 911 if you are in doubt.

- For a simple cut, minor sprain, or a relatively minor injury to an arm or leg—and if none of the danger signs mentioned above are present—urgent care is usually fine. But if it's a fracture in an older person who can't get up, or if an injured limb looks deformed, rotated, or blue, call for an ambulance.

- Urgent care clinics that are affiliated with the larger, higher-volume hospitals are generally going to be staffed by more qualified and experienced practitioners.

- For trauma to the head or torso, lean toward going to the ER. If you have time, call your PCP for advice. This is a judgment call—remember the suggestions from Dr. Simon.

➤

- Learn more about how your local ambulance company functions.

- If the ambulance service isn't optimal, but you have little choice, direct the 911 operator to stay on the call until emergency responders arrive.

- If your injury is not life-threatening, it doesn't hurt to ask the ambulance driver to take you to your preferred hospital, where your PCP has visiting privileges.

- In an emergency, after 911, your next call should be to your primary care physician.

- In the hospital, there's always a **senior administrator in charge** or a **junior administrator**, or what might be referred to as **first on call**. If you are in a serious situation and the staff on hand refuse to help, you can ask to speak to an administrator via the hospital operator.

- If a doctor you've just met, whose experience and background you know nothing about, says he has to do surgery on you immediately—take a deep breath, summon the courage, and start asking questions.

- Always provide medical staff with your full range of symptoms and medical history. Be assertive about your needs and clear about what you think might be the problem.

- Keep a copy of your emergency medical information attached to your driver's license or ID in your wallet, as that's the first place emergency responders will look. It should include your (1) allergies, (2) medications, (3) serious diagnoses past and present, (4) baseline EKG if you can get it, (5) family health history, (6) PCP contact information, and (7) person to contact in an emergency.

- Heart disease is the number one killer of women, but many women do not experience heart attacks as men do. They tend to have more general aches accompanied by cold sweats, shortness of breath, and other symptoms that they underplay.

- Be aware of the symptoms of a heart attack: (1) uncomfortable pressure, squeezing, fullness, or pain in the center of your chest that lasts more than a few minutes, or that goes away and comes back; (2) pain or discomfort in one or both arms, the back, neck, jaw, or stomach; (3) shortness of breath, with or without chest discomfort; and (4) a cold sweat, nausea, or light-headedness. Sometimes, a sudden and inexplicable dizzy spell can be a danger sign if it's coupled with an increased (or markedly *decreased*) pulse rate, a slow heartbeat, or other cardiac symptoms such as clammy, pale skin.

- Be sure to say to emergency responders, "I'm having chest pain," particularly if you are a woman with a known heart condition.

- Research your local ERs ahead of time to find out their pediatric expertise; the number of patients who visit annually (more than 20,000 is ideal); and whether they are ACOS-designated trauma centers (check www.facs.org/trauma/verified.html). At a minimum, find out the hospital(s) where your PCP has visiting privileges. Bear in mind that hospital-to-hospital transfers are very hard to facilitate.

- Children, especially infants, should always go to an ER that has pediatric expertise.

- Being in an ER or a hospital can be a chaotic experience. Constantly listen to your instincts and ask, *Is this right?* In a teaching hospital, know who you are dealing with, and make sure an attending physician sees you.

➤

- Be respectful of how challenging a caregiver's job can be. If you are unhappy with the care you are receiving, be polite but firm and comport yourself like a confident health care consumer.

- Request a copy of your complete records before you leave. The best time to ask for imaging is when you're with the technician.

- Remember that a hospital is a business. If you're unhappy with the service you received, consider contacting the institution's ombudsman and also noting your concerns on the patient satisfaction survey.

- A visit to the emergency department isn't meant to be a substitute for primary care. If you've been seen and released, and a day or two later you're still feeling lousy, work with your internist to find a specialist who can help you figure out the cause of your problem.

PART III

> # What to Do When Serious Illness Strikes

Get to the No-Mistake Zone by following the four steps of Intensive Case Management.

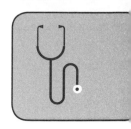

PATIENT, M.D.

*You've got a major health problem. Approach it
like a pro.*

I've been my own client twice. The bunion surgery was the easy case.
The hard one was a few years ago, when I was diagnosed with primary
hyperparathyroidism, an endocrine disease that can cause bone weakening,
kidney stones, gastrointestinal disorders, psychological issues, and a host of
central nervous system ailments.

The main symptom I experienced was fatigue. I'm normally an energetic
guy, but I was taking naps on the weekends and was exhausted by ten p.m.
every night. I assumed it was just part of getting older. Then during a physical exam, my PCP noticed I had had elevated calcium-level readings a few
years running. "This has been going on too long," he said. "It's just mildly
elevated, but we should check your parathyroid hormone levels as well."

There are four parathyroid glands that regulate calcium, the most essential element governing your neurological system. If these glands detect inad-
equate calcium in the bloodstream, they emit parathyroid hormone, or PTH,
signaling your body to release the calcium stored in your bones to the rest
of your body. When you have primary hyperparathyroidism, one or more of
your glands is stuck in the "on" position, mistakenly commanding your body
to leach more calcium than necessary.

Sure enough, my PTH levels were also high, so my PCP referred me to
an endocrinologist at a major teaching hospital. At our appointment a few

days later, the doctor confirmed that I had primary hyperparathyroidism. In fact, tests showed that I had already suffered about 20 percent bone-mineral density loss. The excess calcium in my bloodstream, he said, had been causing the fatigue. Without treatment, I'd eventually suffer from severe calcium depletion, osteoporosis, and further degradation of my entire neurological system. Depression and an inability to concentrate and think analytically were symptoms I could expect even sooner.

"So, the only question now," the doctor continued, "is which bisphosphonate do you want to be on?"

I sat there motionless, like a piece of furniture. This was the first time I'd ever been diagnosed with a serious condition, and I was afraid. I knew that things could go wrong in the health care system. This had to go right. I'd need to follow my own rules.

"What would a bisphosphonate do?" I asked.

"It would tend to ameliorate the calcium leaching from your bones," he said, "and restore some of the bone-mineral density that you lost."

"Okay, so, we do that. What are we going to do about the disease?"

"Well, we usually try a bisphosphonate for eighteen months to two years, and then if it hasn't worked, we do surgery."

"So, a bisphosphonate doesn't do anything to the disease process?"

"That's why we usually end up in surgery," he said.

"Then why do a bisphosphonate at all?"

"That's what we do."

That's what we do was not an answer that inspired confidence. There was zero chance that a bisphosphonate would cure me—it would simply treat one of many symptoms. What this doctor was suggesting seemed crazy to me. I was so upset, I sweated through my entire shirt. As I walked to my car, I thought, *I've got to find the best doctor for me, an expert who spends all their time on my specific condition.* That person turned out to be Dr. John P. Bilezikian.

To find him, I followed the same steps I described in Chapter 6: I immersed myself in the literature (a PubMed search showed that Dr. Bilezikian was a prolific author on the topic); and I called a dozen physicians in Los Angeles, New York, and Boston to ask, "Who's *the* expert on primary hyperparathyroidism?"

Dr. Bilezikian is an endocrinologist at NewYork–Presbyterian Hospital/

Columbia and the chief of the division of endocrinology at Columbia University College of Physicians and Surgeons. From the time he graduated medical school in 1969, he's been focused on my disease. He's also a lead author in the longest case study—116 patients over fifteen years—comparing outcomes for those who had surgery for primary hyperparathyroidism versus those who did not.

I picked up the phone, called his office (his number was easy to find on the school's website), and got his scheduling administrator on the line.

"I've just been diagnosed with primary hyperparathyroidism," I explained. "I'd like to schedule a consultation with Dr. Bilezikian."

"He's booked for four months," she said.

If you have a fast-moving disease like pancreatic cancer, the doctor's staff knows you *cannot* wait. You need to be seen yesterday. If you have primary hyperparathyroidism? It's not a ticking time bomb, and they know you can wait a little longer. But what if you are feeling psychologically desperate for action? To jump ahead in the queue, there are a couple of things you can try. Start by reaching out to any contacts you have at the hospital where the doctor practices, the university where he or she teaches, and current or former patients. Tell this person about your diagnosis, and ask, *Would you call the doctor and help me get in sooner?*

If you have no connections, not even tenuous ones, then just explain your situation fully to the doctor's staff. One easy way to show that you are a sophisticated patient: Mention the physician's articles or the recommendations of colleagues or prior patients that led you here. Then wait your turn. They get cancellations, just as restaurants do, and you can ask them to call you if that happens. Often it just takes a little persistence and confidence. Call, beg, plead. Say, *Look, I'm really scared about this. I'm not sleeping at night. Is there any way I could possibly see Dr. Wells sooner? I'm prepared to come in first thing in the morning. Yes, I understand I may have to wait for three to four hours, that's really not a problem. I can get over there really quickly.*

The people on the other end of the phone line are every bit as human and caring as you are. They *want* to get you in. Listen to them. Get the manager of the doctor's calendar on your side. Explain why you're concerned, and ask what you can do to see the physician sooner. Will this work 100 percent of the time? Of course not. But why not try?

Because Dr. Bilezikian was a semiretired physician, who saw patients only a couple of days a week, he had a pretty stacked schedule. I found a contact at his hospital and asked that person if he would call the doctor on my behalf. It helped shorten my wait time from four months to four weeks.

When I walked into Dr. Bilezikian's office, he'd already read my file—about twenty-five pages, including lab reports and bone scans—which I'd sent in advance of our consultation. He confirmed the diagnosis. And though we discussed different treatment approaches, he felt that surgery was my best option.

Because I had done so much research on my problem, I knew that one of the biggest risks of the procedure was damage to the vocal cords. If the delicate membranes in your throat get nicked, you don't speak anymore. I asked Dr. Bilezikian who he would recommend for my surgery.

"Well," he said, "we have someone here who is very good . . ."

I listened quietly as he gave a persuasive explanation as to why I should use their surgeon. Then I got serious with him.

"Doctor, I appreciate your recommendation. But I traveled twenty-five hundred miles to meet you, and had a friend ask personally if I could see you sooner. You're the world's top expert on my disease. I don't want to hear who your best surgeon here is. I need the very best in the country." It may have made him a little uncomfortable, but I needed to be assertive.

He responded in kind. And that's how I first learned about Dr. Robert Udelsman (the physician who previously described why it's important to shop for the right surgeon when you are having a major procedure). He is chairman of surgery at Yale–New Haven, and he pioneered an approach to parathyroid surgery that has become the gold standard. It involves testing the patient's hormone levels as the operation is happening.

Here's why this technique is so revolutionary: The four parathyroid glands are the size of small peas, and they are located, depending on your physiognomy, somewhere between your jawline and the top of your chest. Finding anything that tiny in the body can be pretty tricky, but there's an additional challenge of figuring out *which* of the four glands is defective. Presurgical imaging can help the surgeon locate enlarged (and therefore presumably overactive) glands, but it's a rough science. The scans don't give 100 percent accuracy.

Because PTH is a short-lived hormone, once the malfunctioning gland is removed, the PTH levels in the blood go back to normal very quickly. In the old days, a surgeon would dig around until he found your overactive gland, remove it, and sew you back up. But sometimes a patient turned out to have more than one bad gland, and the surgeon wouldn't even know about it until he discovered that the hormone levels hadn't gone down. That realization would come *after* the operation—until the advent of a brilliant idea: Why not check the patient's hormone levels on site, during the procedure?

Adjacent to Dr. Udelsman's operating theater is a specialized blood lab. As soon as the first gland is removed, blood samples are sent to the lab every five to ten minutes through a small pass-through window, and technicians begin measuring the patient's PTH levels and calling out the numbers, which should start decreasing once all the diseased glands are removed. It's a significant difference in protocol that ensures he gets out all the defective glands *before* he sews you back up. Dr. Udelsman didn't create this technique, but he refined it to the standard it is today, and he published an incredible study—reviewing the outcomes of 656 of his own patients over eleven years—that heralded a new era for parathyroid surgery. After reading his study, I knew he was the surgeon for me.

Three months after my meeting with Dr. Bilezikian, I was prepped for surgery with Dr. Udelsman. The imaging showed I had two enlarged parathyroids that had to be removed. As I was being wheeled into the surgical suite, Dr. Udelsman said, "All right, I'm going to put you under for a little bit, and then we'll go after these things and get them out."

Normally, I'd be nervous, because I knew what could go wrong. But I had no anxiety at all. In hindsight, I'm sure it was because I did my homework: I had immersed myself in the literature, found a top endocrinologist to consult on my case, gotten an accurate diagnosis, picked the best treatment for me, and found the right surgeon to do it. I was in the No-Mistake Zone.

About an hour later, as I started to come to, I could hear Dr. Udelsman talking with the surgical fellows at the foot of the bed. My PTH numbers were being called out, and they were getting lower: "Fifty-two . . . fifty-one . . . fifty . . ."

When they finally got to 48, I couldn't help myself. "I'm cured!"

Dr. Udelsman walked over, took my hand, and leaned in to whisper in my ear. He didn't want the fellows to hear, because he wanted what was happening to be a learning experience for them.

"Actually, you're not," he said. "They think you are too, but I know you're not. I took out two glands. Your PTH has plateaued, when the numbers should have been dropping faster, which means you still have a bad gland in there. You've got at least one more that needs to come out."

Now I was worried. "Uh-huh. I understand," I said. "Put me out. I can't be here for this."

Most primary hyperparathyroidism cases involve one gland, sometimes two, or maybe all four. Three is a very rare presentation. Finding the two enlarged glands was easy, but now Dr. Udelsman needed to poke around for the third, perhaps a fourth—and the imaging hadn't shown where they were located.

After ninety minutes, he found a gland that looked, based on his experience, to be the culprit. He was right. My numbers went down, and he sewed me back up.

When I woke up from surgery, the most interesting things started to happen. The bedsheets felt incredibly rough on my bare skin; the nurses' voices from across the room were clear and loud; the ceiling lights were intensely bright; colors seemed more saturated; meals needed less salt. I realized how much my entire nervous system had been suppressed. As time passed, my energy levels transformed. Everything changed. I was cured.

Surgical suites are booked for fixed periods of time with little margin for delay. My surgery wound up being two to three times longer than expected, blowing the entire operating schedule for that day, because I was *that* patient, the one with the unexpected anomaly. Being that case makes you prone to medical error, especially if you're in a facility that doesn't have a lot of experience dealing with your specific condition. Thankfully, Dr. Udelsman and the staff at Yale had plenty of experience to anticipate—and masterfully handle—my surgical surprise.

What's more, had I gone to a surgeon who did not use intraoperative PTH testing—or one who did but lacked the wisdom to know that my plateauing numbers meant there was another bad gland—the outcome would have been grim. I'd have been sewn back up, gone through the healing process, and still not been cured. That would have meant more surgery, more sedation, more scar tissue, more anxiety, and more costs. Which is just the kind of terrible experience I want to help you avoid.

In the next chapters, I'm going to teach you how to get to the No-Mistake Zone by following the four steps of Intensive Case Management, which are: Immersion, Diagnosis, Treatment, and Coordination.

By following these steps—that is, by immersing yourself in the illness, reaching an accurate diagnosis, picking the right treatment and provider, and coordinating all aspects of care—you will vastly improve your outcome in any situation. And while I explain the ICM steps in order, you'll find that immersion and coordination are so important that they are practiced at every turning point, not just at the beginning and end of your journey.

Thankfully, my surgery went well, but looking back, I realize that my biggest mistake was letting a couple of years' worth of unexplained elevated calcium go by. I should have been tested sooner. But I didn't recognize my lapse until I was diagnosed. Here I'd been counseling clients that, when you get lab results back, if anything is outside normal limits, and your doctor doesn't address it, you have to ask, "Should we be investigating this, to find out why this number isn't normal?" It's a simple question I should have asked, too.

Over the years, I've seen people dwell in guilt and uncertainty over the decisions they've made in their own care or the care of a family member: *I should have gotten Dad to the doctor the minute he told me he was feeling dizzy. Why did I push Mom to get that surgery? How could I have ignored my symptoms for so long?*

But let's stop worrying about the things we didn't do last year, or the actions we wish we had taken yesterday. Instead, let's focus on where we are *now*. Resolve to move forward, with a clean start, and do all you can today to get the best possible outcomes.

Part of that process involves accepting the reality that you may need help. You might think you can manage everything yourself. But you just don't know how you will react to a scary diagnosis. In my case, I was confident that I could follow my own advice, because I'd guided other people for decades.

If you are facing a serious health crisis, you'll need that steady quarterback described in Chapter 4. Develop a support team to help guide you. If you haven't already asked someone to play this role, start that conversation now with someone you trust. Pick this person wisely and share the steps of Intensive Case Management with them.

QUICK GUIDE

CHAPTER 8. Patient, M.D.

- If you need an expert consultation as soon as possible, but the nature of your disease doesn't typically merit urgent attention, reach out to hospital, university, or patient contacts and see if your PCP can help. Ask, *Would you call the doctor and help me get in sooner?*

- If you have no connections, explain your situation to the doctor's staff, mention the physician's articles, recommendations of colleagues, or prior patients that led you there, and wait your turn. Ask to be notified of cancellations.

- You never know if you will be *that* patient—the one with the unexpected anomaly that makes your procedure suddenly more complicated. Being that case makes you prone to medical error, especially if you're in a facility and/or are being treated by physicians with little experience in your specific condition. The four steps of ICM—Immersion, Diagnosis, Treatment, and Coordination—will help you avoid this problem.

- Focus on the future, even if you've made missteps in the past. Starting today, take the opportunity to better manage decisions, on your own or with support.

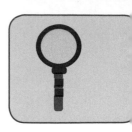

CHAPTER NINE

STEP 1–IMMERSION

*Learn everything you can about your illness and the
doctors who are passionate about it.*

Jessica's problems began when she hit puberty and started to
develop an unusual range and number of maladies: asthma, fever,
pain, rashes, severe allergies, whooping cough, and a distended stomach.
She'd get sick, be treated for her symptoms, and recover. But some months
were worse than others, sending her in and out of the hospital and causing
her to miss more than a year's worth of high school and a year of college.

By her mid-twenties, Jessica had been given almost every diagnosis
under the sun. One doctor even recommended brain surgery to correct what
he suspected was a neurological disorder. Her father, Chandler, a technology executive, took Jessica to specialists in that disorder, and they all agreed
she didn't have it—and that brain surgery was a terrible idea. In fact, Jessica
had been kept safe from bad medical decisions pretty much all her life, by
Chandler's immersing himself in the literature and consulting with experts
at each new, alarming turn of his daughter's illness.

"Most clinicians are so busy seeing patients that they're not home at
night on their computers reading the latest research," Chandler said. "They
go to maybe two conferences a year, but they're not up on all the latest clinical trials and treatments. They may not be up on the latest *anything*."

Steering treatment requires a lot of careful fact-finding, and that's where
Step 1 of Intensive Case Management, Immersion, comes in. Roll up your

sleeves and investigate the data, just as we did with Catherine's Churg-Strauss diagnosis, Rachel's ear surgery, and Sally's hip pain.

Even if all you can do is an hour or two of online research (at PubMed, Expertscape, and the websites of reputable institutions), you will be better educated about your illness than if you do nothing at all. And once you start looking in the right places, it's amazing what you can discover. For instance, many major hospitals and medical institutions are getting savvy about their Web presence, providing video interviews with veteran physicians and researchers as well as patient-friendly summaries of their work. If you've been told you have breast cancer, and you feel uncertain about the diagnosis or the treatment your doctor is prescribing, you can log in to the website of the National Comprehensive Cancer Network (www.nccn.org) and find well-produced, easy-to-understand guidelines that explain the different types of breast cancer, how they're normally detected, and what the current evidence-based (i.e., recognized as best-practice) treatment options are, depending on your age, disease stage, and other factors. Or maybe you're at a later stage of colon cancer, the standard treatment isn't working, and you want to look into some aggressive options. The National Cancer Institute (www.cancer.gov) has a clinical-trials search engine that can be a jumping-off point for a conversation with your oncologist.

In practice, the immersion process looks like this: you (and a trusted helper) mine the online research and seek out the soundest thinking on your condition, the best doctors to consult with, and the most relevant treatment guidelines. And so it goes throughout your illness. It's a continuing education that will also help refine the evolving list of questions you bring to doctor appointments.

The other important part of immersion is revisiting your medical records. Remember that the smallest of clues can sometimes point to the right diagnosis. (Jennifer discovered an early mention of psoriatic arthritis in her medical records; Amanda's blood disorder was detected with help from her mother's history.) But even more important, your physicians need to make decisions based on your past and current health. Doctors may be the only professionals who are regularly asked to provide services and render judgment without comprehensive information—by that, I mean without reviewing a patient's full history. If you are overwhelmed by your own medical situation, it may be time to ask your support team to help you collect and distribute your records.

—————

Chandler had a strong feeling that his daughter's immune system was compromised, but it wasn't until Jessica got older that they got to an accurate diagnosis. One day when she was twenty-five, her bottom lip and tongue started to tingle. They became so inflamed, it looked as if she'd been stung by a bee; then her tongue began to block her airway, making it difficult for her to breathe.

When we get sick, we often think that Symptom A + Symptom B + Symptom C = Diagnosis. But as Jessica and her dad can attest, that's not always the case. The way to solve a medical conundrum is to stay focused, immerse yourself in the data, and seek out experts to guide you along the way. As the disease progresses, it will become easier to figure out.

Chandler had done an amazing job of overseeing his daughter's care, but her problems were becoming overwhelming, and he reached out to me, to be a sounding board. Every few days, he'd call to discuss: *Should we be doing this test? Should I talk to this person? Who else can we call? Where else can we go? What else can we do?*

It took many months of working together like this before he finally got to the heart of Jessica's problem. She had two conditions: idiopathic acquired angioedema (unexplained swelling) and lupus, a chronic autoimmune disease that causes the body to attack its own healthy cells, tissues, and organs, causing inflammation and potential damage to the heart, lungs, joints, brain, kidneys, blood, and skin. About 1.5 million Americans suffer from some form of lupus; 90 percent of them are women. While there is no cure, an increasingly wide array of drugs is available—some that suppress the immune system's attack on the patient's own organs, and others that help to manage the symptoms of lupus flare-ups, which include joint and chest pain, skin rashes, fatigue, fever, and more.

Making matters worse, Jessica appeared to be having an allergic reaction to the prescriptions that were supposed to alleviate her symptoms. Chandler appealed to the specialists for help: *No one has been able to figure this out—I need someone who can think outside the box. Maybe that's you?* An allergist who welcomed the challenge discovered Jessica was sensitive to something called polysorbate 80, an inactive ingredient mostly used as an emulsifying agent and found in minuscule amounts in some foods and medications.

Jessica's father also called doctors around the world to ask if they'd ever seen a combination of lupus and angioedema, and whether anyone had done studies on polysorbate 80 allergies. Chandler developed relationships with Dr. Bruce D. Logan, a skilled internist who tirelessly invested himself in getting to the bottom of Jessica's problem; Dr. Stephen A. Paget, a leading New York rheumatologist; Dr. Jeffrey A. Gelfand at Harvard, who discovered the first medication for angioedema thirty years ago; and Dr. Kenneth C. Kalunian, a renowned lupus specialist, and Dr. Bruce L. Zuraw, a top allergy and angioedema expert, both at UC San Diego.

Meanwhile, Jessica's lupus was getting out of control, and she was put on a very strong immunosuppressant that shut down her hyperactive immune system. Her lupus subsided. But six months later, tests showed that her liver and kidneys were inflamed from the drugs she was on—now she was at great risk of organ damage. As soon as she was taken off the medicine, of course, her lupus came roaring back, causing butterfly rashes across her face and inflamed knee, elbow, hand, and wrist joints. Everything suddenly felt urgent and high-risk, and Chandler was incredibly worried about the next steps in her treatment plan. He called the members of her team—doctors and researchers—and asked, with the passion of a desperate parent, if they would take part in a conference call to discuss her case. After much schedule wrangling, a date was set.

Chandler beamed that day on the line. "Wow," he said. "Are we all on? This is amazing." Getting a dozen clinicians on the phone to discuss a single case is no simple feat. (See Chapter 12 for tips.) But Chandler had worked to bring in people who relished the challenge and wanted to make a difference. One doctor spoke up and asked, politely, if Chandler would please withdraw from the call: "No hard feelings, but we need to have a debate about Jessica's options, and it's better if we don't have to censor ourselves." Chandler didn't mind at all. Anything to help them do their jobs better.

The consensus was that Jessica should start something called plasmapheresis, a process similar to dialysis, in which her blood would be drawn out of her body and put through a machine that separated out the plasma— which contained the inflammatory antibodies that were attacking her system. Then synthetic blood plasma would be put back in, spurring her system to regenerate healthy plasma. Plasmapheresis is a short-term option for lupus patients who don't respond to standard treatments, but it doesn't work for everyone, and there's a risk of blood clots, infection, and worse flare-ups than before.

Jessica would try it for several months, and if all went well, they'd introduce a weaker immunosuppressant drug into her body. Finding one that didn't contain polysorbate 80 was Chandler's next mission. Such a medication didn't seem to exist. He called a pharmaceutical company that made a popular lupus drug and asked if it would create a special batch without this one ingredient. Unfortunately, no one was willing to risk providing a formula that hadn't been safety tested. So Chandler focused instead on finding ways to mitigate the effects of polysorbate 80 on his daughter's system.

Meanwhile Jessica was doing well on her plasmapheresis protocol, and toward the end of the trial, she started taking Imuran, an older immunosuppressant with relatively low toxicity. She was also put on high doses of Benadryl and prednisone to combat any potential allergic reactions. Between the Imuran and the plasmapheresis, her lupus went into remission.

Granted, Chandler is the most committed and tireless advocate I've ever met. Not everyone has the same capacity, but the point is this: You will make great strides if you put in just a fraction of the effort Chandler does. And if you have a helper at your side, the outcome will be twice as good.

"When you're watching your kid suffering, you do whatever you have to do," says Chandler. "You're not going to stop when a doctor says, 'I'm running out of ideas.' You just keep calling experts. Some doctors will see the complexity of your case and say, 'I don't have time for this.' But others will be stimulated by it. Find the ones who say, 'We need to figure this out, and I'm going to talk to every smart colleague I know about it.'"

And as Chandler notes, you needn't ever feel sorry about seeking out more opinions: "If you have a complicated case, there are so many resources: people at NIH who will speak to you; people at pharmaceutical companies who will tell you about what they're trying to do; doctors and researchers and biotech companies and people at disease-based organizations who you can talk to and get more expert names from."

Today Jessica's care is in the hands of some of the leading minds on lupus and angioedema in the country. And Chandler knows that when his daughter has problems that her physicians can't figure out, they can bounce ideas off contacts around the world.

"My daughter's condition is chronic," he says. "We deal with it. She'll be dealing with it until we find a cure."

CHRONIC CONDITIONS: THREE THINGS TO WATCH

Some health problems are discrete: you confirm the diagnosis, find the right physicians and treatments, and hopefully, reach a speedy cure. But for patients, like Jessica, who suffer from chronic conditions—things like lupus, diabetes, asthma, arthritis, chronic obstructive pulmonary disease, fibromyalgia, and more—getting better is a lifelong process. If you have a chronic illness, there are three realms that need vigilant monitoring:

1. Changes in your symptoms
2. Changes in your health that only your physician can detect
3. Changes in science

As a patient, you are the best monitor of number 1, **changes in your symptoms.** Sometimes people think that chronic degenerative disease follows a linear progression in which every year is worse than the last. That's just not true. Biological processes ebb and flow. Do a gut-check on your symptoms as part of a weekly routine: Are you experiencing more or less pain? Greater fatigue, trouble breathing, increased swelling? Tell your doctors. And ask if there are specific symptoms they want you to monitor, and how often you should report them. Remember that as your body matures, internal processes and hormonal shifts can affect the frequency and intensity of your symptoms. Likewise, external factors—such as poor diet, exercise, and sleep patterns—can cause stress, putting a toll on your body and making back pain, autoimmune conditions, or cardiovascular problems more noticeable. Simple respiratory or urinary tract infections can aggravate a condition, because your immune system is working overtime to fight on two fronts. Stay in tune with how you are feeling, and report changes to your doctors so they can help you to feel better, sooner.

Number 2, **changes in your health that only your physician can detect,** are things you may not even be able to perceive, such as cholesterol, hormonal fluctuations, and lung function. If you've got cystic fibrosis, getting precise measurements of your lung function could help your physicians fine-tune treatments while also making sure you aren't showing the early signs of other diseases.

"Often, when you have a chronic disease, there are also comorbidities—fellow-traveler conditions—that frequently associate with the primary disease in question," says Seattle rheumatologist Dr. Philip Mease. "For instance, with psoriatic arthritis, there is a genetic proclivity to having metabolic syndrome, a triad of obesity, hyperlipidemia, and hypertension."

Part of a patient's job is to ask:

Doctor, we've dealt with my skin and joints thus far. How can we attend to the other potential problems—issues that tend to crop up in patients with my disease—that I might experience down the road?
How's my blood pressure today?
I've come in first thing in the morning without having eaten. Can we add a lipid panel to the blood test that you're doing?

Learn more about the disorders associated with your chronic condition, and work with your PCP or specialist (whoever is taking on principal responsibility for the management of your disease) to precisely monitor the signs and symptoms of your illness, as well as its potential fellow travelers.

Finally, number 3, **changes in science.** Keep abreast of the latest and greatest news about your condition and how it is being treated. A couple of quick steps: (1) set up Google alerts on your disease, (2) research the best philanthropies focused on your condition, and sign up for their newsletters and e-mail flashes about important developments, and (3) visit PubMed periodically to read the latest articles from respected journals that focus on your illness.

If, during your research, you find an expert who is especially knowledgeable and approachable, schedule a consult, then stay in

➤

touch. This person may become your go-to specialist, or they may be a physician-researcher in another state with whom you periodically consult, in addition to seeing your local doctor. You can ask to keep the dialogue going in a few different ways:

Thank you so much for your help, doctor. Would it be okay with you if I check back in when there's a change in my symptoms, for better or worse, just to let you know if the treatment is working?

I know you've dedicated a lot of your career to developing more effective and safer treatments for my condition. And I know how busy you are. If I learn about new drugs for my disease, I'd love to check back with you to get your opinion on whether they're right for me.

When you are developing new therapies for this condition, if you think one might be appropriate for me, I'd love to learn more about it. Would it be okay if I kept in touch?

If this feels awkward, remember that your disease is their life's work—they want to know how patients are responding to treatment, what's working and what's not, and the subtle differences among patient populations. I was on a call this morning with a doctor I'd never spoken to before, telling her about a woman who had a painful chronic illness for which this physician was an expert. She remarked, "There are so many wonderful things, right on the horizon, that may be helpful for her. . . . Please have her call me, because I want her to know there's hope out there for her."

My experience is that clinicians at the cutting edge are excited about their work, and they want patients to know what's available to help them. Even a simple check-in, a few times a year, will give you access to their up-to-the-minute expertise.

"The patient should never say that this condition is a fait accompli, written in stone, and nothing is ever going to change. Because knowledge changes, people change, and situations change," says Canadian internist and preventive medicine expert Dr. Sheldon Elman. "Being on top of things as time goes on is the way it goes. For example, there may be a new medication available, but the patient didn't go back to see their doctor because they thought, 'What's he going to tell me? This is the way it is.' No. They should be proactive. I have people who call me regularly and ask, 'What's new?' "

Good specialists are constantly monitoring the research on the drugs they prescribe, because whenever a new drug is approved by the FDA or embraced by the medical community, it's not known yet how it will work in a *much* larger group of patients over a longer period of time. So ask your doctor: *What's the latest learning on my medications? Are researchers recognizing any serious limitations? Drug interactions? Side effects?*

Just as important, inquire if there are new medications you should be trying: *What are their advantages—and disadvantages— over my existing prescription? What are the known side effects? How might they work in someone with my specific illness and other medical problems?*

Keeping tabs on the scientific progress for your condition could become a life-changer for you at some point. But at the least, if your current prescriptions are not controlling your symptoms or you are dealing with very unpleasant side effects, don't hesitate to reach out to the experts you've come to rely on and ask, "What's new?"

Eric, a crisis negotiator of sorts, faced his own crisis several years ago when his internist found an abnormal blood test result during a routine physical. A biopsy confirmed that Eric had prostate cancer. Like Chandler, Eric likes to study every piece of a puzzle until he can solve it. But while Jessica's chronic condition required years of immersion on Chandler's part, Eric's disease had a well-worn path toward a cure.

Prostate cancer is the second most common cause of cancer death in men. (Lung cancer is first.) But while one in seven men will be diagnosed with the disease over a lifetime, only one in thirty-six will die from it. In fact, about 2.5 million Americans are alive today who have had prostate cancer at some point.

Most prostate cancers are discovered after a patient is found to have an elevated amount of prostate-specific antigen, or PSA, circulating in his blood. PSA levels can vary over time for lots of reasons, but if your internist discovers that yours is above a certain number, or increasing at a rapid rate, he may order a biopsy. A pathologist will then study your prostate cells under a high-powered microscope and give them grades, based on a five-point scale. Cells that are close to normal—mostly round and symmetrical—are given a grade of 1; at the opposite end of the spectrum, asymmetrical cancer-riddled cells get a 5. (A grade of 3 or more is considered cancerous.) The pathologist will look for the two most common grade patterns in your cells, list them in order of prevalence, and then add them up to calculate your Gleason score.*

Eric's Gleason was a 7 (3 + 4), meaning most of his cells looked like 3s, with the second most common cells being 4s. This was pretty aggressive prostate cancer for a fifty-two-year-old man.

The day he got his diagnosis, he made two calls. The first was to his wife. She was terrified—they'd been married for nearly twenty years and were each other's soul mates—but she said to him: "We're going to get through this."

His next call was to me. (Eric knew that I had previously served as CEO of the Prostate Cancer Foundation, so that made me another "expert" on his list of people to contact.) There are several different initial courses of treatment, the three most common being surgery, radiation therapy, and watchful

---

*For example, Gleason scores of 9 (5 + 4) or 10 (5 + 5) mean that the cancer is very aggressive; but a score of 6 (3 + 3) indicates a far less serious cancer.

waiting for presentations that don't require immediate intervention. Some patients will follow more than one path depending on their overall health, how aggressive the disease is, and whether it has spread. I had a strong opinion about the specialist Eric should see (Dr. Mark Kawachi, a pioneer in the realm of robotic prostate surgery at City of Hope National Medical Center in Duarte, California) and the treatment (a radical prostatectomy) that would give him the best outcome. But Eric is a data junkie. He needed to go through the immersion process and come to his own decisions.

"Okay, here's the deal," I said. "I know you're going to research this thing to death. And you can't have surgery for five weeks because you need time to heal from your biopsy. So you've got five weeks to do whatever you want. And at the end of that five weeks, you're going to end up with Dr. Kawachi at City of Hope."

Eric had a good laugh about my subtle way with advice. Anything to lend a little emotional support. Logistical support was next. "While I have you on the phone, let's conference in Dr. Kawachi's office and make an appointment to see him, because his schedule is pretty tight. If you decide to go another way, we can cancel it."

Because prostate cancer is so prevalent and progress on the disease has been so great, there was plenty of wisdom and material online for Eric to plunge into. Here are the two main questions he researched during the next five weeks:

1. Do I have the most accurate diagnosis? Eric wanted the best information about his prognosis. He understood the seriousness of his Gleason, but what if the reading had not been accurate? There are many good pathologists who can look at slides and provide a second opinion. Eric went to the top. Dr. Jonathan Epstein, a professor of pathology, urology, and oncology and an attending pathologist at Johns Hopkins Hospital, has probably examined more prostate cancer tissue than any other pathologist. And Eric found him by reading the literature on prostate cancer pathology and asking around for pathologist recommendations.

"I just called him," Eric would later tell me. "He was sitting at his desk. He answered the phone. I told him I had been diagnosed with prostate cancer. 'I want you to read my pathology.' 'Great!' he said. 'Send me the slides.'"

Eric packaged his slides in an overnight envelope and shipped them off. When Dr. Epstein's report came back, he had a new score: Gleason 6 (3 + 3). In effect, it downgraded his cancer's aggressiveness. He had to put the new information in perspective, as just one pathologist's opinion, but it was a big relief to him. Next, he wanted to know:

2. What's the best treatment for me—and who's really good at it? Because the prostate is buried deep within nerves and tissues that control things like bowel movements, urinary function, and sexual response, letting a surgeon dive in there with a knife is a scary prospect. In fact, thirty years ago prostate cancer surgery almost always resulted in extensive bleeding, incontinence, and impotence. The treatment was often worse than the disease. So much has changed.

Every day during his spare moments, Eric studied the websites of the major treatment centers for his condition, places like UC San Francisco, Memorial Sloan Kettering, MD Anderson, and Dana-Farber. He talked a lot about his diagnosis, having no shame in grilling friends and colleagues who had been through it: *What was your surgery? Who was your doctor? How were your symptoms? How are you now?* Pretty quickly, he learned the lexicon of his disease and the names of the innovators in its cure, including Dr. Patrick Walsh, a urologist at Johns Hopkins who, in the early 1980s, developed a nerve-sparing surgical technique that saved men from the devastating side effects.

Eric ultimately came to the conclusion that he needed a radical prostatectomy—the removal of his prostate. But would he go for robotic-assisted surgery, a newish technique at the time, which involved creating small incisions in the abdomen, while using surgical telescopes and tiny instruments? Or should he opt for open surgery, which meant a single, larger incision through which the surgeon would use his hands and tools, allowing for a tactile and visual assessment of the tumor? Eric knew he would heal faster with the robotic option, but there was little data to show which technique provided a better shot at getting all the cancer out, with fewer cases of impotence and incontinence. Eric had, by now, a long list of questions, and it was time to interview specialists.

"What I discovered is that people give you advice based on their experience," Eric said. "The older urologists would tell me, 'You really want to do open surgery, because when I get in there, I can *feel* the tumor.' Then you talk to the guys who are doing robotic, and they say, 'The robotic is so much more sensitive, and I'm looking at the tumor on a high-definition screen.'"

It soon became obvious that if he was going to go robotic—the direction in which he was leaning—he needed a surgeon who'd performed the technique a lot. So he asked every doctor, "How many of these have you done?" Since it was an emerging method, the numbers he was hearing weren't very impressive: *I've done a hundred. I've done two hundred. I've done seventy-five.*

In the meantime, Eric was getting to know Dr. Kawachi.

"I'm not sure he was glad he met me," Eric recalled, "because every day I would write up a memo on my research and send it to him. He would call me back in the evenings, after he got out of surgery, and answer all my unsophisticated questions. I was genuinely interested in the science, and he was committed to this new technology, so we developed a rapport."

He asked Dr. Kawachi, "How many robotic radical prostatectomies have you done?"

The answer: *2,700.*

"That's a good number," Eric said.

In the spring of 2008, Eric underwent a four-and-a-half-hour procedure with Dr. Kawachi. There were no complications. He went in for surgery on a Friday and returned to work the following Thursday. Shortly afterward he called me to share some news: The biopsy had come back with negative margins. They got all the cancer.

"What do you think this means?" he asked. It meant he was *cured.* Hearing that word made him a little nervous, as if a bullet had just whizzed by his head. Recalling the moment years later, he had some interesting observations about how the Immersion step had saved him from panicking.

"When I was in the game, I was so focused on data, I found comfort in research," he said. "I couldn't just sit on a bench and worry. I needed to do whatever I could do to learn and to move this process forward—to fix my problem. So that's what I did. I didn't spend a lot of time in fear. Not that I'm not a fearful guy, but that emotion didn't crop up."

Seven years later Eric is still cancer free. The day he got his diagnosis, he told his wife that there had to be a silver lining somewhere in this frightening situation. And there was: understanding the importance of family and close friends.

"When you're staring in the face of cancer or some other life-threatening issue, that becomes very clear," he said. His advice for people going through a similar health crisis? Let a friend be a friend. "Lean on your support system," he said. "People want to be there for you. It's not a burden—it's an opportunity. Don't steal their opportunity to help you."

T hough he came to realize how much his personal network meant to him, Eric was one of the rare patients who needed very little help. Most people, when they get sick, try to go it alone—but I think that's a mistake. Few can push down the raw emotion that springs up inside them and stick to the facts in order to make thoughtful and objective decisions.

How will you react when a distressing diagnosis comes your way? Everyone, and I mean *everyone*, can doubt their instincts and become passive in the face of unexpected illness.

Take the almost-identical case of Patrick, a sixty-five-year-old retired detective on Long Island, New York, who was having a routine physical exam when his primary care physician discovered that his PSA blood levels had tripled in the last eighteen months. A biopsy confirmed he had prostate cancer. Although his prognosis was very similar to Eric's, Patrick made a few missteps at the outset that almost put him on a path toward disaster.

To start, he went to a general urologist at his small-town hospital, even though he was just a train ride away from Memorial Sloan Kettering Cancer Center in New York City, one of the best hospitals for cancer in America. Patrick's local doctor shook his head and told him it didn't look good. He could remove Patrick's prostate, but he recommended three months of aggressive chemotherapy first to shrink the tumor.

"We can start your chemo tomorrow," the doctor said. (*Tomorrow!*) Chemotherapy affects patients in different ways, but Patrick wasn't ready for the possibility of nausea, vomiting, hair loss, a compromised immune system, and other painful side effects. Plus, it was the holidays. He asked for more time. The doctor grumbled about not wanting to wait too long, then acquiesced. "Fine," he told Patrick, "but in the meantime, let's schedule a bone scan to determine if the cancer has metastasized."

Three days before Christmas, Patrick and his wife went to the hospital for his bone scan. "If I were you, I wouldn't be very optimistic," the doctor warned. Luckily, the scan was negative, but Patrick's wife had had enough. She had been doing some reading on prostate cancer, and from what she could tell, chemotherapy seemed to be what you turn to when all else has failed.

"How many times have you done this chemotherapy-first protocol?" she asked.

Ten times.

Later at home, she begged Patrick to get a second opinion: Maybe he should call someone at Sloan Kettering?

No, he told her, that place was a big, cold cancer center, and besides, he didn't want to hurt his doctor's feelings.

Patrick is a smart guy. As a detective, he did good work by digging deep, asking tough questions, and taking the time to root out the truth. Yet he didn't investigate his own case. When patients are under stress and feeling vulnerable, they may want to stick close to home. (As a caretaker of a spouse or relative, you may want to *let* them stay snuggled up in bed with a bowl of chicken noodle soup.) But if the diagnosis is serious or complicated, you owe it to yourself and the people who love you to seek out better care than you can get at the local infirmary. You don't have to fly all over the world, but you ought to, at a minimum, do three things:

1. Educate yourself about your disease.

2. If you are considering a small hospital, ask: "How many patients a year do you admit with my specific condition?"

3. Ask your physician: "How many times have you done this procedure/protocol?"

Volume—that is, the number of times a surgeon has performed a procedure, or a hospital has cared for patients with a specific illness—is critically important for certain complex operations, including heart and aneurysm surgeries, and surgery for cancers of the pancreas, esophagus, ovaries, and prostate. The more your doctor has done, the better the outcome you are likely to have.

"If I were interviewing a surgeon," says Wisconsin oncologist Dr. George Wilding, "I would just ask: 'How many of these do you do a year? How long have you been doing it? What is your training, background, track record, morbidity, side effects?' I think it's good to get a sense of frequency. If it's a difficult, complicated procedure—like cutting out the pancreas and a number of other organs, which takes a tremendous amount of experience and skill—if someone said, 'No problem, I do four or five of these a year,' I just don't know about that. On the other hand, you don't want someone who claims they're doing so many that, if you do the math, you think 'How are you getting this done?' Or for something like robotic surgery for prostate cancer, you don't want to be among the first fifty or one hundred cases that person ever did. There's definitely a learning curve there."

To test this idea—that a doctor's surgical volume makes a difference in a patient's outcome—researchers reviewed the cases of more than 5,100 men with prostate cancer who had undergone radical prostatectomies between 1996 and 2003 at four of the nation's top hospitals. They discovered that patients who were treated by rookies—doctors with fewer than 50 surgeries under their belts—had a 24 percent chance of the disease returning within five years. They also found that it took about 250 surgeries for a doctor to get really proficient (reducing the disease recurrence to 13 percent). When you got to the real pros, surgeons who'd done more than 1,000 procedures, the probability of the cancer returning dropped to about 8 percent. So if you make the mistake—and it *is* a mistake—of going to someone who hasn't done enough prostatectomies to become good at it, you are tripling the odds that your disease will come back.

Women face similar dangers. In a 2014 *Gynecologic Oncology* article, researchers studied the survival outcomes of nearly 12,000 California women with late-stage ovarian cancer, comparing factors such as the patient's race and socioeconomic status and, most important, the experience levels of the hospitals and physicians who treated them. Physicians who treated ten or more ovarian-cancer patients a year, and hospitals that admitted twenty or more ovarian-cancer patients annually, were considered "high volume"; those with fewer were deemed "low volume." As one might expect, women who were cared for by a high-volume physician at a high-volume hospital had a 31 percent higher survival rate than patients who were seen by low-volume doctors at low-volume hospitals. Astoundingly, only 4.3 percent of all patients, regardless of race or wealth, obtained that winning high-volume combination. The majority (53 percent) passively accepted the bad hand of being seen by a low-volume physician at a low-volume hospital.

You don't have to settle for the poorer outcomes associated with low-volume care. **To avoid becoming a statistic, seek out hospitals that have entire departments devoted to your condition, and ask your doctors,**

How many times have you done this surgery/seen patients with my specific disease?

A few days before Patrick was to start chemotherapy, he got in touch with me, at the urging of his wife. His story appalled me. Although the chemo-first, surgery-second approach is commonly used in some other cancers, like breast cancer, this approach—called neoadjuvant chemotherapy—would be highly unorthodox for Patrick's presentation of prostate cancer. As his wife had seen with just a bit of reading and research, chemo is typically employed for prostate cancers after surgery and radiation therapy have failed—which was not Patrick's case at all. *Starting* his treatment with chemo was akin to recommending amputation for a sprained ankle.

Cutting to the chase, I pointed Patrick in the direction of Dr. Peter T. Scardino, chairman of the department of surgery at Memorial Sloan Kettering (and author of the foreword to this book) and a coauthor of the study that found better outcomes for prostate cancer patients who had high-volume surgeons. Patrick would later admit that he showed up for his appointment with a chip on his shoulder, figuring this legendary institution and its star surgeon would be full of themselves.

"But when I walked through the door, everyone was so nice," he said. "Dr. Scardino was warm and charming. He explained all my options without judgment."

So how do you fire Doctor A when you've decided that going with Doctor B is a much better option? If you're a guy like Patrick, you don't beat around the bush. He simply told his local urologist, "I've got the opportunity to be seen by a world-class surgeon, and I'm going to take it. Thanks for all you've done."

Dr. Scardino performed the surgery in early 2012. I got a call from Patrick three days later. "I'm strolling up York Avenue, and man, I feel really good," he said. "I guess cancer agrees with me, but I wouldn't recommend it for everyone!"

Of course, his doctors will need to monitor him, as his disease can always return. But the last time we spoke, Patrick reported that his most recent PSA test was a zero. "I think I'm in the clear," he said. "I really do."

I admire Patrick. He's a soft-on-the-inside, hard-on-the-outside guy who spent time in Vietnam as a younger man. The kind of person you could stay up all night in a bar with, trading war stories. He's seen more disturbing things than many of us can imagine. Yet his cancer diagnosis completely disarmed him. Luckily, his wife was able to get him thinking, *Maybe I need another opinion?* This was one of the few times in his life when he needed to ask for help.

Patrick learned pretty quickly that he would have better outcomes at a "big, cold cancer center." But I once knew a guy who drove every day from a small Pennsylvania suburb to his job in Philadelphia, and when his mother developed esophageal cancer, he sent her to the local community hospital for surgery. He was a very bright man who loved his mother dearly, yet it never occurred to him that she would get better care at the Hospital of the University of Pennsylvania, which he passed on his commute six days a week. He probably thought she would be more comfortable in a small hospital close to home.

Community hospitals are terrific institutions that can do great things, but this was a difficult and risky procedure, which should be done only by a surgeon at a hospital that has a high volume of similar cases. In this woman's case, there *was* a complication after surgery—a mucus plug clogged her esophagus. Presumably, in a larger institution, the medical staff would have detected and resolved it rapidly, because it's not an uncommon issue. But hers was missed, and her brain was deprived of oxygen for too long. She suffered irreversible brain damage.

Even if you think your surgery is a cinch, you don't know if you're going to have an anatomical anomaly that can't be predicted. You want to be at an institution where the experience and resources are in place, so that if a complication presents itself, there's a likelihood the staff has seen and managed it before—and even if they haven't, they've got the expertise to figure it out. Had I not had Dr. Udelsman and his team overseeing my parathyroid surgery, I would have been in a terrible situation. Luckily, he spotted my problem. Even better, it didn't cost more to have the surgeon-in-chief on my case. If you wanted the best lawyer in New York City, you'd have to pay a fortune to get him. In medicine, it frequently doesn't cost any extra to get *that* guy. Academic medical centers take Medicare and most insurance plans, and they have the most experienced physicians. Consciously exploit this any time you can.

"For the more dangerous and complex operations like pancreatic, esoph-ageal, neurosurgery, perhaps lung surgery, big cancer operations, endocrine surgery, cardiac operations," says Dr. Udelsman, "there's no question that you want an institution that does high volumes, with a wealth of expertise, and intensive care units staffed by full-time, board-certified intensivists who are in-house, twenty-four hours a day. So that when a patient has a cardiac arrest in the middle of the night, it's not a physician's assistant all alone try-ing to pump that patient's chest, but a doctor who's been through this before and knows what to do. That's a big deal. All the major hospitals will have intensivists, but if you're at a small place, they can't always afford it because it's too expensive, and it's not a requirement."

Dr. Anthony D'Amico, a professor of radiation oncology at Harvard Med-ical School and the chief of genitourinary radiation oncology at the Brigham and Women's Hospital and Dana-Farber Cancer Institute, is a methodical physician and educator. Here are his thoughts on the maxim of major hospi-tals for major problems:

"If you have appendicitis, a gallbladder that needs to be removed, hyper-tension, or a tendency toward high glucose—but not frank diabetes—these are things that can be managed just about anywhere. But if you've got can-cer, significant heart disease, complications of diabetes—these are life-threatening issues, and you don't want any unexpected situations to get in the way of expert care. So you have to go somewhere where that's what they do," Dr. D'Amico says. "For example, all I treat is prostate cancer—that's what I do. I've seen tens of thousands of cases and all the variations on a theme. It doesn't mean something new can't come along, but it's unusual that I haven't seen something *like* it before. So you want to go to where you're *not* the unusual case, you're of the more common, garden variety of what goes on day to day, and there's less chance for error."

Which is not to say that community hospitals don't do good work. But what you want is a winning combination of a skilled high-volume special-ist *and* a well-equipped, high-volume hospital. There are some very good doctors who leave large institutions in favor of small community hospitals because they want to focus on patient care, without the pressures of being in a large, publish-or-perish bureaucracy. But the only way to know that you've already got an expert in your own backyard is to do your homework on the physician and his or her institution. Ask about volume and track records. Here's Dr. Udelsman again:

"Some community hospitals are really good," he says, "especially the ones that have a Level I trauma center. And you can just ask, *Are you a Level I or not?* That means they've got well-equipped ICUs and intensivists on staff. I think orthopedic surgery done at a quality community hospital with quality surgeons is probably fine. Hernias—local inguinal hernias, umbilical hernias—those can be done at the local hospital. Fixing a ruptured appendix in the middle of the night, routine colon surgery—all probably okay; but again, you never know when the easiest operation can turn into something horrific. And when you're the doctor in the operating room, you're kind of stuck. You've got to either know what to do or have the right people there to help you."

All of which brings us back to the question Dr. Roboz posed earlier: *What are all the things that could go wrong during my operation?* The institution and doctors you select need to have a lot of practice in your procedure, because practice makes perfect.

"Think about a surgeon like a musician," Dr. Udelsman says. "A professional violinist practices every day, for hours. And then when they go to a major concert, they've walked in with thousands of hours of practice—for *one* concert. Good surgeons do the same thing."

I liked this analogy so much, I tracked down Martin Chalifour, the principal concertmaster of the Los Angeles Philharmonic who took up the violin at age four, to ask him, "How do you get ready for a performance?"

"When I'm preparing for a concert it never leaves my mind," Chalifour says. This means up to six hours a day of practice, listening to and deftly leading the entire violin section, calibrating the sound to complement the natural acoustics of the hall, maintaining his instrument and making sure that it has fresh strings.

And while there are the rare exceptions, the world's best violinists are focused solely on their instrument and musical style. "You *have* to concentrate on one to become the best you can," Chalifour says.

A surgeon has the same responsibilities to her practical skills, her operating room team, and her instruments. And while there are the rare surgeons who achieve excellence in more than one realm of medicine, you will find that the best physician for you is the one who is focused almost entirely on your specific procedure, and who can perform it at a well-equipped institution that enables him to do his best work.

QUICK GUIDE

CHAPTER 9. **Step 1—Immersion**

- Mine the online research, seek out the soundest thinking on your condition, and find the best doctors to consult with and the most relevant treatment guidelines.

- Collect your medical records and distribute them to your physicians.

- For chronic illness, the three realms that need vigilant monitoring are (1) changes in your symptoms, (2) changes in your health that only your physician can detect, and (3) changes in the science.

- Find an expert who is especially knowledgeable and approachable, schedule a consult, and stay in touch.

- Keep tabs on the scientific progress—it could become a life-changer for you at some point.

- Seek out hospitals that have entire departments devoted to your condition, and ask your doctors: *How many times have you done this surgery/seen patients with my specific disease?*

- Remember that it doesn't frequently cost any extra to be seen by high-volume specialists at high-volume academic medical centers, because they take Medicare and most insurance plans.

- Choose a hospital where the experience and resources are in place, so that if a complication presents itself, there's a likelihood the staff has seen and managed it before.

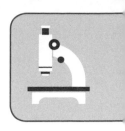

CHAPTER TEN

STEP 2–DIAGNOSIS

How to be sure you've been correctly diagnosed? Follow the carpenter's rule: Measure twice, cut once.

*D*o *you have a minute? I have your test results, and they're not good.* Every day someone who thought they were fine listens to a devastating medical verdict. If it happens to you, I'm asking you to take a deep breath and summon up more strength than you thought you had.

Step 2 of Intensive Case Management is getting to the right diagnosis before you agree to surgery or other invasive treatments. You'll notice this has been a theme in many of our case studies. This is crucial. I know how emotionally overwhelming this experience can be, and I hope this book gives you the confidence and courage to tell your doctor you'd like to get another opinion, and bestows on you the energy to do the research on your condition. Because that's really what you need to do. Please understand that an incorrect diagnosis isn't just inconvenient and frustrating—unnecessary treatment can seriously harm or even kill you.

Diagnostic error exists at alarming rates in the United States. A 2015 report from the Institute of Medicine found that diagnostic mistakes contributed to 10 percent of all American deaths. It is also well established in current medical literature that missed diagnoses alone (i.e., undiagnosed illnesses) may lead to 40,000 to 80,000 preventable deaths per year. When you broaden the scope of error and include patients who survive diagnostic missteps but suffer significant permanent injuries, the figure doubles to 80,000 to 160,000 patients annually, according to a 2013 Johns Hopkins investigation. To come to this number, researchers analyzed paid malpractice claims over a twenty-five-year period to discover that diagnostic error was the most common, costly, and dangerous of all medical mistakes, amounting to an inflation-adjusted $39 billion in malpractice payments. The three most common types of blunders were a failure to diagnose (54 percent); a delay in diagnosis (20 percent); and a wrong diagnosis (10 percent). In my line of work, I see these sorts of slipups—and their often-fatal consequences—all the time.

Claire, a vibrant wife and dedicated mother to three children, was facing an uncertain future in which others would have to care for her. She had been diagnosed, at one of the world's most esteemed hospitals, with a type of sinus cancer. She received chemotherapy treatment and radiation, but the cancer kept recurring—and quickly. What was going on? Her family came to me for help. After collecting her tissues and having them reviewed by independent experts, the problem became fairly easy to see. Claire had been misdiagnosed. She actually had another type of very rare cancer, for which the chemo she got was simply wrong. We were able to get her on the right treatment path for her disease, but we couldn't make up for the six months that had been lost while she was on the wrong therapy. Claire died a couple years later, at the age of fifty-two.

Tommy was the robust patriarch of his family. In his late fifties, he developed anemia, and his primary care physician put him on iron supplements. Over a period of eight months, he was also plagued by a runny nose and nasal irritation. Tommy's PCP referred him to an ENT, who scheduled exploratory sinus surgery to get a better look. That's when Tommy's family got in touch with me. When we stepped back to look at Tommy's medical records and his collection of symptoms (something his PCP had failed to do), the big picture we saw was pretty grim. No one had noticed that Tommy had slowly lost about twenty-five pounds in the last year—and he wasn't dieting. We sent him to a top oncologist in a major teaching hospital near his home. Cancel the surgery, the doctor told him. Your problem isn't in your sinuses; you have renal cell carcinoma (kidney cancer). It was a devastating outcome. Tommy had a partial kidney resection. He was well for about six months before the disease returned. He had the best care one can get and lived about another eighteen months. But I often wonder what would have happened if we had seen him earlier.

Dana was also diagnosed with kidney cancer and had part of her kidney removed. I got involved in her case afterward, to help manage her care when she seemed to be at death's door. Unfortunately, she was overwhelmed and not very assertive when it came to her health. One day an associate of mine got a phone message from her, in which she apologized for not returning our calls. She had been so busy, she said, because she was dealing with a recurrence of her disease—the very thing we were there to help her with. *By the way*, she said in her message, *I'm having the entire kidney removed tomorrow*. Since we hadn't been given the opportunity to secure another opinion for her, all we could do was gather her pre- and postsurgical tissue pathology to have it reread by an expert on renal cell carcinoma. Bad news: It wasn't a relapse; it was something new. Dana had cancer of the renal pelvis, the funnel-shaped upper end of the ureter, which carries urine from the kidney to the bladder. She hadn't needed her kidney to be taken out, and she certainly didn't need the type of chemo she was on. We were able to get her doctors to switch her to an appropriate treatment after showing them evidence of their diagnostic error. But Dana never fully recovered from that second surgery. She died six months later.

The other day I was on the phone with internist Dr. Neda Pakdaman, a clinical assistant professor in the department of medicine at Stanford and the medical director of Stanford's Concierge and Executive Medicine programs. I asked Dr. Pakdaman a hypothetical question: If *you* were facing a serious diagnosis, would you get another opinion?

"The funny thing is, I had a situation where I had to have surgery, but I had so many other things going on in my life that I just asked a colleague to recommend a surgeon and had it done. That was probably *not* the best way to do it," she admitted with a laugh. "Because now whenever that part of my body acts up, I'm like, 'Maybe I should've seen a couple of more people just to make sure.'"

I appreciate her candor! Doctors are busy and only human, like us. But the truth is, Dr. Pakdaman knew to get down to business when the diagnosis was serious: "I did end up having another procedure that was a bigger deal," she continued. "There was a physician I thought very highly of, whom I've seen do procedures, and whom I trust implicitly. But even with all that, I did get a second opinion just to make sure that I was doing the right thing. I ended up going with the first doctor, but it was just one of those things where it was a big enough decision, and a big enough intervention, where . . . You know, I'm a mom; I have a husband. You don't want to go under the knife or go in for a procedure that maybe you didn't need, because what happens if something goes wrong, and now you're not there for your family?"

And yet that's what most people do. Why is it that so many of us, when in the presence of doctors, shirk our responsibility to seek out additional information?

An intriguing study out of Emory University may shed some light. In the experiment, participants were asked to make a risky financial decision. Subjects in one group had to make the choice on their own, while those in the other group were counseled by a financial expert. Researchers studied the participants' brain activity, using functional MRI machines. Can you guess what they discovered? While in the presence of an expert, many subjects essentially shut down parts of their brain that weighed and calculated their options, thereby offloading the decision-making process to the professional. In essence, having an expert in the room makes many of us go a little unconscious.

"If there's any doubt in a patient's mind, or if I have a doubt, I will often suggest a second opinion," says Dr. Elman, the Montreal internist. "Because, hey, we're all human. Getting a concurrence from another brain or set of eyes is not a bad thing. Invariably, you get the question, 'Am I going to anger my treating physician?' to which I say, 'If he or she is upset about you getting another opinion, then you have the wrong doctor taking care of you.'"

When a doctor tells you that he or she wants to cut into your body, pump you full of chemotherapy, or zap you with radiation, that is the time to snap to and summon your decision-making capabilities. I'm saying this not to make doctors sound like mad scientists but to remind you of the gravity of what you are signing up for. Be sure you are being treated for the right problem before you say yes. Just as Jim learned when he wrongly self-diagnosed a heart problem and was given unnecessary stents, it's a terrible mistake to rush into powerful therapies.

This is especially true when it comes to cancer. "Cancer is a life-threatening illness," says the Harvard radiation oncologist Dr. D'Amico, "and it's important that the patient is completely satisfied that what they are about to embark upon is the best course—and also that they trust the doctor and the team they're working with. Even if the first doctor is who they end up with, a second opinion provides peace of mind that they've done their homework, and sometimes it provides important information that they didn't get at the first encounter."

Researchers interested in learning more about the rate of cancer-related diagnostic error performed an exhaustive review of the existing medical literature on the topic, going all the way back to 1967. Data from autopsy studies pointed to an overall error rate of 4 to 44 percent, meaning that up to 44 percent of the time, people died from a cancer that was missed or misinterpreted. When they reviewed the literature on oncology malpractice claims, missed breast cancer was one of the most frequent allegations; malignant melanoma was second. That seems to square with an alarming 2006 white paper from Susan G. Komen for the Cure, in which experts estimated that every year as many as 5,000 to 10,000 patients who were diagnosed with invasive or in situ breast cancer may have been misdiagnosed and inappropriately treated. And in a 2012 *Wall Street Journal* investigation of the medical value of second opinions, the vice president of medical operations at MD Anderson, a prominent cancer center at the University of Texas, noted that as many as 25 percent of patients who arrived at his institution with diagnoses for certain cancers such as lymphoma ultimately received a different finding.

How do diagnostic flubs happen? There are many instigating factors, but the most common ones will sound familiar to you by now: doctors getting only fragments of a patient's medical record history, causing them to miss important pieces of the disease puzzle; patients failing to disclose all their symptoms, thereby delaying a correct diagnosis; radiology images and pathology slides being misinterpreted, mishandled, or never reported to the patient; physicians latching onto an incorrect diagnosis without having the time to investigate or consider other possible causes.

The good news is that these are all problems you can anticipate and work to avoid, using the steps of Intensive Case Management. As we've seen, Step 1, Immersion, in which you collect all your medical records, will provide your physicians with the full picture. Step 2, Diagnosis, will help you avoid pathology misreads, confirmation bias, and other diagnostic errors.

What I'm asking you to do here is get independent expert opinions and have your results reread, just as we did with Dana and Claire's tissues, just as Eric did when he sent out the slides of his prostate cancer, and just as Chandler did when he consulted with experts before letting a neurosurgeon operate on his daughter.

Although it's common to use the phrase *second opinion* when we talk about putting additional brains on a problem, what this step really requires is getting an *expert opinion*. You don't necessarily need a *second* opinion—you need the *right* opinion. Your local specialists may be very good, and they may have the right opinions. But if you're facing a potentially show-stopping issue, and your community-based physician is a general ob-gyn (as opposed to a specialist in high-risk pregnancies) or a general neurologist (instead of a multiple sclerosis expert), you don't really need a second opinion from another general practitioner at a larger institution. What you want is an expert opinion from someone who can provide the best perspective, based on his or her in-depth experience with and study of your specific condition.

If your diagnosis was arrived at from a reading of pathology reports and/or imaging, it's a good idea to have those reread too. Most people are under the impression that diagnostic tools have evolved to the point where we can just run a blood test, examine cells on a slide, or look at images and have 99.9 percent accuracy, like the smoking gun of DNA evidence in a courtroom. But the reality is that much of diagnostic medicine relies on human judgment, which can vary based on a practitioner's training and experience—and even workload. Imagine you're a staff radiologist who's expected to review twenty sets of images an hour. You have *three minutes* per case. How easy it would be to make a mistake! You know three minutes is not enough time for some of the conditions you're reviewing, but you do the best you can. This is the reality for much of the imaging readings and pathology that gets done today. We falsely assume that test results are always accurate, and that the process that provided those results is a solid science. But that science is being practiced by *people* operating *machines*—two proven sources of error.

In a 2009 *Cancer Cytopathology* study of 742 patients who got a second opinion of their pathology reports and slides, there was "major diagnostic disagreement" in 69 cases (9 percent)—in other words, a different diagnosis. In a larger study the following year, researchers discovered that a lab technician's ability to accurately interpret a pap test culture for cell abnormalities (which could point to cervical cancer) often ebbed and flowed depending on the time and day the reading was done. The authors examined the work of four cytotechnologists, with varying years of experience and speed, who read nearly 25,000 slides over an eight-month period. They found two fascinating patterns that presumably pointed to a technologist's deteriorating performance. Three of the four workers detected significantly more abnormal results on Fridays than on Mondays; and two reported far fewer abnormal results in the late afternoon than they had in the morning. What does this mean to you, the patient? Imagine that it's three p.m. on a Friday, and across town a technician is about to pull up your slides. You have a greater chance of getting an incorrect diagnosis because the technician's rate of accuracy is falling.

As the patient, you can't control human error that you are unaware of. But you can follow a simple formula: Measure twice, cut once. That's a basic rule of carpentry—and the only thing at stake is a piece of wood. Shouldn't it be a basic precept of medicine as well?

If you've been diagnosed with cancer, my best estimate of the minimum it will cost for treatment (i.e., the amount your insurance provider will be charged) is $50,000. Why not spend another $150 to $300 to have the pathology reread in order to make sure you're treating the right cancer? Why not meet with an expert on your specific type of cancer, at least to hear if he or she has a different take on your disease progression and treatment options? Health insurers regularly cover second opinions. In fact, some even require them before a major surgery. In most cases, if you are seeing a specialist at a teaching hospital or major medical institution, your extra costs will simply be copayments. But even if your insurer won't cover another opinion or reread—or the expert you want doesn't take your insurance— how much would you be willing to spend to ensure you're getting the correct diagnosis? It's important to think about these issues *before* we get sick. A phone consultation could cost as much as $500 if you find your insurance won't cover it. That's a lot of money for most people, but it's far cheaper than the cost of surgery, drugs, and unnecessary treatments, not to mention the pain and suffering involved, if your initial diagnosis is wrong.

The process of finding a good radiologist or pathologist to review your imaging and/or lab results is similar to the process of finding an expert. Start by looking at the websites of the centers of excellence in your specific diagnosis. So let's say you need your lung cancer pathology reread. Look up the pathology departments of the top teaching hospitals and institutions near you, and see who is focused on your disease by reading up on those pathologists' research areas. Or call the department, explain your condition, and ask for a referral. Remember, if you're only getting a reread of your results, then this isn't necessarily a search for a doctor you will meet with regularly, so you needn't find someone in your town or city. You can have your slides, images, and tissues sent express delivery to some of the better-known hospitals across the nation, many of which have second-opinion forms online.

Another way to protect yourself from diagnostic error is to be on your guard against confirmation bias—that's the tendency, when you already think something is true, to pay more attention to evidence that confirms your belief. We've all fallen prey to this kind of thinking at one time or another, in innocent ways: Your foodie friend raved about a restaurant, so it barely registers with you that the chicken is served cold and the chardonnay warm; a favorite mentor lends you one of his beloved books and you dutifully study it for meaning, even though you'd probably never finish it had you simply found it on your own. Confirmation bias also happens when a really smart, interesting friend tells you how amazing her cardiologist is, so you chalk up the doctor's curt bedside manner to quirky genius. Likewise, if you already think you have compromised heart function, and your doctor sees a small amount of blockage—that may confirm your false belief that you have a cardiac problem.

Physicians sometimes struggle with confirmation bias because they don't have time to sort through complicated cases. So once you are diagnosed as having ovarian cancer, and get sent down the line to a specialist, a surgeon, and more experts, everyone accepts the finding because they aren't given the time or incentive to rethink it. *Two doctors have already labeled this as ovarian cancer, and I'm treating it as ovarian cancer, because they're my colleagues, and they are capable clinicians who probably don't make mistakes.* (Seeking expert opinions from practitioners who operate outside the first doctor's orbit may help you avoid this.) All too often patients compound the problem by failing to ask assertive questions. Tommy, for instance, had a history of low red blood cell counts. When his doctor gave him iron supplements, he accepted that as an adequate response, never exploring the possibility that anemia wasn't his ultimate, underlying problem.

But Tommy's internist also didn't ask the questions *Why is my patient anemic? Couple that anemia with his weight loss and other symptoms, and is there a diagnosis I'm missing here?* This is the state of medicine today. That's why, when a diagnosis is unclear or uncertain, you need to keep searching and seeking expert opinions, until you are satisfied that you have the best answer. Consult your trusted support team, explain your predicament, and ask them if they can assist you in your research. You need to know: Who are the top experts on this condition? Let your team help you get this step right.

HOW TO QUESTION YOUR DIAGNOSIS

Diagnostic error is common, costly, and dangerous. Here are the questions to ask your doctor to be sure yours is accurate.

I understand that you believe I have this disease, but how confident are you in the diagnosis?

Is there anything else this could be?

Are there more tests that can be done to confirm this diagnosis?

Was the lab test sample good/the imaging clear? Would it make sense to get a second read?

Have you read all my medical records to get the full picture of my symptoms? Would it help if I went over them with you?

You say I have an abnormal blood test/a lab abnormality and that we can treat it with medication. But is it possible that this is indicative of a bigger problem? Are there other tests we should be doing to rule out serious diseases?

Before we move forward with treatment, are you confident we've explored all my options?

I appreciate what you're saying, and it sounds very serious. I'd like to get my lab reports/imaging/medical records in order to get a second opinion.

A WORD FROM THE DOCTORS: SHOULD YOU GET A SECOND OPINION?

Be very cautious about a doctor who is inexplicably dismissive about a second opinion. Good physicians will not only respect your request, they may even help you find someone with more experience in the realm of your disease than they possess.

> "I encourage patients to seek out second opinions. Medicine is very dynamic, and things change all the time. I frequently send patients to the Mayo Clinic, or Cleveland Clinic, or other world-renowned hospitals to get other opinions or to see what might be a different approach than what I'm recommending—or to agree with it. I'll also refer patients to specialists within my cardiology group because they are the real experts and I trust them. But if something is over-the-top complicated and there's no clear answer—no clear right-or-wrong decision—then it can be good to get an outside opinion. Any time you have a potentially life-threatening issue, getting another opinion is really important. I've had patients tell me they came to see me because their first doctor told them they shouldn't get a second opinion—and they didn't like hearing that. Some doctors maybe haven't gotten the message, but that type of answer never really works, in my opinion."
> —Michael H. Davidson, M.D., F.A.C.C. (Chicago)

> "A doctor that doesn't like second opinions? That patient should go find another doctor right away. I know it exists, but it still just amazes me when someone says, 'You don't need a second opinion. This is a straightforward situation.' Now, someone might ask me, 'Do you think I need a second opinion?' That's a complex question. I always encourage any patient who raises the question to avail themselves of that option. And more often than not, I will help facilitate it. I'll

give you an example. We just had a situation . . . there's a certain kind of cardiovascular intervention we do, and it's not simple stuff; it's complicated. I asked [my colleagues], 'Who do you think has the largest volume in the United States?' Then I called the patient and said, 'We're very, very good, but we're second highest in volume on this procedure. Cedars-Sinai in L.A. has the highest volume.' Lots of people focus on volume alone, which is not always correct, but it's one of the things that guides you toward picking a specialist. That's how we dealt with that situation. . . . If I don't know the answers, I ask questions. You talk to people. You search the literature. I don't know any other way to do it but to be persistent."

—Eugene J. Sayfie, M.D.,
F.A.C.C., F.A.C.P. (Miami)

"There are really good reasons for getting second opinions, and one that's obvious is if both you and your physician know that there is an aspect of your disease that another physician is going to be more expert in or has more experience with. It would be great if physicians' egos weren't threatened by that sort of thing and would be open to it. I think everyone would be better off if there could be acknowledgment that some physicians just know more about a certain area and that it's going to be valuable to get an opinion about that. . . . Even if the second opinion yields exactly the same input and advice and assesses the person the same way, it's valuable to get that confirmation. It gives the patient confidence that they are moving in a proper direction."

—Philip Mease, M.D., F.A.C.R., F.A.C.P. (Seattle)

"Sometimes having a fresh pair of eyes on your case can make a huge difference. You can always go back to the same person, feeling more informed, like, 'Okay, I really trust my first doctor and I want to go with what they're saying.' Or your eyes might open to alternatives. Even supersmart doctors do things different ways. It needs to be right for the patient too. Getting another opinion gives you more information, so you can make an educated decision."

—Katy M. Setoodeh, M.D.,
F.A.C.R. (Santa Monica, CA)

"As an internist, if a patient has an issue that I feel pretty comfortable dealing with, but they still want to see someone who's in an academic center, I welcome that. Their health is my greatest concern, and their peace of mind is really important. If the consultant agrees with what I have been doing, then I've won. If the consultant disagrees, and has a good reason, then I've learned something new, and I've won. It's a no-lose situation for me. . . . Other times, when a patient feels that their specialist might be offended that they want a second opinion, I'll say to them, 'Have the [expert] call us, and we'll send over your records, slides, or whatever they need.' Or I'll just say, 'Tell your doctor that I was the one who felt it was important for you to get this second opinion,' so that it's all on me, so I'm the bad guy."

—Bryan J. Arling, M.D. (Washington, D.C.)

"Facing a really big decision—be it surgery, chemotherapy, or any significant treatment course—there is great value in getting a second opinion. If anything, it brings peace of mind to know that you did your due diligence. I'm always open to that. There are times when patients have come to me [as an internist] and said, 'This is what I've been told.' Maybe it's something very clear cut, like a completely occluded coronary artery. They need a bypass. I don't think there are many people out there who are going to tell them they don't need bypass surgery. I can give them that perspective, and then I can also tell them, 'You're in the hands of one of the best cardiac surgeons there is. It's up to you if you want to get a second opinion, but this person is amazing.' Or I can give them the opportunity to go to a larger medical center and see someone who's done a higher volume of cases. At the end of the day, it's about this patient's life. We want to make sure that when they look back on it, they feel 100 percent comfortable about the decision that they made."

—Neda Pakdaman, M.D. (Palo Alto, CA)

QUICK GUIDE

CHAPTER 10. Step 2—Diagnosis

- Get to the right diagnosis *before* you agree to surgery or other invasive treatments.

- Be mindful of the three most common types of diagnostic blunders, which are: a failure to diagnose, a delay in diagnosis, and a wrong diagnosis.

- Try not to rush into powerful therapies, especially when it comes to cancer, which is often misinterpreted.

- Remember that diagnostic errors may be caused by: doctors getting fragments of a patient's medical history; patients failing to disclose symptoms; radiology images and pathology slides being misinterpreted, mishandled, or never reported to the patient or the physicians; physicians latching onto an incorrect diagnosis.

- You don't necessarily need a *second* opinion—you need the *right* opinion. Seek out an expert (as opposed to a general practitioner) with in-depth experience in your specific condition.

- If your diagnosis was arrived at from a reading of pathology reports and/or a study of imaging, it's a good idea to have those reviewed too. Check the websites of the better-known hospitals across the nation, many of which have second-opinion forms online.

➤

- Physicians can be subject to confirmation bias when they don't have time to sort through complicated cases. Seeking expert opinions from practitioners who operate outside your first doctor's orbit may help avoid this.

- When a diagnosis remains uncertain, continue to seek expert opinions until you are satisfied that you have the best answer. Consult your trusted support team for help in finding the right experts.

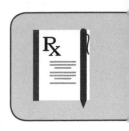

CHAPTER ELEVEN

STEP 3—TREATMENT

How to identify the right treatment plan—and the best doctor for you

Y ou've immersed yourself in the language of your condition. You've consulted several experts. You have confidence in your diagnosis. Now it's time to focus on which doctor and treatment plan is right for you. Although you probably want to put this problem behind you as quickly as possible, try to refrain from rushing toward the very first proposal you hear.

I think most people intuitively know to avoid that rush, but sometimes it's hard to see what your alternatives might be. That was how Marissa, fifty-four, felt when her doctor called to give her some bad news about a sunspot on her face.

Since her early forties, Marissa had had an unremarkable freckle, no larger in diameter than a pencil eraser, in the center of her left cheek. It was symmetrical and tan, with normal borders that never really changed. In other words, nothing suspicious.

An attractive New Yorker who made a living as a sales rep, Marissa was sensitive to the industry perception that her looks affected her bottom line. So she had a dermatologist laser off the blemish. It returned a year later. A second try faded the mark but only a little. Undaunted, her dermatologist said, "I've got all kinds of tricks up my sleeve. Let's get this." He tried a chemical peel. Two months later her freckle was bigger and darker. *This may be a sunspot I'm going to have to live with for the rest of my life*, Marissa decided.

When she turned fifty, Marissa found a different dermatologist and treated herself to another round of expensive cosmetic procedures to *get that spot*. But after thousands of dollars' worth of lasers and acid treatments, the blemish still didn't budge, so her doctor suggested trying a procedure that he normally used to remove tattoos. *If this doesn't work, nothing will*, he said. *But let's do a biopsy first, just to be safe.* Marissa wondered if that was even necessary. After all, several dermatologists had seen her sunspot, and none of them had ever worried about it. But she agreed to do it.

A week later the doctor rang with her results. It wasn't just a sunspot, he said. It might be cancerous. They'd know more after it was removed, and he wanted that done *immediately*.

"What's immediately?" Marissa asked.

Three weeks.

Marissa's doctor specialized in Botox, hair removal, collagen—all the latest and greatest cosmetic fixes. So he referred her to a doctor in his office who was trained in something called Mohs surgery, in which the skin lesion is sliced away in stages and studied under a microscope between each stage, with more layers being removed until the entire cancerous area is gone. The doctor told Marissa she'd need to find a plastic surgeon—or they could recommend one—who would close up the hole that surgery would make in her face.

This woman must be out of her mind, Marissa thought to herself as she sat listening to the doctor talk. *They're going to make a hole in my face? And it's going to stay open until I see a plastic surgeon?* Now she was spooked. And determined to get another opinion.

It was a smart move on Marissa's part, because at that moment she was at the very beginning of her Intensive Case Management journey and many miles from the No-Mistake Zone. How do we know this? Her diagnosis was vague (or at least, she wasn't clear on the specifics of her condition); she was having a gut-level rejection of the surgeon; and she wasn't convinced that Mohs was the correct treatment.

In Step 3, Treatment, you should focus on two key questions:

> *What is the best course of treatment for my specific disease?*
> *Who is/are the best doctor(s) to administer that treatment/*
> *perform my surgery/oversee my therapy?*

You may find the answers simultaneously, as very often the physician who presents the most thoughtful, evidence-based plan of therapy is also the practitioner you want carrying out that plan.

But if your instinct is telling you something's not right, or if you're feeling unnecessarily rushed, you might want to pause, seek out more information, and consult with an expert.

Marissa rightfully believed her condition was serious, and she wanted to consult with a skin cancer expert. She started her search online, but that led nowhere. She next asked friends for referrals and eventually was connected to a nurse practitioner who was able to recommend a few excellent doctors to her. They were all dermatologists, trained in surgery, and on staff at major New York hospitals. Truthfully, Marissa was already a savvy enough consumer that she could have found a doctor on her own with just a bit of guidance. To recap, here's what she could have done, and what you can do too:

1. Go to the websites of the best major hospitals in the largest cities near you, click through to the department that fits the realm of your condition, and read the bios of the dozen or so specialists and surgeons who focus on your disease (for example, the skin cancer experts within the cancer program).

2. Call the doctors whose expertise most clearly fits your needs.

3. If you're unsure which doctor to consult, or if you're unable to secure a timely appointment with the one you want, there is almost always a phone number, e-mail contact, or online physician referral feature to get help from a hospital staff member.

"It just didn't occur to me to look to these places," Marissa said later. "I never thought of it. I should have, but it didn't come to me."

Marissa ultimately chose Dr. Erica H. Lee, a board-certified dermatologist at Memorial Sloan Kettering. Why? Because Dr. Lee works at a high-volume hospital for melanoma, and her background exactly fit Marissa's needs: she specializes in Mohs, dermatologic, and laser surgery, with an expertise in the management of basal cell and squamous cell carcinomas, early-stage melanoma, and rare skin tumors.

When Marissa called for an appointment, she was given one for later the same week. The scheduling assistant told her they needed to reread Marissa's biopsy slides, as they would not accept the pathology interpretation of another doctor.

"But why?" Marissa asked.

The reply: *Because we're Memorial Sloan Kettering. That's what we do.*

Pathology is an art. Rather than rely on an outside doctor's take, Marissa's new dermatologist wanted to see the slides for herself.

When Marissa showed up for her appointment on a Friday, Dr. Lee explained that they had studied the slides many times over. She believed Marissa's correct diagnosis was in fact a slow-growing melanoma that looked to be between Stage I and Stage II. Dr. Lee did not believe that Mohs surgery was the right procedure for Marissa's cancer. Instead, she recommended a full surgical excision, removing sections of the skin and tissue in Marissa's left cheek, examining them overnight, and then going back in to get more if the margins weren't clear. Marissa would still need a plastic surgeon to repair the hole, using skin grafts.

Her new diagnosis and treatment plan was even scarier than the first. But now she knew exactly what she had, and she was relieved to be in the care of a high-volume cancer center. She scheduled a surgery date and secured a plastic surgeon.

Because Marissa had a slow-growing melanoma (her first dermatologist's urgency was based more on caution than on evidence), she could have taken the time to consult with a third doctor. Maybe she'd have gotten a different perspective on her diagnosis and treatment. But in her case, I think Marissa was already in the No-Mistake Zone: she felt confident about the diagnosis, she had found a skilled specialist, and they'd come up with a treatment plan she believed in. When Marissa asked herself, *Is this the best treatment for my disease, and is this the doctor I want doing my surgery?* she could answer yes to both.

For that, she is now cancer-free. She got *much better* health care because she did additional legwork and didn't rush toward the very first treatment plan proposed.

GETTING TO THE NO-MISTAKE ZONE

Think about the times when you had to make life-changing decisions—like accepting or turning down a job, moving across the country or staying put, asking someone to marry you or breaking up with that person. I suspect you've made some decisions very well and others not so carefully. Try to remember how you conducted yourself in the situations that worked out the best, and bring the same process and skills to this undertaking. Here's how you will know when you are in the No-Mistake Zone:

1. **Your diagnosis is specific and confirmed.** By specific, I mean it's not that you simply have "shoulder pain"—you know that you have a torn rotator cuff. Or it's not just "breast cancer," it's HER2-positive breast cancer. Know precisely what you are dealing with.

2. **You're convinced about when and why you need to be treated.** For the majority of conditions, you need to factor in the correct intensity and timing of treatment. With back pain, for example, you typically move slowly through various approaches to alleviate distress, first trying rest, then physical therapy, and then maybe steroidal injections to see if the pain subsides. You'd resort to surgery last, and only when absolutely necessary. Pancreatic cancer that's surgically removable would be at the opposite end of the spectrum: you want that done *now*. To be in the No-Mistake Zone, you should have a clear understanding of the importance of waiting or acting in your specific circumstances. Ask your doctor: *When does treatment need to begin? What happens if we don't start at that time?* Unless you need to act *now*, take the time to get a second opinion. Even in emergency situations, you still may have time to pause and ask if this is the right procedure and specialist for you, just as Tracey's family asked after she fainted in the shower and injured her spine.

➤

3. **You've explored the most promising treatment options and understand their benefits and risks.** For virtually every disease, the number of possible treatments is limited. You have spoken to several physicians who specialize in the different options, and you've immersed yourself in the research. You can say with authority: *Here are my choices, and here are the benefits and risks of each.* If you've been thorough, you'll hit a point where additional research and discussion doesn't add much to what you already know.

4. **You've met with experienced physicians who can carry out the treatment plan at an institution that's appropriate for the care you need.** If you have appendicitis, your small community hospital is just great. If you need abdominal aortic repair, it's not. You can't be in the No-Mistake Zone unless you've aligned the caliber of the institution with the magnitude of your problem.

5. **You can visualize your treatment plan and how the various steps will be coordinated.** This is when your proposed course of therapy evolves from a foggy vortex of confusing information that's barreling toward you . . . into a *clear,* executable framework in which things line up and make sense to you.

6. **Your gut is telling you:** *This is the treatment for me, and this is the physician I want to carry it out.* Congratulations. You are now in the No-Mistake Zone. Act with confidence.

Sometimes I see people do a really nice job managing their own case: they read up, meet with experts, explore treatments. But then when it's decision time, and two or three excellent opportunities are laid out before them, they freeze up, unable to choose. One consequence of doing your homework is that you may discover several wonderful doctors who can carry out your therapy! It's okay to be nervous about your decision, but if you feel confident about numbers 1 through 5, you are already in the No-Mistake Zone. You have a bounty of good options, so move forward knowing that whichever one you choose will be right.

M arissa's melanoma had a pretty clear road to a cure, but when
you're dealing with conditions for which there are an array of
treatments, the information-gathering process takes longer. It may sometimes feel dizzying, but you will come through it so much better if you follow the steps of ICM. And as Eric says, let a friend be a friend during this
time. Because even the most driven, checklist-making person doesn't know
how he or she will react to an earthshaking diagnosis.

Samantha, a thirty-nine-year-old health technology executive from the
New England area, comes to mind when I think of people who can accomplish just about anything yet couldn't manage their own illness, let alone
collect information that would help them make a proper treatment decision.
In Samantha's case, she had a very interesting backstory that was having a
subtle but significant effect on her actions.

Her ordeal began in April 2011, when she was having a CT scan of her
neck for a problem sore throat. Her doctor saw something troubling on the
film: a shadow, possibly a cancerous growth, in her brain. They would need
to do an MRI to get a clearer picture.

Samantha lay incredibly still inside the claustrophobic machine as technicians covered her with blankets and played soft music in the headphones
around her ears. As the apparatus fired up, whirring, humming, and knock-
ing like a mega-size washing machine on the fritz, Samantha lost herself in
morbid thoughts. Her sister-in-law had died, at thirty-two, from a glioblastoma, a very aggressive brain tumor. It too had been discovered after an MRI,
and she was immediately wheeled into surgery. She died five months after
her diagnosis.

As the machine droned on, taking detailed images of her brain, Samantha went down a checklist: *Have I been a good mother? A good wife? Do I
believe in my work? Am I living an intentional life?* A resounding *yes* came
back to her, bouncing off the walls of the machine and flooding her body
with a feeling of peace. *If this is the end,* she thought, *I have no regrets.*

Thankfully, it was not. A top neurologist at the hospital—the same physician who had treated her late sister-in-law—looked at her imaging and told
her she could go home. *We think this is a meningioma,* he said, *a very slow-
growing tumor on the outer membrane of the brain. They are almost always
benign and rarely metastatic.*

Watchful waiting was the best course for Samantha. She would have a scan every three months, and if it looked like the tumor was growing, then they would consider surgery. Her doctor said that some people undergo radiation therapy instead, to shrink and kill the tumor, but she wasn't really a candidate for that.

Samantha nodded dutifully and made an appointment for the next scan. Three months later: no change.

A friend of Samantha's had a connection at Johns Hopkins and begged her to use it: "Just call this person, tell them you'd like to get a second opinion." "No, no," Samantha said. "I'm fine. Really." But her friend wouldn't relent.

Embarrassed, and not wanting anyone to worry about her, Samantha made the call. A Johns Hopkins neurosurgeon reviewed her scans and agreed that it was a benign meningioma. Samantha didn't ask him any questions about treatment options. Nor did she do any research on her problem. She decided not to discuss her condition with anyone else.

At her six-month appointment, her tumor looked different—it had grown slightly. Her neurologist recommended surgical removal. She thanked him, set a surgery date for the first week of January, went back to work, and forgot about the whole thing.

"I just didn't want to spend any energy on it, because it's terrifying," she recalled later. "I didn't ask for any help because I didn't want to be a burden. I didn't want anyone to ever think about me as someone they should pity."

At her husband's urging, Samantha promised she would do some research. Two months before her surgery, the couple took a romantic trip together. "How is your research going?" he asked.

Samantha was caught off guard. She turned away sheepishly, as if she'd just been exposed as a cheat. "Let's talk about that later," she said. "We're on vacation!"

"No," he said. "Let's talk about it *now*."

Samantha froze. She couldn't admit that she was failing herself—which meant failing him, failing their children. Instead, she fell apart, in a sobbing, can't-catch-your-breath meltdown.

"I haven't done *any* research," she finally said through tears. "I can't do it. I feel so lonely. I don't know who to talk to, I don't know what to say, and I don't know what to do."

It's hard to admit to your partner that you feel lonely and isolated, because you know that it's not his or her fault. Samantha, like so many patients at this juncture, had been locked inside herself. And what she said next surprised them both: "I don't want the same doctor doing my surgery."

Samantha admitted that she had been having flashbacks to the day she and her husband sat in the waiting room, waiting for his sister's operation to be over, only to have the neurologist—now Samantha's doctor—deliver the terrible news: "I'm sorry. It didn't work." She needed to start over and find a new surgeon, but that felt like an insurmountable task.

If it had been her husband or one of her children in the same predicament, Samantha would have dropped everything, dived into the literature, gotten third and fourth opinions on treatments and doctors, and tracked down the authors of the latest studies to pick their brains about treatment outcomes.

"But because it was my diagnosis, I was absolutely paralyzed," she admitted. "I work in the health care space and am better equipped than anybody to manage my own care. But I was the biggest idiot you can imagine in terms of how I was dealing with this."

Her husband, who knew when to let her be in charge and when to push, was warm and caring as she talked out her fears. He could tell she desperately needed help. He had the courage but not the competence in this realm, so he reached out to my team. I would be her quarterback. From that point forward, Samantha would follow the four steps of ICM—the same steps that you will follow, with a little help from your support team, if you find yourself in a medical crisis. For Samantha, ICM looked like this:

Step 1. **Immersion** in her case, which involved (a) researching the literature on meningiomas and taking note of the names of the most passionate experts on this condition, and (b) collecting and distributing her medical records (with a Medical Summary) to each new specialist she met;

Step 2. Independent confirmation of her **Diagnosis**, which meant sending her MRIs to three additional radiologists for rereads (one of whom, incidentally, found an additional, smaller, meningioma, which turned out to be inconsequential, but it gave Samantha more information);

Step 3. Consultations on the best course of **Treatment** for her specific illness with physicians who had a high level of volume and skill in treating meningiomas; and

Step 4. **Coordination** of her records, appointments, and care (more on coordination in the next chapter).

BETTER ONLINE RESEARCH: TREATMENT GUIDELINES

Your treatment decisions will be guided by the advice of your doctors, but it's up to you to do homework. That means searching the medical literature on the course of action being proposed, and seeking out the treatment guidelines for your disease. Treatment guidelines represent the agreed-upon thinking among disease-specialty organizations of the best, evidence-based therapies for your specific condition. You can usually find them by searching, say, "treatment guidelines diabetes" or "treatment guidelines atrial fibrillation."

Check the About Us page of the organization that wrote the guidelines: Is it a reputable institution (i.e., affiliated with the professional organizations and disease associations)? Are the authors based at established academic medical centers and institutions? Are the guidelines described as being federally approved, and therefore vetted by the U.S. Department of Health and Human Services (HHS)?

You can also start at HHS's National Guideline Clearinghouse (**www.guideline.gov**), where you can search by disease or medical topic to find the most recent recommendations on a variety of conditions and protocols. These guidelines are written by and for specialists, so the material may be trying at first. But as you immerse yourself, you will become more comfortable with the language, and you will encounter the same concepts and recommendations again and again.

If you have cancer, the National Comprehensive Cancer Network (**www.nccn.org**), a nonprofit alliance of some of the world's leading cancer centers, has a must-visit website for treatment guidelines, video libraries, patient advocacy resources, and practical information. The site is bifurcated: One branch serves patients and their caregivers (**www.nccn.org/patients**); the other is a physician resource (**www.nccn.org/professionals**); also a fascinating read if you feel up to it. But the aim is the same: the promotion of better cancer care, education, and research. As a patient, you can summon up e-booklets that give intelligent overviews of the tests and treatments related to your disease, pointed questions to ask your doctors, and a step-by-step review of the standard treatment steps for your condition.

If *all* you did was pore through the NCCN guidelines, I am certain you would have a better grasp of the proper course of therapy for your cancer. And at this stage of Intensive Case Management, if your physician is suggesting a course of treatment that veers far from the guidelines, you can ask, *What about this? The NCCN guidelines say* X *is the usual first-line treatment for cancer at my stage and presentation. Can you tell me what you think about* X? *And help me understand better why you are suggesting* Y?

———

Let's skip right to Step 3. After learning more about her condition and its most devoted practitioners, Samantha began to consult with a series of neurologists—specifically, meningioma experts—to discuss her treatment choices. This was her information-gathering process, a listening tour of sorts. Or "data collection," as I like to call it.

"I didn't like it," Samantha recalls now, laughing. "Because every time you meet with a new doctor, they pull up your scans and look at them in front of you, and you're sure they're going to find something else—that it's really a glioblastoma or some other terrible type of brain cancer."

Still, Samantha was stoic throughout this arduous process. We didn't let her take a break—we set up new appointments for her every week. "I felt I couldn't *not* go to these doctor meetings," she recalls. "Even though I just wanted to crawl back under my rock, I was like, 'Okay, what's next?'"

In Samantha's case, we knew she had the energy for it, and we couldn't risk letting her use a busy work calendar as an excuse not to go. But the right frequency and pace of data collection is a judgment call that you and your quarterback will have to determine together. And this is when giving those four points of support—clinical, intellectual, logistical, and emotional—can really help a patient to feel whole and steady.

Here again, because I think they are so important, are the must-ask questions for when you are consulting with experts and gathering information about a treatment plan. You should supplement them with ones that speak to your specific condition and personal concerns.

Tell me more about yourself, doctor:

"What portion of your time as a cardiologist/oncologist/pulmonologist do you spend on this specific type of condition/illness/procedure?"

"How long has this been a specialty for you?"

"You told me you spend about 70 percent of your time on this procedure. I'm sure there's an enormous amount of research and literature on the topic. What do you do to stay on top of the rapidly advancing science?"

"Have you yourself published any research on it?"

I have some questions about this treatment:

"Why is this surgery/drug/test necessary?"

"When does treatment have to begin?"

"What are the risks/side effects? Are they reversible?"

"How long is the recovery period and what will it involve?"

"How many times have you done this surgery/used this protocol, and have you had any complications?"

"What will happen if we don't do it?"

"Are there nonsurgical/less aggressive options we should try first?"

"How do they compare to my surgical/more aggressive options?"

"Patients need both the knowledge and the guts to ask questions," notes Dr. Elman. "Unfortunately, the vast majority will take whatever their physician says—'Now we're going to do this procedure' or 'We're going to give you this treatment'—without asking any questions. If you've done the proper research, it makes me a better physician. Personally, I love the informed health care consumer. It's much better than having a patient who just follows blindly. Is it more work? Yes. More challenging? Yes. But it's often more rewarding."

By consulting with experts and asking informed questions, Samantha learned that despite her first doctor's recommendation of surgery, she really had three approaches to consider. Waiting and watching was still on the table because her tumor was not growing rapidly. (It had grown a tiny bit and then stopped.) Second, she was a candidate for stereotactic radiation therapy—also sometimes referred to as Gamma Knife radiosurgery—a technology that, despite its name, isn't a knife at all but rather a noninvasive technique to treat tumors and other abnormalities of the brain. But she also needed more information about the pros and cons of that treatment versus her third option: surgery.

Samantha became an expert on her condition over the next few weeks. For instance, she learned that Gamma Knife delivers short, powerful, highly targeted bursts of radiation that kill only the tumor. It requires just one session, and patients typically experience a quick recovery. Although it would save her from an operation, there were two drawbacks: First, the dead tumor would remain in her head. Second, if the radiation didn't work, or the tumor came back, they'd have to cut into her brain after all.

She also discovered that if she chose a surgical path, she would need a brain surgeon who was an expert in removing meningiomas from the atrium of the lateral ventricle—where hers was located—which is about as deep and central in the brain as you can get. In fact, the best way to reach her tumor was by cutting through the part of the brain that controls speech and field of vision. Her surgery had to go right.

Over the course of several months, Samantha met with a series of excellent neurosurgeons, some of whom were Gamma Knife experts. As you might expect, the traditional surgeons made the case for surgery, while the Gamma Knife experts advocated radiation.

"Every additional perspective that I got, I felt stronger," she said. "I even got to a place where I *thought* I knew what the answer for me was going to be"—radiation—"but then I talked to one more surgeon who spoke convincingly about its risks"—a very small chance of developing radiation-induced cancer, ten or more years out—"and I felt incredibly confused. I got stuck. I was so frustrated. How is it possible to have such conflicting views?"

At some point, you will probably come to this same place. Feeling confused and uncertain during this process is completely normal. You've got a lot to consider. Here's what you need to do in order to stay sane:

Separate the Data Collection from the Decision Making.

By that, I mean divide the process into two phases. Gather information first, without drawing any final conclusions; then, only after all the facts are in, make an informed decision.

Very often, people want to resolve an issue and put it in the rearview mirror. It's human nature to say, *Okay, here's the thesis as to what I've got and what I should do,* and then look at each new piece of information that comes in as evidence that either *increases* or *decreases* the probability that your original thesis is correct. Instead, I want you to stay neutral while you are collecting the facts. You will learn more about your choices, feel less stress, and make better treatment choices.

When clients are spinning from information overload, desperate to make a decision, I tell them what I told Samantha: *Picture yourself standing firmly, weight distributed equally on both feet. Don't lean forward, and don't lean backward. Your only job right now is to collect data and remain perfectly balanced.*

"Yes, I can do that," Samantha said. She had made an assumption (*brain surgery is bad*) that she was trying to support or refute. I asked her to very intentionally and aggressively stay in the middle—to not have an opinion yet.

Samantha liked hearing that data collection was her only job—that she didn't have to press the decision button yet. She's natively the kind of person who doesn't want to commit to something until she has all the facts. You, like Samantha, have permission to *stay neutral.*

My other recommendation for clients who are in the process of deciding on treatment is this: *Don't go too far into the weeds.* There are matters on which you will be able to render judgment, and some that will crush your spirit if you insist on trying. For instance, you probably won't be able to intelligently engage with an oncologist about the nuances of different chemotherapy regimens or with a brain surgeon about which surgical tools are best. And that's really okay.

"A story comes to mind of a *very* educated patient who needed a bone marrow transplant, and wanted to consult with six of the major transplant centers to hear what everybody had to say. I cautioned her against it," recalls Dr. Roboz. "By the time she got to the third place, she called me in tears: 'I should never have done this.'. . . . Sometimes there are distinctions without a difference, which can be enormously confusing for patients and very disruptive to them getting care, resulting in delays and anxiety."

If a master chef changes the brand of knife he uses in his kitchen, do we start betting against his success? No. We judge him on his skills, talent, and ability to adapt to the environment in front of him. It's the same for a great surgeon. If you sincerely believe in your surgeon's track record—in her skills, talent, and ability to adapt—then let her figure out which tools and methods she is going to use. Don't worry about things you would need a medical degree to understand. What you *can* understand and judge is this:

> *How often does she do my specific surgery?*
> *Is it the primary (or only) thing she does?*
> *Does she have any reported results?*
> *What can she lead me to expect about her results?*

Listen to the answers you receive, then trust your gut. Have you gotten the truth here? Is this somebody you feel comfortable with? Get a sense of the physician, the institution, and the very important measurable factors like volume and complication rates.

For Samantha, the decision of whether to go with radiation or surgery also sparked some soul searching. She discovered that she had unexplored fears about radiation. Before she was born, her mother had taken diethylstilbestrol, or DES, a drug prescribed to prevent miscarriages. It was banned in 1971, when it was found to cause rare vaginal cancers and infertility in the female children of its users—who learned of the risk only when they reached their childbearing years. Until Samantha had children of her own, her mother had been wracked with guilt at the possibility that she had done her daughter irreparable harm. Five to ten million children were exposed to DES in the thirty years it was on the market, so when people talk about novel therapies, Samantha is rightfully wary.

"I know it sometimes takes a really long time to figure out that they don't work," she said. "I don't want to live a life where every day I'm waiting for the study to come out that proves that getting radiation on your brain doubles your chance of developing brain cancer twenty years later. With stereotactic radiation therapy, the numbers show it's a low risk. But there aren't a lot of people who have it done when they're forty, like me. I know it might never happen, but it's an unknown I can't deal with."

Samantha ultimately came to the decision that surgery would be the right choice for her. After having met with six surgeons, she trusted her gut and picked her guy. What tipped the scales in his favor? He was the only one who had suggested she additionally undergo a functional MRI (so her language and vision processes could be better mapped, helping him to pinpoint the best surgical entry route) as well as a CT scan to review her brain's blood flow.

But here's the interesting twist: she also decided to put the brakes on surgery. Her tumor wasn't growing anymore, so there was no real rush to begin treatment. Now that she had the right doctor and plan, she could monitor her condition with the confidence that she would know what to do when the time came to act. It was her decision entirely. She was back in control.

"In the old days, I couldn't talk about my condition without crying. But now I'm so educated about my specific circumstances and all the different ways you can treat it. People look concerned and I say, 'You can't worry about me because *I'm* not worried for me,'" she says. "I can live my life again. I don't feel like I'm at the end of a set of decisions that have been made *about* me *without* me. I'm an incredibly informed, intentional master of my own domain."

Indeed, she is. Still, it bears repeating: Even if you are the most accomplished person in your family, let them help you when the time comes. See if a friend will assist in researching your treatment options; ask your spouse to accompany you on doctor visits to ask the hard questions you may not be thinking of. Do this even if, like Samantha, you are sure you can handle everything yourself.

"I see now that I needed you guys to be on me, checking in every single week until, eventually, I learned the skills for myself," Samantha says. "People really do need to appoint the CEO of their process and give them permission to be the boss. Because if you don't, you'll keep reverting back to your default state, which is to do nothing. And that leaves you a victim."

Navigating the health care system is not easy, and patients often feel that they have to figure everything out on their own. Over the years, my colleagues and I have helped thousands of individuals go through the process of deciding on a course of treatment. And we've found that people from all walks of life often face common issues, even in widely divergent cases. Here are four talking (and thinking) points to consider during this phase of ICM—inside tips from our practice. Discussing these issues with your doctors and support team will be helpful to everyone involved.

1. SOMETIMES THE WAY TO A CURE ISN'T A ROAD, BUT A BRIDGE.

Despite a daily barrage of bad news, the truth is that you will still get the finest possible health care in the United States, where we are living in an extraordinary age of medical accomplishment. For the first time ever, when you are diagnosed with a fatal disease, if you can hang on long enough, you may live to see a cure for your condition, or at least a life-prolonging treatment. In 1964, for instance, the five-year survival rate for the most common childhood leukemia was 3 percent. Today it's about 92 percent. Or think about the basketball great Magic Johnson. When he announced on November 7, 1991, that he was HIV positive, nobody thought he'd be alive in five years. Nearly a quarter-century later, with the help of a daily multidrug cocktail, he can still beat anyone his age one-on-one on a basketball court. Disease affects everyone differently, but for Johnson—as for many with HIV—his "bridges" may keep the disease in check forever.

I often ask clients to embrace the concept that we are building a bridge to a bridge to a bridge. In other words, their treatment won't necessarily cure them, but it can often buy them another six months, three years, five years, whatever the case may be, until new and better drugs for their condition become available. This is especially true for cancer, which can be a relentless enemy, coming back harder than before.

Biomedical research is advancing at an unprecedented rate, helping us to develop a deeper understanding of what causes disease, better and more precise diagnostics, and safer and more effective therapeutics. Immunotherapy, for example, is an exciting new approach to cancer treatment that harnesses the patient's own immune system to identify and destroy cancerous cells. As of this writing, clinical trials in which immunotherapy has been used for patients suffering from previously untreatable cancers—such as advanced melanoma, lymphoma, and leukemia—have shown impressive results, with some patients having their disease held in check for as long as fifteen years. Because of these promising findings, biomedical companies are developing many potentially effective new drugs on an expedited basis. But these sorts of therapies aren't routinely prescribed, and it's important to discuss immunotherapy with your oncologist, as there may be specialized tests they can recommend to help determine whether your cancer will respond to this hopeful new therapy.

Another very promising approach is targeted therapy for cancer. In fact, whenever we take on a cancer client, we ask the physician to send his patient's biopsy tissue for testing to one of the commercial molecular profiling companies. (Foundation Medicine, Caris Life Sciences, OncoPlexDx, NantHealth, and Guardant Health are well-known firms, and their services are typically covered by insurance.) Depending on the test, the profiling company analyzes your cancer tissue for known genetic mutations or abnormal levels of certain proteins. Then it sends a report directly to your doctor, to be shared with you. In some cases, there are already drugs on the market, or in clinical trials, that specifically target the abnormality in your tumor. (In general, only licensed clinicians—your oncologist or PCP, for instance—can order these tests. While the information can be confusing to a layperson and should be interpreted by a doctor, it's important to remember that these reports, like all your medical records, belong to you, and you should ask for a copy.)

For example, we recently had a client with inoperable non-small-cell lung cancer that had spread to his spine. The test showed that his cancer had an EGFR mutation, which gave us a wonderful new therapeutic option with a drug called Tarceva, which specifically targets EGFR mutations. Since it's an oral drug, the patient could take a pill and live his life.

For some cancer diagnoses, molecular testing is always the first step because the results help oncologists determine whether the patient can benefit from targeted therapies—like EGFR-targeting Tarceva for certain lung cancers and HER2-targeting Herceptin for some types of breast cancers. In most cases, these drugs are *better* than traditional chemo, with far fewer side effects.

But because there are so many different types of molecular abnormalities in different cancers, the intelligence gleaned from these reports might serve as a helpful backup arsenal in case a first- or second-line therapy stops being effective.

That's what Matthew, a patient in his early seventies, did when he ran out of options for late-stage papillary thyroid cancer. His family was told to begin hospice care, but we thought there might still be some outside-the-box therapies that could help him. We got Matthew's tumor profiled and learned his cancer had something called a BRAF mutation, which is relatively common in papillary thyroid cancer *and* metastatic melanoma. A drug, Zelboraf, had just been approved for the treatment of metastatic melanoma with BRAF mutations.

Could Zelboraf help Matthew? The president of my company, Gregg Britt, went with him to his next oncologist consult. It was a sensitive situation, as Gregg didn't want to alienate Matthew's doctor. He approached the issue very honestly. "Matthew's in a tough situation, and his family asked us to look at all potential therapeutic options. So, let me share with you what we did. . . .

"As you know, BRAF mutations are not uncommon in papillary thyroid cancer, and now we know that Matthew's cancer has them," Gregg continued. "And as you may know, Zelboraf was just approved last week for metastatic melanoma."

Matthew's doctor had never heard of Zelboraf, but he was open-minded and examined the package insert. Gregg was able to present sound evidence that an FDA-approved drug targeted Matthew's specific mutation. "If Matthew's game to try it, I am too," the doctor said.

We'd laid the foundation; the next challenge was getting Matthew's insurance company to sign off on prescription coverage. If a tried-and-true drug that's been FDA-approved for one disease has a track record of use and effectiveness for a *different* disease, the likelihood that insurance will cover a prescription for someone with the second disease is high. But Matthew was using this brand-new (and very expensive) drug for an off-label purpose (i.e., not for melanoma) that hadn't been widely established yet. The likelihood of coverage was low.

What do you do in a situation like this? There's an 800 number printed on every health insurance card. Start by calling your carrier to request an exception. Anticipate that it will need to be persuaded. Next, recruit your physician to make the professional and clinical arguments for this treatment. Matthew's doctor explained to the insurance company that they had exhausted all other avenues; he presented the cancer's DNA profile; he described how the drug is meant to target BRAF mutations; and he impressed upon them that denying Matthew this drug would be a death sentence. The insurance company said yes, but it took a couple of weeks.

By the way, you can also get your pharmacist, your family members, and the drug company to call and write letters to your insurer. Don't be afraid to ask—everyone's interests are aligned. Your doctor wants you to have the drug because it may help you; the pharmaceutical company and the pharmacy want you to have it because this is their business.

Matthew responded well to Zelboraf and began to feel a little better. He started eating again and taking walks with his wife. But after a while, he developed side effects that were unpleasant, so he went off the drug and succumbed to his disease. His bridge ended up being a short one, about four months long, but his family cherished the extra time.

"I think it's a laudable goal that we all should be striving for, to do this precision medicine, to implement genomics more, to use it to design and target therapy," says oncologist Dr. Wilding. "Of course, we're not at the point where everyone should have their genome on a stick drive, walking around with it for their diabetes or cancer or whatnot. But I think someday that's where we're going to be."

Many physicians are dismissive of the value of tumor profiling. Sometimes that's because they lack familiarity with the science behind it. Other times—and this is something patients need to understand—it's because the information gleaned is likely to have no effect on a course of treatment. The truth is, for all the testing we order for clients, game-changing discoveries are few. But we know that the trajectory of benefit will only rise, because molecular profiling technology is developing at warp speed. For now, the idea behind tumor profiling is that if one bridge is ending, it may help you select another treatment and erect another bridge to a cure. As a data junkie, I always want more information—especially if there's a chance it will make a difference. But the decision of whether to test is a judgment call that patients must make with their doctors.

If you have cancer and want to have it profiled, you will need to ask your doctor (typically, your lead oncologist) to facilitate it. This is a very reasonable request, but you may want to prepare before approaching your physician. Read articles from reputable newspapers or medical journals about tumor profiling for your cancer, and print the About Us pages from the companies that perform these services. Bring them to your next oncology appointment, and say:

I know that a lot of cancers are caused by genetic mutations. There's this technology I've been reading about. I think it might be helpful over time to have my tissue biopsied. What do you think?

Or if you want to take a more aggressive approach:

It looks to me like this is the technology of the future. I see we're making progress in defeating a lot of different cancers by understanding the mutations that cause them. And the day may come when I'm going to need a clinical trial to try a new drug that targets my disease's specific mutations. I'd like to send my biopsy tissue to be profiled. I think it would be good to know what we're dealing with.

Don't be upset if you get some resistance. Your doctor may not be comfortable with the technology. But if you have been comporting yourself as a well-informed and courageous patient, he or she will more than likely listen to your request and respect your wishes.

2. BE ON THE CUTTING EDGE OF TECHNOLOGY.

Targeted drugs, immunotherapy, laparoscopic surgery—these are just a few realms of medicine that are rigorously tested before they become available to the general public. If you are considering a clinical trial for an experimental treatment, or even one that is already FDA-approved, you want to be sure it's right for you. The answer will depend on your health status (*Physically, would you be a good candidate for this treatment?*), your personal values (*Are you, like Samantha, wary of newer innovations?*), and your data collection (*Have you done your homework on this technology and asked your doctor about the risks and rewards involved?*).

I am a devout believer in FDA-sanctioned clinical trials. They are tightly regulated; the sponsors developing the drugs invest a ton of money in them; patients typically get a very high level of medical attention because they must be monitored very carefully; and once a patient is enrolled in a clinical trial, it is his or her choice at any time, any day, for any reason or no reason at all, to withdraw without questions.

The main risk, in my experience, is that most doctors don't consider it part of their job to do a nationwide, or even a regional, search to find the best match for their patient. Typically, they don't look beyond their own hospital's clinical trials, or maybe they're recommending a trial at another institution because a colleague is involved. They rarely do a systematic search for your specific problem. Maybe they're suggesting a certain trial because it's buzzing in their orbit. And it could be great! But is it necessarily the best one for you? Maybe, or maybe not.

I don't blame doctors. They just don't have time to do countless hours of research on www.clinicaltrials.gov (the NIH registry that catalogs clinical trials) and other resources. Or to make the dozens of phone calls to the principal investigator (the clinician running the trial), and sometimes to the drug companies, to confirm that they are still recruiting; to find out if there's a trial opening closer to the patient; to learn the process for enrollment, the eligibility requirements, and (if the trial is full) whether there's a waiting list. And those are just the steps needed to get to the point of sending in the patient's medical records and having her undergo a head-to-toe physical exam in order to determine if she is even eligible.

For patients, seeking out clinical trials on their own is a frustrating, full-time job, performed in a foreign language. I don't encourage anyone to try this at home. But what you *can* and should do is to proactively engage in the process with your specialists. If your doctor is suggesting a trial:

- Read the trial's informed-consent documents, which always list someone to call if you have questions.
- Search for the trial at www.clinicaltrials.gov for more information.
- Call the leading disease-research foundations to see if they are enthusiastic about it or have others to recommend.
- Check the treatment guidelines for your condition to find out how the proposed experimental protocol compares to the standard therapies for your disease.

Most important, ask your physician:

"Why do you think this trial is right for me?"

"Have you looked at trials at other hospitals or in other cities?"

"Am I a good candidate for this trial given the other problems [diabetes, heart disease, pulmonary conditions, etc.] I have?"

"What are the results of prior trials of this treatment? What were the benefits and complications? How did the patients fare?" (You may find specific data on previous trials at www.clinicaltrials.gov.)

"Does it make more sense for me to try the standard therapies for my disease first? Why are you recommending this trial instead of a standard therapy?"

It's very tricky to be at the cutting edge of new technologies. But your doctor's level of knowledge about a new treatment's results will tell you a lot about their personal investment in your condition. If you hear *I don't keep track,* or *I can't remember,* that's problematic. You want somebody who is continuously studying the latest developments. You now are a different breed of patient. You know the kinds of questions to ask. If what comes back is *I don't know,* ask yourself, *Then why is this treatment for me—and why are you the doctor for me?*

3. KNOW YOUR LIMITATIONS, AND FACTOR THEM INTO YOUR TREATMENT DECISIONS.

If a doctor does not consider the entire human being in front of him, he is apt to give less than optimal care. When eighty-year-old Sally was told she needed an immediate artificial hip replacement, her orthopedic surgeon didn't consider that another physical factor (the twisting of her body to compensate for vision loss) might have been causing her pain. And that's not surprising. But what is troubling is that he failed to consider her advancing age and how this major surgery would affect her life.

I recently met a woman with end-stage cancer, whose husband wanted to fly her to Mexico to pursue all sorts of unproven therapies. His attitude was, "What's the downside?" Don't get me started. Besides the heartbreak that these kinds of futile treatments can bring, there are serious dangers involved. I suggested to the husband, sensitively, "Your wife is very weak, and I hate to be morbid, but what if she has an adverse reaction in a strange place? What if she ends up dying in a hotel room in Tijuana while you're off pursuing her next oxygen-treatment appointment?"

Although I generally encourage people to travel as far as necessary for the best treatment when it matters most, you still have to consider the risks. If you're thinking about crossing the country for surgery, are you stable enough to fly? How long will your recovery be? Are you prepared for the extra costs and inconveniences if there are complications and you get stuck there for a while?

If you need to regularly visit a hospital or clinic for chemotherapy and/or radiation treatments, choosing a place where you feel comfortable and safe can give you the additional resolve you need to get through it. On the other hand, if you're enduring eight weeks of radiation, and it's a ninety-minute drive every day, you may want to find a place closer to home. Getting stuck in traffic, finding parking, waiting in the lobby—all those things can wear you down.

When Hal, an active man in his late seventies, was diagnosed with acute myeloid leukemia, his local oncologist wanted to begin chemotherapy immediately. But Hal's son persuaded him to see a specialist in nearby Cleveland for a second opinion. As soon as the doctor met Hal, she knew that this train was headed in the wrong direction. Hal wasn't feeling the full brunt of his disease yet; in fact, he was barely symptomatic. But he *would* feel the powerful side effects of the proposed treatment. They would come on hard and strong, like a freight train crashing through his front door.

The optimal strategy for Hal was blood transfusions that would abate his fatigue and help keep him functioning at a high level. When that stopped working, as one day it would, then he would need to decide whether to resort to a very intensive, two-week in-patient chemo regimen in which the doctors would, in effect, do a hard reset of his entire immune system. That in turn would leave him vulnerable to all kinds of infections that would require aggressive treatment on top of the chemo. If he survived the treatment, he could enjoy eighteen months or more of remission and health as good as if he didn't have the disease at all. And who knows? Perhaps more medical bridges would be built in that time frame.

With this new information, Hal and his family decided to hold off on chemotherapy for as long as possible, because that would be a brutal option. When the time comes for a therapy like that, you either decide that you are going to go for it, or you opt for palliative or hospice care instead, so you can be as comfortable as possible during the time you have left.

Be honest with yourself. Are you in the right shape for this treatment? Are there mental, physical, or emotional factors that will make your recovery more unpredictable, more risky? And ask your doctor:

ASK

"Why is this surgery/drug/test necessary?"

"What are the risks/side effects of this procedure?"

"Is there anything we can do to minimize the side effects?"

"How long is the recovery period and what will it involve?"

"What will happen if we don't do this?"

"Are there nonsurgical/less aggressive options we can try first?"

"How do they compare to my surgical/more aggressive options?"

If you hear *There's a range of side effects*, ask, *What's most probable for me? For someone my age, and with my specific disease stage?* Ask your doctors to speak honestly with you about the risks and benefits, so that you're making intelligent decisions—so that you can be, as Samantha put it, an incredibly informed, intentional master of your own domain.

4. BE SURE YOUR TEAM IS CLEAR ABOUT YOUR HEALTH GOALS AND VALUES.

Economists call it a coordination game. When all the players' interests are aligned, and everyone makes mutually consistent decisions, the outcome will be good. In health care, if you don't articulate your interests to your caregivers, how can you be sure that everyone is aiming for the same goal?

Many years ago we were involved in the case of Joan, a seventy-five-year-old woman with advanced bladder cancer. When surgeons first operated on her, they discovered that her bladder was literally sticking to her pelvic wall in a hard, fibrotic mass of tissue. It was much worse than they had thought. They took some tissue to biopsy and sewed her back up. Joan was at death's door and suffering terrible pain, mostly due to the stress on her kidneys from the swelling and urinary obstruction caused by the cancer. "Anything we do now," her doctors told the family, "may be more harmful than helpful. Let's just make her as comfortable as possible."

Joan's daughter called my team. "This hospital is giving up on Mom," she said. "That's not acceptable." We were able to get top bladder cancer experts consulting on her case by phone. Because Joan's cancer appeared to be very aggressive, they felt it might respond well to chemotherapy. We got Joan transferred to a center that was willing to try an intensive course. "This might not work," we warned the family, "but let's give it a try."

In fact, the chemo worked so well that Joan's cancer receded, along with her fibrotic tissue and the stress on her kidneys. In the middle of her regimen, she was discharged from the hospital. She started taking her dog for long walks and talked about picking tennis back up.

Given her success, we explored the idea of trying another operation, to remove more of the cancer. The family consulted with a top bladder cancer surgeon, who agreed that Joan was a candidate for potentially curative surgery. Although it might not work—and there were risks, including death—Joan and her family had already accepted that she would probably succumb to her disease. They wanted to swing for the fences. The surgery took six intense hours, as the doctor cut away at the dead tissue and removed part of Joan's bladder. Afterward she was declared cancer free, which lasted more than a year.

Eventually and inevitably, Joan's cancer returned. It stopped responding to therapy, and nothing more helped. But her aggressive approach had gained her another full eighteen months of life. That might not seem like much, but it was enough for Joan to see the birth of another grandchild and spend two more Christmases with her loved ones.

Joan's original doctors had done nothing wrong, by the way. Given the late stage of her aggressive disease and its unusual presentation, they believed nothing more could be done, and it was their duty to protect her from drugs and operations that could cause more pain. But their views were not aligned with Joan's and her family's.

Treatment approaches vary widely. Some patients prefer to forgo interventions and accept the disease progression; others want to try the standard protocols, but if their disease advances beyond hope, they reject further risky (and costly) treatments. Then there are those, like Joan, who take an aggressive, go-for-broke approach—and fight to the end.

The more serious your condition, the more important it is to have everyone's goals in alignment. One way of making your wishes explicit—and enforceable—is to complete a health care advance directive, a multipage document in which you, the patient, provide basic instructions for your care. It often includes a living will, which states treatment preferences if you are no longer able to make decisions or speak for yourself, and a health care power of attorney, in which you appoint a proxy to make decisions on your behalf if you cannot. The nonprofit organization Caring Connections (www .caringinfo.org) provides state-by-state advance directive forms that you can fill out. Those diagnosed with terminal illnesses may also want to complete a more detailed Physician Orders for Life-Sustaining Treatment (POLST) form, which patient and caregiver discuss and complete together. A POLST carefully spells out preferences for such medical interventions as CPR, tube feeding, antibiotics, do-not-resuscitate orders, and comfort. (You can find your state's POLST form at www.polst.org.)

Decide what you want across the treatment spectrum as early as possible, and have a conversation about your choices with the people who are most involved in your care:

> *I know this is a hard topic, but I want everyone to understand what my wishes are. I know you may have different views, and I'm happy to talk about them now. But please understand that it will make it much easier for me to go through this treatment if I know that you understand what my goals are, and if I know you are going to respect them.*

When families are facing end-of-life issues, having a trusted internist weigh in can be helpful. They've been down this road before and can sometimes bring sage medical advice. "When I'm meeting with a family at the hospital, and it looks as though someone doesn't have very long to live, I try to get everybody involved and have everybody's opinion in the open," says Washington, D.C., internist Dr. Bryan Arling. "If the family wants an additional consult, every hospital has a team that may include an intensivist, a psychiatrist, a nurse, or an administrator. They can look at these cases and help to determine a prognosis, to help make decisions as to whether this is the time to let go."

As Dr. Arling notes, that decision exists in a bit of a gray zone, and it can change over time—which is why it's advisable to hear everyone out. Sleep on it for a day or two. "Try to think of what the loved one would be coming back to in terms of quality of life," he says. "Sometimes, I will say, 'If this were my loved one, knowing what we know about the chance for a meaningful recovery, the kindest thing we could do is to withdraw all diagnostic and therapeutic interventions and allow a natural death'—so the decision is all on me. Because family members shouldn't have to be in a situation of telling the hospital, 'Stop taking care of my relative.'"

In these cases, Dr. Arling will also stamp the patient's charts AND, for Allow Natural Death, instead of DNR, Do Not Resuscitate. "A DNR order sounds as though you're about to resuscitate, poised over the patient's sternum to do CPR, but you just withhold it," he says. "DNR is a term I've never really embraced nearly as much as AND, allowing a natural death."

As a patient, as long as you are making informed and thoughtful choices about what you want, there is no wrong approach. The decision of how and when (or if) to treat is yours alone. And it can change with the circumstances. But it's important that your caregivers and family members are clear about your wishes ahead of time, so that they are never in a position of having to make painful guesses about what's best for you. Give them that clarity.

QUICK GUIDE

CHAPTER II. **Step 3—Treatment**

- Try to refrain from rushing toward the very first treatment proposal you hear.

- Focus on two questions: (1) What is the best course of treatment for my specific disease? and (2) Who is/are the best doctor(s) to administer that treatment/perform my surgery/oversee my therapy?

- You will know you are in the No-Mistake Zone when (1) your diagnosis is specific and confirmed; (2) you're convinced about when and why you need to be treated; (3) you've explored the most promising treatment options; (4) you've met with experienced physicians who practice at institutions appropriate for the care you need; (5) you can visualize the steps of your treatment plan; (6) your gut is telling you, *This is the treatment for me, and this is the physician I want carrying it out.*

- Review the must-ask questions when consulting with specialists and gathering information about a treatment plan (see pages 224 and 225).

- Separate the data collection from the decision making. You don't have to make a decision yet. Remain neutral until all the data are in.

- Don't obsess over the things you would need a medical degree to understand. Instead, get a sense of the physician, the institution, and the very important measurable factors like volume and complication rates.

- Lean on your support team for help with research and to accompany you on doctor visits to ask questions you may not be thinking of.

- Seek out treatment guidelines from reputable organizations such as the U.S. Department of Health and Human Services (www.guideline.gov) and the National Comprehensive Cancer Network (www.nccn.org).

- For patients with cancer, getting your tumor tissue molecularly profiled may provide useful information. Research reputable journals to find out how this technology is being used for your specific cancer, and ask your oncologist to facilitate a test.

- Proactively engage with your specialists and the disease philanthropies to learn as much as possible about FDA-sanctioned clinical trials that might be right for you.

- Be honest about your readiness for a therapy. Factor your mental, physical, and emotional limitations into your treatment decisions—especially if you intend to travel for care.

- Ensure that your team is clear about your health goals and values. If appropriate, complete a health care advance directive (available at www.caringinfo.org) or a Physician Orders for Life-Sustaining Treatment form (www.polst.org).

- When families are facing end-of-life issues, having a trusted internist weigh in can be helpful. PCPs, who have been down this road before, bring sage medical wisdom.

- The decision of how and when (or if) to treat is yours alone. Have a conversation about your choices with your caregivers and family members so they will have clarity about what's best for you.

STEP 4—COORDINATION

How to make sure your doctors are performing like a team

Hospital horror stories abound. Perhaps the most famous is that of Willie King, a fifty-one-year-old heavy-equipment operator and father of three, who had suffered for years from diabetes. By 1995, his right foot and leg were so infected with gangrene that he would probably die if they weren't removed. At his doctor's urging, he made an appointment for below-the-knee amputation, or BKA surgery, at a community hospital in Tampa, Florida. When King arrived, an admitting clerk entered his personal information into the computer system and put him on the surgical schedule, but with one grave error: he was listed for a *left* BKA.

An astute floor nurse caught the mix-up on the paper schedule and corrected it by hand—*right* BKA—but no one fixed it in the computer system. Another nurse spoke with King about his surgery, correctly identified his right leg as the surgical target, and noted it on her record too. As she wheeled him toward the operating room, King joked, "You know which one it is, don't you? I don't want to wake up and find the wrong one gone!" And yet that's exactly what happened. An OR nurse, shaking and in tears, caught the mistake and immediately brought it to the surgeon's attention, but he had already cut through the wrong leg. Of course, King's diseased right leg still had to be taken.

Trial testimony revealed that a series of coordination mistakes were made that day. Despite the fact that two nurses had caught the error, it remained in the computer system, on the blackboard in the operating room, and on the OR schedule. By the time King's doctor arrived in the operating suite, the wrong leg had been prepped for surgery. And no one checked King's consent form or medical history, both of which were readily available in the operating room. King was awarded $1.125 million for the hospital's systemic coordination and communication failures that left him a double amputee.

Called a never-event (because it never should have happened), King's case sparked intense research and review of our nation's patient safety protocols. Today, if he were to check into a hospital, he'd likely have to sign a consent form that provided his name, medical status, reason for surgery, and risks of the operation. Virtually every staff member he interacted with would repeat the same information to him: "Hello, Mr. King. I see you're having below-the-knee amputation today on your right leg, is that correct? And you are a diabetic, right? Are you on any medication?" Another health care professional would use permanent marker on his leg to indicate the incision site (by writing YES, or getting it signed by the doctor or patient), so that King could confirm it was the correct limb. The surgeon would review his chart and, in some cases, call a "time out," during which the entire surgical team would discuss King's condition and the planned treatment, so that everyone was on the same page, and anyone who had different information could speak up.

Thankfully, never-events like King's botched amputation (also called a wrong-site surgery) are fairly rare, causing minimal injury (a scar, a delayed recovery) but hardly ever the kind of permanent damage King experienced.

And yet *other* sorts of never-events exact serious trauma and costs. In a 2013 study, researchers examined two decades' worth (from 1990 to 2010) of paid malpractice settlements to find 9,744 surgical never-events (totaling $1.3 billion in paid claims), in which 155 patients died and 184 suffered permanent injuries. The most common never-event, according to the study, was a "retained foreign body" (49.8 percent)—as in the accidental leaving behind in a patient's body of a sponge, a tool, or in the case of one Canadian woman who didn't understand why she kept setting off metal detectors, a thirteen-inch-long retractor. The next most common never-events included surgeons doing the wrong procedure (25.1 percent), operating on the wrong site or limb (24.8 percent), and operating on the wrong patient (0.3 percent). Being rare isn't enough. Never-events should *never* happen to you.

I've yet to have a client experience a never-event on my watch, but we've certainly had people come to us after a hospital debacle that occurred due to poor coordination and communication, or when a medical team lacked the necessary depth of skill and volume of practice to anticipate and guard against terrible blunders. The good news is that medical institutions take patient safety very seriously. And *you* will be even better protected: when the time comes that you need to go to a hospital for serious medical care, you will have done your homework on your condition, selected the best possible treatment, and found the specialist and institution most capable of carrying it out. Most important, you'll have a trusted support person at your side—someone who will help communicate and coordinate your needs and health status, serving as a crucial backup check for your safety.

Step 4, Coordination, may be the most important responsibility a health care quarterback can take on. This step starts long before you go to the hospital, and it doesn't end until after you have returned home and recovered to the point that you can manage on your own again. For example, record collection and distribution—the groundwork of Intensive Case Management—requires small feats of coordination. Having a methodical friend who can help you with it will prove so valuable. When you are confirming a diagnosis and collecting data in order to make decisions about a treatment plan, you'll likely need help scheduling (and confirming) appointments with experts; double-checking that they've received your records in advance of a consult; and taking notes (or recording meetings) in order to remember what each doctor says.

But then there are times when coordination is *crucial* to your safety, when having a helper to be your eyes, ears, and voice may well protect you from becoming a victim of medical error. Those times are (1) during the course of treatment, and (2) at the "intersections" of care, including during and after a hospital stay.

COORDINATION DURING THE COURSE OF TREATMENT

This will be essential no matter whether you are having a onetime surgical procedure or enduring months of therapy. Coordination is especially important when you have multiple chronic conditions, several treating doctors, and a blitz of medications to schedule or are being cared for by more than one facility. With a cancer diagnosis, for instance, you might have a surgeon, a radiation specialist, a medical oncologist, a neurologist, a nutritionist, a psychologist, a physical therapist, and more.

"There's so much information, you can't possibly take it all in, and you need to have another set of eyes and ears there," says Stanford internist Dr. Neda Pakdaman. "It's also really valuable, if you're going through a variety of clinics, appointments, or settings, to have someone who can be a record-keeper, to carry information—be it in a paper binder or in electronic format—on all your medications and relevant records, just to make sure it's all there. That person can be an important part of a system of checks and balances."

During the treatment stage, ask your coordination helper to (1) join you during important treatment meetings, (2) be your record-keeper, and (3) update your Medical Summary and distribute it to your doctors. Your Medical Summary is like a time line of your symptoms, diagnoses, interventions, medications, and changes in your condition or care. Sadly, most physicians never get this kind of full-data capture from patients.

If you have multiple health problems that require attention from specialists in different realms of medicine, physicians need to know what you've been up to when you're not in their world. For instance, you're not going to know how certain prescriptions you're taking will interact with one another over time. Even commonly used medications, such as aspirin, anti-inflammatories, erectile dysfunction medications, birth control pills, and drugs that control stomach acid can have serious interactions with a treatment, sometimes increasing or decreasing its intended effects and unintended side effects.

Another example: A patient learns she has a chronic hepatitis B infection. But because she never develops the symptoms—and she perceives herself to be in excellent health—she decides to forgo treatment and regular follow-ups with a hepatologist. Many years later she develops cancer. She starts chemotherapy, which suppresses her immune system, in turn causing her hepatitis B to become active, leading to severe liver dysfunction. Had her oncologist screened for hepatitis B, or communicated with the patient's internist or hepatologist beforehand, this terrible and potentially fatal turn of events could have been prevented by giving her antiviral therapy before starting chemotherapy.

Doctors have gotten used to rendering judgment and making recommendations based on incomplete information. But it doesn't have to be that way. Why trust your memory to share important medical clues about your health? Add them to your Medical Summary, and share it with your doctors. When we provide these records to physicians, they are thrilled to get them. It's something they almost never receive.

Several years ago Dr. Pakdaman found herself in the support role when her mother was diagnosed with metastatic cancer. She or her father accompanied her mom on every medical visit. And whenever relevant issues transpired, Dr. Pakdaman made sure that her mom's oncologist was informed about it and weighed in if needed. "We would just send a communication saying, 'We saw doctor so-and-so today, and this is what came up,'" she recalls. Keeping your doctors in the loop is an easy way to stay on track, yet it can do wonders for the doctor-patient partnership. "Everybody collaborated really beautifully together," she recalls. "We ended up having a more open and productive relationship with her whole care team as a result of those conversations."

As Dr. Pakdaman can attest, it's very easy for care to get fragmented, for communication to break down. "I always tell my own patients: 'Even though I try to be very much on top of it, if you're going to go see another specialist, please make sure I know about it. If you have an appointment that I didn't coordinate for you, please send me an e-mail, so I can make sure to get the doctor's notes.'" The other thing she asks patients to do is send her an update afterward, "just to give me their perspective of what transpired," she says. "It allows me to pick up on things, like 'Wait, what the physician said in his notes versus what the patient told me are different. There needs to be clarification.' It makes care more seamless when everyone is on the same page."

If your quarterback is managing your appointments, ask her to help you relay important developments to your other doctors. Because, as Dr. Pakdaman says, "if you're the one who's sick—maybe you're on medications that make it difficult to think straight, or you're physically exhausted—you're not going to have the bandwidth to do it all yourself."

Even with the best intentions, at some point during treatment you may suddenly find yourself adrift. Frequently in medicine, patients feel as if their care has become conductorless. No one is really in charge.

You could have the best physicians in the world, but if they're working alone and in the dark, getting you better won't be easy. Historically, it was the job of the primary care physician to be the conductor, but as I noted earlier, that rarely happens anymore. Let your support team help you to make sure that your talented caregivers are working in concert. One way for him or her to do that is to ask the doctors to get on a call. For example:

> *Dr. Adams, I'm concerned that the beta-blocker Mom is taking for her heart disease is aggravating her psoriasis. As her dermatologist, you've seen how bad it's gotten. But her cardiologist says she really needs to stay on this drug. And I know you're worried about your ability to get her psoriasis under control while she's on it. Mom doesn't really know what to do, and I'm not sure we really understand all the nuances of this problem. Would it be possible to get on a quick conference call with me and Mom's cardiologist? Just fifteen minutes to figure out a solution? I'm more than happy to speak with your scheduling assistant and find a time that works best for you.*

When nobody is coordinating care and patients are wading through dangerous waters alone, a seemingly small problem can suddenly become huge. But sometimes just getting doctors to talk to one another can turn a case around. That's what happened to Taylor, twenty-five, who developed sharp pain in the upper part of her abdomen after a frightening car accident.

As far as the emergency room doctors could tell, she was scuffed up and scared but had no internal injuries. She saw her internist right away. He prescribed painkillers and heartburn medication, but they didn't fix Taylor's aches. In fact, the pain got so bad, she checked herself back into the ER, where she was given more X-rays and pain meds. Her internist next referred her to a gastroenterologist, who did an upper endoscopy but didn't find anything wrong. Next, she was sent to a pain management specialist, only to be sent away with another prescription, but no answers.

Taylor had consultations with a half-dozen specialists, but none seemed to be able to figure out the cause of her pain. She had missed two semesters of business school and was in danger of losing her place if she didn't return in the fall. Her father finally stepped up to manage her case. First, he collected all of Taylor's medical records and created a Medical Summary. Next, he called her internist, with Taylor on the line:

Dr. Greene, Taylor and I have serious concerns about her health. She's been struggling with this pain for almost a year now. I've collected all her medical files and created a time line of her condition, and I'd like to send it to you. Taylor is now in danger of being expelled from school. Everything she has worked so hard for will be lost. All I'm asking is, would you review her records, and then get on a conference call with her pain management doctor and GI specialist? I can facilitate the call. If I can get the three of you to put your heads together, do a little problem solving, for just thirty minutes, it would be tremendous. Because Taylor is spiraling right now. I really need your help.

He made a similar impassioned plea to the other two doctors, and they all agreed to put in the time to discuss her case. If you have a strong bond with your internist, you can ask if he or she can facilitate a conference call. But if the relationship isn't there, or your PCP has dropped the ball, it's perfectly fine to make the call yourself, or to ask a trusted friend or family member to do it. She doesn't need to yell or make a fuss. She shouldn't blame or accuse. She just needs to approach your doctors respectfully, as a caring person, with concerns about a problem that she truly believes they can help solve.

In Taylor's case, her doctors reviewed the records her father sent in advance of their conference call. While the internist took the lead on the call, Taylor and her dad sat in, offering information and asking questions when necessary. They came to discover—thanks to the Medical Summary—that Taylor had been prescribed a wide and vast number of pain medications. Further, because she felt as if she had to deal with her pain alone, Taylor had been self-medicating: She'd piggyback prescriptions, double up dosages when one dose didn't work, and refill as often as possible. She was addicted to eight different narcotics. She could barely make it through the day, let alone go back to school. It was clear that her health problems had become increasingly complicated due to her fragmented care, and her doctors were genuinely saddened and concerned by her struggles. They devised a new plan of care for her.

A month later Taylor's life was slowly getting back on track. She was on a single pain medication, time-released through a patch. She was seeing a psychotherapist, who was helping her cope with the trauma of her accident and subsequent addiction. Her internist, who determined that her aches were probably not GI-related, was working to get her into the right realm of medicine, to get to the bottom of her pain. Best of all, she was starting class again in the fall. Thanks to her father's legwork, her doctors were acting like a team again.

COORDINATION AT THE INTERSECTIONS OF CARE

Some 40 percent of the 5.8 million car crashes that occur in the United States each year are at intersections. You can imagine the most common reasons: being distracted, failing to watch for hazards, assuming incorrectly what the other driver is going to do. The same is true in health care. Patients are most vulnerable to harm at medical intersections—maybe when they are being transferred from an emergency room to surgery on a different floor with an entirely different team; or during the handoff from the night shift to the morning staff; or when they're being sent home to recuperate.

"Patients and their families need to be aware that hospitals are dangerous places. They really shouldn't be there any longer than they need to be," says Dr. George Wilding, the Wisconsin oncologist. "The biggest problem in the health care system in this country is communication. And it's well documented that the points of concentration where you look for potential communication problems are the handoffs: between nurses ending shifts, between doctors, between one human to another. Patients and their family members need to have a sense of awareness of what's happening. Talk to people. If things don't jibe, raise questions."

And if you still aren't getting the information you need? Do what doctors do: ask for a family meeting.

When Jonathan, at forty, suddenly had a stroke, he was taken by ambulance to the emergency room of a large university hospital. Tests showed that the cause was a previously undetected heart flutter that had been causing small blood clots. A CT scan of his chest also revealed suspicious lesions in his lungs, possibly cancerous.

Jonathan's sister, Hannah, shared his complete medical records with the hospital and quarterbacked his case, but she couldn't figure out who to talk to. A stream of medical professionals were in and out of his room: nurses, hospitalists, residents, fellows, a cardiologist, an oncologist, a neurologist. It seemed as if he had ten different doctors consulting, but nobody was in charge.

Oftentimes the attending physician—the one responsible for coordinating care and providing the family with reports—does her rounds, and then she's in surgery, or is gone for the rest of the day, and the patient's family misses a chance to communicate with the lead doctor. If you find yourself in a similar situation, and you need real-time information, just ask the charge nurse: *Who is the attending physician, and what time does he or she make her rounds this week?*

Sometimes a patient's care plan is a mystery to the family, even though it makes sense to the clinicians. In Jonathan's case, he had so many medical issues that Hannah needed to have an in-depth conversation with the lead doctor. She went to the charge nurse and said, "My brother has never been in the hospital before. He's facing some difficult challenges and decisions, and he's going to need my help. But I feel like I'm really unclear about what the next steps are in his treatment plan. It would really help us, as a family, to better understand the care plan for my brother. Can you help us set up a family meeting with the attending physician? We can be available at any time."

Physicians typically initiate family meetings when there's serious news to impart, but you have every right to call one if, say, there's been a serious change in the patient's condition, or maybe it's time to consider withdrawing care, or there's simply been a gap in communication and you need to ask, "What's the plan, doctor?" You can arrange a family meeting through the head nurse or a social worker. The speed with which a meeting occurs will depend on the attending physician's schedule, but your request should be treated with attention and respect.

Hannah learned during their family meeting that Jonathan needed to stabilize before they could begin rehab for his stroke. A cardiologist and oncologist were consulting on his heart and lung issues, but he was still too sick to begin treatment, so those problems were being monitored until he was better. Hannah now had a handle on who was in charge and what the next steps were for her brother.

If you (or a loved one) are about to start a hospital stay, be sure you have a support person at the ready who can effectively communicate with your medical team to ensure you're getting safe, high-quality care at every stage. Here are some specific actions you can take both during and after your stay.

TWO WAYS TO STAY SAFE DURING A HOSPITAL STAY

1. Let your caregivers know more about you. When you arrive, find out who is in charge of your care when your attending physician is not there, and introduce yourself and your team leader to that person. If you're being seen by hospitalists—who change from one shift to the next—don't assume they've fully communicated with one another about your current medical status. Ask to speak to the charge nurse, and let him or her know that you've got a support person with you. Provide your helper's cell phone number in case of an emergency. Share any forms—HIPAA release, power of attorney— that formally grant your helper rights with regard to your care. Not sure how to start this conversation? It might go a little like this:

> *I want to introduce you to my dear friend Laurie. I know I'm not going to have the clarity or the energy that I need to be an effective patient, but Laurie is committed to helping me through this. And I want you to know that when she speaks, she speaks for me; and when you speak to her, you can count on her to communicate all of it to me. Her job is to help me be the best patient I can possibly be and to help you guys be the best care providers you can be, because I know how hard you work and how tough it can be sometimes.*

Your caregivers really want to help you, but the pressures of the system often make it harder for them to do their job as thoughtfully and effectively as they want to. When you acknowledge the difficulty of what they do, and let them know that you've got a caring quarterback who's there to provide support, it changes how people see you. You *get* it, and you're helping them achieve exactly what they want: getting you better.

Another way to be remembered as a patient is to bring three specific categories of information with you to the hospital. These are:

- **Medical information.** Tape a list next to your bed that spells out in large type the following: your diagnosis, any medications you are on, any allergies you may have, and any major medical issues or secondary diagnoses that might be relevant to your current condition. For instance, have you had a splenectomy? Are you diabetic? Do you have a stent in your heart? Has your hip been replaced? Any one of these could become a factor if you have complications.

- **Organizational information.** Post a phone and e-mail contact list of your physicians and family members; a photocopy of your insurance card; the place you were born; and your religious affiliation, if that applies. Those last two items are optional, but I think they make you more approachable. Learning where someone was born often sparks personal memories: "My mother was born in Detroit, too," or "I've always wanted to visit Hawaii—what's it like?" The reason to note your religion is that in every hospital of substantial size, there are clergy of all denominations who rotate through the wards to check on patients and give them support. If you'd like that, just say so. They'd love to do it.

- **Personal information.** You really don't want to be the patient in West 16B who had spine surgery—you want to be thought of and cared for as a human being. How do you achieve that? One way is to bring in photos to set on your bedside table or tape on the wall. *Here's my family: I've got an eighteen-year-old daughter, a sixteen-year-old son, and a ten-year-old dog named Buckley.* Or maybe you display a snap of you skiing with your girlfriend, or watching a football game at Lambeau Field. When my mother was recovering from a hip injury, I had a photo of our entire family made into a large poster that I taped to the wall, so she could see it from her bed. She loved it, and all the nurses got to know the life stories and accomplishments of her grandchildren. To them, she became the proud grandmother, rather than just the lady in 12B with a broken hip.

What else do you like to do in your spare time? Bring your favorite books and music, your knitting materials, your sketch pad, your deck of cards—whatever will make you feel more at home. This needs to be *your* room. Every person who enters will see you differently for it (and you'll make an otherwise antiseptic space more comfortable). The nurse who stops in to deliver your pills will say, "I just finished that book, it's terrific!" The anesthesiologist who drops by to introduce himself before your procedure will ask, "Don't you just love Bach's violin concertos? I like to play music for my patients during surgery—do you have any special requests?" The orderly who brings your soggy fish filet and fruit cup will say, "My father did card tricks. Let's see if you know this one." Your relationships with your caregivers will transcend the ordinary.

The second way to stay safe in the hospital is to . . .

2. Work to proactively prevent hospital-acquired conditions. These are anything that make you sick as a result of being treated in a health care setting. That means adverse drug reactions, falls, infections, pressure ulcers, pneumonia associated with ventilator use, and more—and they occur in about 12 out of every 100 patients. Here are some areas that deserve special attention—and things you can say and do to prevent a hospital-acquired condition:

- **Drug information.** Before you swallow the pills brought to you or accept any new medications, ask the nurse what the drug is and what it's for. If you have a complicated regimen, a simple way to avoid errors is to create a schedule and tape it to the wall. I've done this numerous times for people. Across the top row, list the days of the week; down each day's column write times, medications, and dosages. Whenever you take something, have the nurse check it off. If there are any changes to your schedule, ask your doctor to make sure it's properly authorized and accurate.

- **Treatment information.** Be alert to, and ask questions about, seemingly unnecessary tests or treatments. If you are in a teaching hospital, for example, you will likely be seen by many very capable medical residents—but you still need to check with your attending physician before agreeing to any new drugs or procedures. If someone wants to wheel you away for a procedure you haven't been informed about, insist that it be confirmed first with your doctor. Just say: *I understand that we're going in for another MRI. I had one yesterday. I was unaware that this is happening. I'm frankly scared about it, and I really don't want to have any additional testing done until we can talk to my doctor. Let's just get him on the phone and see what he has to say.*

- Symptom information. It's easier to treat infections if they are caught early. So be aware of your body. Tell your nurse promptly if the dressing around a wound or the entrance site of a catheter loosens, gets wet, or is causing pain. If you develop a rash, a fever, or new swelling, or if you feel a different kind of pain, you may be getting an infection. Let your nurses and physicians know as soon as possible. Say, *I've never felt this kind of pain before. Please, can you make sure that the hospitalist sees me during her shift so we can have a discussion about this?* Or *My whole leg is red. I've never seen that before. It worries me. How can we make sure it's not something that needs to be treated right now?*
- Clean hands. Unclean hands are one of the main culprits in the spread of infection in hospitals. Don't be afraid to remind doctors and nurses about washing their hands before working with you.
- Medical information. Make sure that new caregivers who come to treat you are aware of your condition, your medications, and any allergies you have.
- Your chart. Finally, don't hesitate to ask to see your chart. Is your name spelled correctly? Is your date of birth accurate? Are your allergies noted? Is there any missing information? You have a right, as a patient, to review your chart and have any errors corrected. Remember, you're in a vulnerable position. You're going to have a significant medical procedure, with a lot of different people involved. Don't be reluctant to convey your feelings of vulnerability. Just politely and respectfully say to whomever is caring for you:

  I have some very specific allergies that are quite significant. I'd sleep much better tonight if I knew that they were in my chart. Can you do me a favor and just let me take a look at it?

  Or maybe it's:

  I'm on a lot of different medications and I want to make sure that you have all of them. It would be really helpful to me if I could see my chart.

  If the hospital uses electronic records, you can ask:

  I know this is all digitized in the computer. Could you just hit the "print" button and let me see the state of my chart since I got here yesterday morning?

The point is not to bark: *Let me see my chart!* Instead, reach for your commonality as human beings. People respond favorably when you're disclosing a well-founded fear.

Sometimes a hospital stay can be so stressful and exhausting, it's just too hard for patients to advocate for themselves or accurately convey to family members what's happening with their care. Having someone stay around the clock with the patient can be a tremendous safeguard, and a comfort. This is especially true for patients who are elderly, frail, extremely ill, or on pain medications or drugs that compromise their mental acuity.

DISCHARGE ORDERS: KEEPING SAFE AFTER YOU LEAVE THE HOSPITAL

According to a *New England Journal of Medicine* study, nearly one-fifth of Medicare patients discharged from a hospital—that's about 2.6 million seniors a year—develop an acute medical problem within the first thirty days that will necessitate *another* hospitalization. Called posthospital syndrome, these problems affect patients of all ages and commonly include heart failure, pneumonia, bronchitis and emphysema, infection, gastrointestinal conditions, mental illness, metabolic disorders, and trauma.

Don't underestimate the toll that a hospital stay takes. You're deprived of sleep because you're constantly being awakened for medication or treatment; you're probably poorly nourished; you're under a lot of mental, emotional, and physical stress, not to mention the pain that can kick in postsurgery. Your support person needs to be hyperalert to your symptoms and activities after a hospital stay.

The best way to guard against posthospital syndrome and other complications is to get a full briefing before or during your discharge instructions. (Unfortunately, some patients aren't even given discharge instructions—a recipe for medical disaster. Insist upon getting them before you leave.) The following is a comprehensive list of questions to ask during discharge. At the end of a hospital stay, you're probably going to be tired, distracted, and eager to go home. Let your quarterback take these on, so you can focus on getting some rest.

THE TEN THINGS YOU NEED TO ASK BEFORE YOU LEAVE THE HOSPITAL

1. Has my diagnosis changed? You went in to have, say, a cancerous lump or tumor removed, and there was a hypothesis about what it would be. Now that it's out, ask, *What was it? Was our theory correct? We thought I had Stage II lung cancer, but is it really a Stage III? Has it metastasized?* Find out more about your condition.

2. What was the ultimate treatment? What did the doctors do while they were operating on you? *Was it a partial or a full removal of the organ? Did they have to take out lymph nodes? Were there any surprises or complications?* It's very important to ask for a copy of your surgical report, too. Every surgery has one. You may need it for myriad reasons, not least of which is that it will become an important part of your medical history. (The answer to your request, by the way, should always be yes.)

3. What should I expect during my recovery? Find out how to navigate the first couple of days, the next week, and the weeks after that. Ask, *Where will I be physically, and what are the symptoms I need to watch for? What's urgent to attend to, and what's something I can alert you to at our next visit?* For example, if you have a fever, let your physician know immediately, because it means you may have an infection. But what about a rash? Shortness of breath? Discharge? Particular kinds of pain? Ask, *What level of pain should I expect? Is there a different sort of pain—sensation, location, duration—that would be of concern?* If you're feeling something burning and sharp in your abdomen, it's important to know whether (a) that's a normal effect of your surgery, (b) this requires a call to your physician during business hours, or (c) this is a "911—let's go!" kind of problem.

4. What sort of equipment will I need? The transition from hospital to home requires logistical organization, which is why so many patients end up feeling unprepared. Just ask, *What do we need at home?* You may need a wheelchair for a few days, or a walker, or a

cane. You may need oxygen for a period of time. If you've had a hip replacement, you may need a raised toilet seat, because you won't be able to sit that low. Are there stairs leading to your house or apartment? Is there a way for you to get up them?

5. **What activities should I avoid, and what do I need to do?** Even after something as mundane as bunion surgery, you have to spend the first couple of days in bed with your foot elevated. No walking anywhere but to the commode. If you've had abdominal surgery, there will be restrictions about lifting and bending. This is the time when you are most vulnerable to reinjuries and falls, so ask, *What are the limitations on my activities? When can I drive? When can I walk up and down steps? When is it safe for me to carry a bag of groceries?*

   Conversely, what are your obligatory activities? Maybe it's icing the site for twenty minutes, six times a day. Maybe it's using a pulley device or large rubber bands every night and every morning to restore full range of motion in your repaired joints. Find out.

6. **Are there any dietary restrictions I need to follow?** Perhaps you need to continue on a liquid diet, moving to a semisolid diet after five days, and then to a solid diet at the end of the week. *Are there special foods we should buy on the way home? Are there salt, sugar, or alcohol limitations I must heed? How much is too much? What will happen if I get it wrong?*

7. **How do I properly care for wounds and incision sites?** If there is a wound, find out how often the bandages need to be changed. Also: *Are there colors or odors to be concerned about? What kind of bandages do I need? Can I shower? Can I go in the sun?*

8. **How do I reach medical personnel?** Because complications don't happen on a schedule, you need to know how you can get in touch with the physician, or her aides, 24/7, for immediate help if something does happen. This question is essential. Get a phone number and a name to ask for.

9. When's my next appointment? Ask, *When should I come back to see you or my attending physician? What should I bring with me?*

10. What's my medication schedule? This may be one of the most important pieces of information you receive at discharge. If you need to take medications, what are they? Get both generic and brand names. *What are the dosages? What's the timing? How long do I take them for?* Get written prescriptions for all your drugs, and ask if they can call them in to your local pharmacy, so you don't have to wait to pick them up. Get your medication schedule in writing so it can be charted on a sheet of paper, with you or someone else making a check mark every time you swallow a pill. When you're in a post-hospital fog and time is amorphous, this is essential. Let's say you're in the bathroom, during your morning routine, and the phone rings. After you hang up, you're going to wonder, *Did I take that pill or not? I was reaching for the phone, and now I don't recall . . .* Now you risk taking no medication or twice the dosage you should have. Don't trust it to memory. Someone close to you ought to know exactly what your medication regimen should be and the warning signs and symptoms of an adverse reaction.

Pharmacies use computerized systems that flag when you are asking for medications that are dangerous for you (based on your profile) or that may be harmful to take in combination with another drug you are on. So it's a good idea to always go to the same pharmacy or chain. The National Patient Safety Foundation (www.npsf.org) has a helpful "Pharmacy Safety and Service" page with guidance on how to work with your pharmacist, who can be a very reliable resource for additional information on a drug's dosage, side effects, and whether it should be taken with food.

Paula, a breast cancer survivor, specifically recalls struggling to fit all her pills, with their various restrictions, into a single day.

"When you're getting chemo, you are being given a ton of medications: *This* one you're supposed to take three times a day, with food. *That* one is seven times a day on an empty stomach. There were, like, thirteen of these, and I remember just sitting down and crying, thinking, *I'm a words girl, not a numbers girl, and I will never be able to figure out the math of my medication schedule.* I researched for hours online, looking for an app to help me do it. I was so fuzzy with chemo-brain. But I was not going to be calm until I got control of the situation. I finally found a pillbox that had teeny compartments for the different hours, and you could label it. That was a lifesaver for me. Then I plugged reminders into my digital calendar that would go off: 'Take this pill. Take that pill with water . . .' I made a complete schedule for myself for every day."

Charts, pillboxes, digital reminders, apps—do what you need to do to make sure you are following your medication schedule correctly. (There are, finally, numerous apps for a variety of operating systems; a "pill reminder" search at www.appcrawlr.com will bring up the most up-to-date products.) And don't hesitate to call on your personal team, to help coordinate care or communicate for you when things slip through the cracks. You shouldn't have to suffer needlessly. You've already been through a tremendous ordeal—now is when the healing begins.

Anyone who's conquered a potentially fatal illness comes back a changed person. The crisis of confidence you may go through can take years to process. Reconnecting with friends, family members, and social groups will help you regain strength. And the best part is, they want to hear from you—they've been waiting to take you back into the fold.

I frequently hear from clients about how grateful they are for the friends who, like devoted sherpas, brought them soup, urged them on, kept them comfortable, and made them laugh. Sometimes patients get so entrenched in the logistical and clinical details that they fail to express their gratitude to these people. (On the other hand, even the most dedicated pals sometimes don't know how to react when a friend gets ill.) But by sharing these memorable moments—times when they've been helped or when they came to the aid of a sick person—they remind all of us to stay connected to one another.

I can't remember my surgery. Our minds are amazing; they close off so much of the pain. Afterward, I remember [a friend] came to the hospital. Everybody else in my family was acting a little crazy. But he was as calm as could be. He explained what was going on. As did the doctors. The healing part was painful. But he assured me I'd be well taken care of. And I was. I had two nurses who were like angels from heaven. I've met a lot of people in my ninety years, never met people like the two of them. They were superconfident, extremely knowledgeable, respectful of the doctor, and respectful of me. I don't know where they came from. And truth be told, they disappeared as they came. I never saw them again.

—Andrea, 89, obstructed-bowel surgery

Hearing from people, getting a note in the mail—it made all the difference in the world to me. But I had a couple of friends who wanted to talk on the telephone. It's one thing to call and pass along your sentiments; it's another thing to start getting mad because I'm not calling you back. People should understand that for this little window of time, it's going to have to be more of a one-way friendship. Your efforts get registered and will be paid off, but I just don't have the energy right now. When you're going through chemo, your world becomes very small. You don't leave the house except for medical appointments or a short walk. So be available for your friends, but make it loose. I loved when friends e-mailed: "Tell me a good time to come over and walk with you." Or "When can I bring you lunch?" That was so helpful. Those check-ins make you feel really good.

—Paula, 57, breast cancer

After my melanoma scare, I was told my face could never see the sun again. I'm a sun worshipper, but those days are over. A lot of friends bought me hats. One girlfriend put together a basket of lotions and products with an SPF-50 base. My mother still calls all the time, asks me how I am, and says, "Don't go in the sun. You're not going in the sun, right?" "No, mom. I'm not going in the sun. You don't have to ask me again." "Oh!" she says. "But I'm your mother. And I will."

—Marissa, 50, melanoma

Sometimes as quarterback your role is to take part in proactive dialogue with the doctors, but other times it's as small as asking, "Okay, when is your next treatment? So you're going to be feeling terrible Wednesday, Thursday, and Friday. This Saturday—I know you love Ojai—we're going to go to Ojai." Because what they want more than anything else is to have their life back. I can assure you, all the clutter gets thrown out the window in about a nanosecond, and all they want are the little things. They may forget that they love having a night away, or that they want to see a play, or that they crave a certain meal—whatever it is, help to give them back the jewels of their life whenever possible.

—Jack, 40, devoted quarterback to
mother-in-law with metastatic melanoma

Once you start to tackle the medical components of your disease, do not dismiss the emotional components. And don't let anyone tell you to "put that on the back burner, you'll deal with that later." I'd make it a part of the mix from the very beginning. Maybe line up a psychologist. Because it's really very emotional.

—Susan, 38, ovarian cancer

You can never have enough information or ask too many questions. Don't be afraid to challenge a doctor, or a hospital, and their decisions. I think it's important, before any surgery, that the family members and the patient have a conversation about what their wishes would be if, God forbid, something goes wrong. Would they want the family to fight for as long as they can? Is there a certain period of time when you just know that it's time? Everyone has to understand the wishes of the patient and be prepared to have to make the hardest decision of your life.

—Kelly, 27, helped navigate her father's recovery
from a botched heart surgery

My wife had metastatic breast cancer, and she was going back to the hospital for a short stay for a procedure. She was still on chemo and miserable. So I asked, "Need anything while you're away? What can I get you?" I'm thinking along the lines of "a book," whatever, something trivial. She says, "A new bed." Okay! I called one of her very closest friends. "I got it," she says, "don't worry about it." The next day my brother-in-law and his wife are running around, asking, "What can we do? Does she need new sheets?" We got it all delivered, set up, cleaned up her room. She came back home and went to her new bed. "What do you think?" I asked. She said one word: "Heaven."

—Seth, 49, loving spouse

There's a dog park where my wife and I take our dogs every day. After my surgery, I said, "Honey, can you pick up the dog's poop? I'd like to, but I have cancer." I played that for all it was worth for a while.

—Patrick, 65, prostate cancer

A friend kept sending me these ridiculous, funny images of animals. I'm not an animal person, but they were really goofy. I would get them once a week in an e-mail. It didn't require a conversation. It was just: "This guy loves me, and is thinking of me, and wants to make me smile."

—Jenna, 29, leukemia

If I had not had this problem, I wouldn't have retired. Now my wife and I wake up happy. We take morning walks. We eat almost all our meals together because she loves to cook, and I'm a great table setter. We play together. I could have done it ten years ago, but I didn't know how. I'm not Jewish, but I've been to Passover seders, and I love the story about freedom. The way our friend tells it is that the Jews were at the water's edge, the pharaoh was coming back, and not everybody went into the sea. Some said, "I'm going to go back into slavery because I feel comfortable with what I know." Some said, "I'm not going back to slavery for any reason," and they jumped into the water. The sea only parted after they jumped into the water. Which is to say: You have to make the decision to let go. But it's not easy, because there's no model of how to do it. I've had a successful thirty-year career—now it's time to reinvent myself? Turn it off, and start over again? That's a hard transition. For ten years, I had one foot in and one foot out. But this episode finally made me say: Jump.

—Jim, 65, lung disease

QUICK GUIDE

CHAPTER 12. Step 4—Coordination

- Coordination begins long before you go to the hospital, and it doesn't end until after you have returned home and recovered to the point that you can manage on your own again.

- Ask your support person to help you with appointments; with record distribution in advance of a consult; and with note taking during meetings.

- Be mindful of the times when coordination is crucial to your safety: (1) during the course of treatment, and (2) at the "intersections" of care, including during and after a hospital stay.

- Update your Medical Summary and distribute it to your doctors. Communicating with your physicians about your health history, medications, and any changes will give them the opportunity to better care for you.

- When necessary, ask your PCP or a trusted advocate to initiate a conference call with your doctors to get your care back on track.

- If your care starts to feel conductorless during a hospital stay, ask the charge nurse to facilitate a family meeting with the attending physician.

- In a hospital, you are most vulnerable to harm at medical intersections, i.e., when you are being transferred from an emergency room to surgery on a different floor with a new team; during the hand-off from the night shift to the morning staff;

or when you're being sent home to recuperate. Effective communication at these junctures can help keep you safe.

- At the beginning of your hospital admission, (1) introduce yourself and your support person to your caregivers and provide them with his or her cell phone number, and any forms that grant them legal rights over your care; (2) bring medical, organizational, and personal information with you that will make you stand out as a patient and help prevent medical errors.

- Work to proactively prevent hospital-acquired conditions and medical errors by (1) inquiring about any new drugs you are given; (2) being alert to seemingly unnecessary tests or treatments; (3) communicating any new symptoms or signs of an infection quickly to your caregivers; (4) reminding doctors and nurses to wash their hands before working with you, if you think they haven't; (5) making sure caregivers know your health status, including allergies; and (6) checking your chart to be sure your information is accurate.

- The ten things you need to ask before you leave the hospital are: (1) Has my diagnosis changed? (2) What was the ultimate treatment? (3) What should I expect during my recovery? (4) What sort of equipment will I need? (5) What activities should I avoid and what do I need to do? (6) Are there any dietary restrictions I need to follow? (7) How do I properly care for wounds and incision sites? (8) How do I reach medical personnel? (9) When's my next appointment? (10) and very important: What's my medication schedule?

- The crisis of confidence some people go through after a serious illness can take years to process. Reconnect with friends, family members, and social groups to regain your strength.

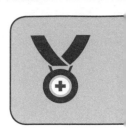

CHAPTER THIRTEEN

COMPETENCE AND COURAGE

Now that you've got it, lead the way.

Some people mistakenly believe that being rich is a safeguard against receiving poor care. Having worked with some pretty wealthy folks, I can tell you it just isn't so. The most well-connected and resourced patients often get terrible care. The reasons are many: they rush to treatment without asking enough questions or getting expert opinions; they go to their small community hospital for big, complicated procedures; or they commit their well-being to a trendy, brand-name doctor, even when their gut is telling them that this person has little investment in their care.

Even worse, I've seen desperate patients, with plenty of means but little judgment, fall for false-hope purveyors who promise easy, "natural" cures that actually do more harm than help. Steve Jobs is a prime example of a man whose intelligence and fortune were useless to him when it came to choosing appropriate treatment.

In October 2003, during a CT scan of his kidneys (he'd had problems with kidney stones), doctors unexpectedly found a shadow on the Apple cofounder's pancreas. "Incidental findings"—things that show up when you're not looking for them—often are a gift: The disease is caught even before the patient has symptoms, when it is more likely to be curable. In Jobs's case, the shadowy finding turned out to be a pancreatic neuroendocrine tumor, a rare and slow-growing type of cancer for which every single competent physician (Jobs's included) would have recommended surgery.

But Jobs was an independent thinker, for better and for worse. Despite the urging of his physicians, friends, and family, he decided not to have the tumor removed. Instead, he tried to heal himself with diet, meditation, and "natural healing" techniques that included juice fasts and colon hydrotherapy. Nine months later the tumor had grown. He finally agreed to surgery, but by then the opportunity for a cure had been squandered. His surgeons found three liver metastases, meaning that his cancer had spread. In 2009 Jobs had a liver transplant. By October 2011 he was dead. It's impossible to know for certain, but there is every reason to believe that his tragic demise at age fifty-six could have been avoided. His biographer, Walter Isaacson, noted a hint of regret in Jobs's voice when he described his early treatment decisions.

You do not need wealth to get excellent medical care. What you really need—and what you now have—is competence and courage. You will be a far smarter patient for following the lessons in this book. You have power as a health care consumer.

My greatest passion in life is helping people from all walks of life get better care. As a much younger man, I spent some years in the trenches of government, hitting my head against the wall trying to reform the health care system. God bless! I cry *uncle*. Now I help real people with real medical problems to get the best care from a broken system. And I'm so much happier for it. The truth is, I couldn't change *anything* back in the day. Every administration from Eisenhower to Obama has tried.

John T. James, the founder of Patient Safety America and a former chief toxicologist for NASA, testified before Congress in 2014 about his exhaustive study that revealed that preventable harm in our hospitals contributes to 400,000 deaths a year. He was counting his son Alex among those lives lost: At nineteen, Alex collapsed during a run and never recovered. As James slowly pieced together the events, he came to believe that grievous medical errors and negligence had contributed to Alex's tragic death.

James has since devoted his life to educating people about the dangers they face anytime they seek out medical care. "You've got to do your homework going in, and you really need an advocate," he says. "If you are not able to advocate for yourself, you need to bring somebody with you who's assertive, knowledgeable, and doesn't take BS for explanations."

James's thorough review of the literature and updated figures on medical error have been lauded by veteran patient-safety experts, who agree that too many people are still being harmed by medical care. Sadly, it's a decades-old problem that's seen little improvement.

"My opinion," says James, "is everybody is trying to fix the system from within, so you have all these hospital checklists and people saying, 'We're going to have a safety culture,' and so forth—but it's not working. What you've got to do is really and truly empower patients to be smart consumers. You've got to just blow the system wide open. . . . If you empower the patient, the system will fix itself. But that's a major change."

Call me a dreamer, but I believe that major change is possible. And it starts with you. By developing a strong bond with a primary care physician, you are investing in your future health and signaling to the medical community that you take your own care seriously. By researching your condition, asking pertinent questions about treatment plans, and getting opinions from specialists who have deep expertise in your specific illness, you're keeping doctors on their toes and exercising your right to make better, more informed choices.

And if a day comes when you face a hard diagnosis, by thoughtfully following the steps of Intensive Case Management, you will impress upon caregivers and hospital staff that you *get it*—you understand how difficult their jobs are, you are aware of the challenges and risks, you know that care can become fragmented. Yet you are staying in charge. You're partnering with your medical team in a way that ensures that *your* expectations, goals, and values are being met. If everyone did this, it would bring about a profound change in the relationships between patients and their physicians, nurses, and caregivers. And that's the only way the health care system will ever truly change.

➤ One Final Thought

Elie Wiesel, the Nobel Peace Prize winner, educator, and humanitarian, was an emaciated teenager on the brink of death when he was liberated from the concentration camp at Buchenwald in April 1945. His parents and a sister had already perished in the Holocaust. Asked once by an interviewer if it was a burden to have been chosen by God to go on living, he replied, "I say to myself, since I did survive, my duty is to do something with my survival. I try. I'm not sure I've succeeded, but I try."

If anyone deserved to retreat into a quiet, simple existence and never speak again of horrific suffering endured, it's Wiesel. Yet he bravely spoke out on behalf of victims of genocide and civil war. He wrote books, taught, and ran a foundation that combats indifference, intolerance, and injustice around the world.

If you have come through a life-threatening illness, the best way to do something with *your* survival is simple: Use your experience to help someone else. This is not to imply in any way that beating cancer, heart failure, or some other health crisis is akin to surviving Buchenwald. It is Wiesel's *spirit* of duty—of taking pain and suffering and turning it into something helpful for others—that speaks to our power to seize a dark chapter of our lives and infuse it with light.

There are times when I've assisted a friend or family member with a complex medical situation, and after their recovery, they ask how they can return the favor. My response is always the same: Would you speak with another patient who is battling the same illness? In some Christian ministries this kind of support is called "coming alongside."

You are in a unique position, no matter your religious beliefs, to come alongside another person who is suffering. You've been entrenched in the health care system. You've had surprises, good and bad. Sometimes your care was far better than you dreamed possible and other times far worse. You know what you wished others had warned you about. You understand how powerful the nausea and fatigue of chemotherapy can be; what it's like to see more and more of your hair in the shower drain; and how conflicted you were—*Am I doing more harm to my body than good?*—each time you went back for another radiation treatment. The fact that you have prevailed over your disease may help another person envision his or her own successful recovery.

How does one begin? It depends on your talents, your time, and where you are in your life. But it can be as simple as reaching out to someone who has recently received a similar diagnosis and letting them know you're there, if they want to talk. Every disease has a philanthropy that needs volunteers. The hospital where you received treatment likely has a support group that you can join to share your experience and lend an ear to patients who are confused or upset.

Some people take great pleasure volunteering for the arts programs at the hospitals that treated them. Others write insightful blogs, of the kind you may have referred to during your illness. When a patient learns that the spot on her face is Stage II melanoma, reading a three-year chronicle of someone else's surgery, complete with untouched recovery photos, is a great reducer of fear. I also invite you to visit www.PatientsPlaybook.com, to share your story. (You'll find as well valuable resources including my "No-Mistake Zone" podcast, links to helpful websites, questions to ask your physicians, forms to get your medical records binder started, and much more.)

However you decide to engage, do so without judgment. If, for instance, a friend opts for a course of treatment that's different from the one you chose (and which you may not think is right for him), show restraint and respect for his decision. There is no one-size-fits-all healing plan. Listen carefully, so you can hear what he really needs from you.

When you've come through the worst of your illness, and you're finally feeling better about the future, I challenge you to sit down and think about how to help somebody else. You'll receive tremendous satisfaction and a greater degree of closure on this chapter of your life if you are able to give back—if you *do* something with your survival.

ACKNOWLEDGMENTS

This book reflects my life's work. And it wouldn't have been possible without Beth, my wife of thirty-six years and the most important person in my life. Her steadfast support, love, and unwavering belief in me are well beyond anything I deserve. Over the many years, she and my daughters, Laura Michelson and Julia Richter, and my son-in-law Ian Richter, have graciously endured my being late to, or called away early from, dinners, soccer games, and important events by patients who needed my help. Along with my sister, Randy Michelson, my family has served as a full-service support team, reviewing manuscripts, refining my thinking, and giving me courage. This book truly has been a family effort, with even my parents serving as my first "patients."

Lisa Sweetingham has been my full-time collaborator for more than two years. She is an indispensable writing partner and deserves the most special recognition and gratitude for her exceptional work. Lisa spent months studying my approaches to health care; sorted through complex information from multiple sources; and conducted interviews with many physicians and patients to find key messages and convey them to readers with clarity, emotion, and encouragement.

In 1988, Dr. Robert Brook, then the head of health research at RAND, took me under his wing and spent years helping me understand how health services researchers think and how their discoveries could be used by patients to obtain higher-quality medical care. His guidance enabled me to incorporate this enormous and insightful body of knowledge into my work.

I also want to thank the extraordinary practicing physicians who found innovative ways to engage patients as integral participants in their own care. Without them, I'd have had no models to emulate. The late Dr. David Rimoin, one of the first medical genetics experts, was one of my most important mentors. An outstanding clinician, researcher, and teacher, he is the standard by which I measure others. Dr. Bryan Arling, my internist when I lived in Washington, D.C., taught me the core importance of primary care, while proving that it can be provided thoroughly, thoughtfully, and efficiently. The data-driven Dr. Bob Oye, my internist now, and the executive vice chair of clinical services at UCLA, showed me how research findings can be used to improve clinical practice—even in a busy, urban teaching hospital like UCLA. Dr. Anthony D'Amico, the chief of genitourinary radiation oncology at Dana-Farber Cancer Institute and the Brigham and Women's Hospital, has an encyclopedic mastery of the literature on prostate cancer, and a remarkable ability to apply research findings to individual cases while being acutely sensitive to each patient's anxiety and concerns.

The incomparable Dr. Bob Simon, who serves as medical director of my company, Private Health Management, understands how all of the body's systems interact and has an uncommon capacity to care for people in every sense of the word. Dr. Simon is proudly old-fashioned, conducting the most meticulous physical exams imaginable (a vanishing art, sadly). He has made life-saving findings in minutes or hours—diagnoses other physicians missed over months and years. I wish all physicians could learn Dr. Simon's skills. Dr. Bruce Logan, an internist and former hospital CEO in New York City, has also solved numerous complex cases that legions of other physicians could not figure. A devout believer in the importance of prevention, especially for cardiovascular issues, Dr. Logan takes a very comprehensive approach and does everything possible to encourage his patients to lead healthier lives.

I am especially grateful to Dr. Peter Scardino, the chairman of surgery and urology at Memorial Sloan Kettering Cancer Center, for his willingness to write the foreword to this book. His surgical practice functions at the highest level, with a distinct culture of excellence in both clinical care and patient service. Dr. Scardino's credentials are among the most impressive in all of medicine, yet he is one of the most down-to-earth, earnest, and unassuming people I know. Two exceptional physicians, Dr. Gail Roboz, professor of medicine and director of the leukemia program at the Weill Medical College of Cornell University and the NewYork–Presbyterian Hospital, and Dr. Albert Knapp, clinical professor of gastroenterology at the New York University School of Medicine, took the time to generously provide insightful feedback on the manuscript, for which I am very thankful.

I also want to thank the many talented physicians, caregivers, and other experts in their fields who provided inspiration or agreed to be interviewed for the book: Dr. Sonu Ahluwalia, Dr. C. Noel Bairey Merz, Dr. Christopher Barley, Dr. John Bilezikian, Dr. James Blake, Dr. Philip Bretsky, Dr. Michael Callahan, Dr. Peter Carroll, Dr. Carrie Carter, Martin Chalifour, Diana Clark, Dr. Don Coffey, Dr. Ken Cohen, Dr. Ram Dandillaya, Dr. Michael Davidson, Patricia Donovan, Dr. Anthony El-Khoueiry, Dr. Sheldon Elman, Dr. Justin Fagan, Dr. Jonathan Fielding, Dr. Michael Friedman, Dr. Jeffrey Gelfand, Eva Gordon, Tom Gordon, Dr. Michelle Israel, John T. James, Dr. Peter Julien, Dr. Andrew Klein, Dr. Michael Levine, Dr. Mark Litwin, Dr. Chris Logothetis, Antonia Maioni, Dr. Philip Mease, Dr. Mark Moyad, Dr. David Ng, Dr. Allyson Ocean, Arden O'Connor, Dr. Neda Pakdaman, Jennifer Peña, Dr. Ed Phillips, Dr. Dan Plotkin, Dr. Eugene Sayfie, Dr. Ted Schaeffer, Dr. Howard Scher, Dr. Marc Selner, Dr. Katy Setoodeh, Dr. Michael Sucher, Dr. Joe Sugarman, Dr. Steven Tabak, Dr. Shi-Ming Tu, Dr. Robert Udelsman, Dr. Andy von Eschenbach, Dr. Michael Wechsler, Dr. George Wilding, and Dr. Lorraine Young.

I have spent decades helping countless people get better care, and without that experience I would not have learned enough to write this book. I am so grateful to those who put their trust in me, especially at the outset when I lacked experience and could offer only my commitment to work as hard as I could and to care as much as my heart would allow. Managing their cases enabled me to see the patterns, develop the techniques, and provide the insights reflected here.

As part of our research, we conducted interviews with nearly three dozen patients and/or their family members to ensure that we captured their experiences accurately. Without exception, each person spoke in great detail, generously giving as much time as needed. I would like to thank every one by name, but out of respect for their privacy, I will thank each individually.

Elise O'Shaughnessy, the formidable *Vanity Fair* editor and writer, was invaluable from the beginning. She brought her red pen and sharp wit to the proposal and early drafts of the manuscript, along with a title suggestion—*The Patient's Playbook*—that won us all over. Health care journalist Shira Berman provided expert research and feedback. Before I started working on this book, Jill Posnick and Tania Pantoja helped me find my writing voice and draw attention to early versions of the teachings in this book.

Lyn Benjamin was one of my first advisers, enabling me to benefit from her experience and expertise in building businesses in the rapidly evolving media world. Lyn has been a source of consistent reassurance, bolstering my confidence whenever it wavered.

Special thanks to Mike Milken, Dr. Skip Holden, Andy Grove, and the other members of the board of the Prostate Cancer Foundation (PCF) who gave me an opportunity to serve as CEO of that extraordinary organization. I have little doubt that PCF and the research community it supports will one day transform the disease into a chronic nonfatal condition for most men. During my tenure, I saw the difference in outcomes when top physician-scientists who are driving research also treat cancer patients. Their talent and dedication was one of my motivations to undertake this project.

When I first began thinking about a book, many authors told me that I would be disappointed in my agent and my publisher, no matter who I selected. My experience has been the exact opposite: I cannot imagine how any agent or publisher could have been more helpful, productive, and committed than Kathy Robbins and Anne Messitte of Alfred A. Knopf.

About ten minutes into our first meeting I asked Kathy if she was "in." She responded, "More than I could imagine," and she delivered. Kathy patiently taught me about the publishing industry, coached me on how to become an author, and diligently read every draft of the manuscript. She used her practical experience to prepare me for each milestone, her emotional intelligence to keep me in balance, her business skills to identify the optimal publisher, and her fundamental decency and integrity to create an outstanding partnership. David Halpern, her fellow agent, provided deeply perceptive advice and guidance throughout the process, and the entire Robbins Office team lent comprehensive support beyond anything I could have reasonably expected.

Anne Messitte, the executive vice president of Knopf Doubleday and publisher of Vintage Anchor Books, has been nothing short of remarkable. Her extensive experience and superior skills have been pivotal in making the book engaging and actionable. Anne believed this book could improve the lives and well-being of countless readers, and harnessed Knopf's considerable talent, power, and resources to make our shared vision a reality. She and Edward Kastenmeier, the vice president and executive editor of Vintage Books, both meticulously and elegantly edited numerous drafts of the manuscript and worked very closely with Lisa and me to get the tone, structure, and balance exactly right.

I should be envied by every author for having the caliber of the Knopf team at my side. Tony Chirico, Paul Bogaards, Chris Gillespie, Anne-Lise Spitzer, Sara Eagle, and Jessica Purcell were there from the outset, implementing creative and innovative strategies and programs to introduce and establish the book. Peter Mendelsund, an insightful and talented designer, developed a distinctive cover that succinctly creates an ideal entry into the book and created the icons inside. Claudia Martinez designed an elegant interior layout that helps structure the content so that readers can rapidly and easily understand it. And when it was time to launch the paperback edition, Vintage picked up the torch and reignited the fire. I owe deep appreciation to Beth Lamb, Russell Perreault, Barbara Richard, Paige Smith, Jessica Deitcher, and Jennifer Marshall, who provided just the expertise, enthusiasm, and energy we needed. Jaime de Pablos, Ingrid Paredes, and Felipe Silva of Vintage Español ensured that our message is readily available to the tens of millions of native Spanish speakers in the U.S. Special thanks to Kim Thornton Ingenito and Tiffany Tomlin of the Penguin Random House Speakers Bureau for giving me a bigger soapbox. And to Eliza Hanson, who has deftly managed lots of complex logistics.

Over the years, the team at Private Health Management has helped put my ideas into practice and improve them immeasurably. Gregg Britt, Debbie Bohnett, Jennifer Peña, Eva Gordon, Tom Compere, and Dr. Simon all arrived at our innovative company with very different backgrounds. None of us really knew what we were getting into, but all of us were unconditionally bound to helping patients and took the risk that we would figure it out. They in turn recruited a cadre of top-notch clinicians, researchers, and administrators, including Carolina Rodriguez, Carrie Davis, Jessica Zambelli, Laura Kusminsky, Kelly Bernard, Monica Arevalos, and many others who work without stint to provide our clients with uncompromising care.

Gregg Britt, my cofounder, business partner, and friend beyond compare, deserves an entire acknowledgment section of his own. Gregg has been most influential in extending my ideas, simplifying them, and converting them into practice, while generating his own invaluable insights. The staff, patients, and physicians we work with rely on and respect him tremendously. Gregg knows more about how to get the best medical care than anyone I know.

Special notice must be given to Melissa Handy, my phenomenal executive assistant. My work style is quite intense and Melissa has the rare ability to coordinate complicated logistics, juggle competing priorities, and keep track of everything, all while maintaining a sunny, calm disposition. I am remarkably fortunate to work with her.

Among my most precious blessings are my many wonderful friends who have provided invaluable inspiration, support, and stimulation. I hope you all know how grateful I am for your commitment to me, my work, and my family. I have also benefited from the personal attention of talented and caring teachers, including Nick Wellner and Oliver Young in Union, New Jersey; Professor Maurice Mandelbaum and Dr. Robert Athanasiou at the Johns Hopkins University; and the JHU medical school faculty and staff, who inspired my career direction. At Yale Law School, virtually every professor was brilliant and, although it was never easy, each taught me something that is reflected in this book. I want to pay special thanks to Judge Guido Calabresi, who gave me the courage and competence to investigate facts in order to discover new truths. I use his teachings every day.

The long journey to this publication marks a beginning, not an ending. Which is why I need also to acknowledge you, the reader, for the persistence and energy you bring to becoming a more effective patient. As you inspire loved ones, friends, and coworkers to find the courage and competence to get the best medical care, you are bringing about a much-needed cultural shift that will improve the lives of people everywhere for generations to come. Thank you.

APPENDIX

RESOURCES TO HELP YOU ACHIEVE
A LIFETIME OF BETTER HEALTH

How to Make Your Medical Records Binder: Step by Step

Medical Records Binder Cover Sheet

Medical Summary

Medical Records Worksheet

Family Health History

Emergency Information

Standard HIPAA Release Form

My Pill Inventory

The Six Websites You Need to Know About for Serious Illnesses

HOW TO MAKE YOUR MEDICAL RECORDS BINDER: STEP BY STEP

It's so important to be prepared for the day when medical issues arise. The worksheets in this appendix are designed to help you complete three practical steps you can take now to achieve better health preparedness. Those steps are:

1. Collect your medical records and organize them into a binder.
2. Create a family health history.
3. Make an emergency information card to keep in your wallet or purse.

The inside of your medical records binder is composed of four main parts:

- Cover Page
- Medical Summary
- Medical Records
- Family Health History

First Steps:

1. You'll need:
   - A thick (at least two inches), sturdy binder with a clear-sleeve cover, plus sleeves on the inside to hold copies of imaging disks
   - Tab dividers
   - Three-hole-punch paper for copies and/or a manual hole-puncher
2. Add a cover page to the sleeve on the front of your binder. See page 287 for an example. You can use the cover page included at the end of these instructions or create your own. Be sure that the words "Medical Records," the patient's name, and the appropriate contact information are printed on the cover page.
3. Your first tab divider is your "Medical Summary," which provides physicians with a picture of your health status. See page 289 for guidance on how to create yours.
4. Next is your "Medical Records" tab. See page 291 for an example. This section includes an inventory of all of your physician consultation files and hospital records. Gather your medical records using the detailed

instructions provided in Chapter 3, and the Medical Records Worksheet that follows this section. Your records should be tab-organized by medical specialty (in alphabetical order), then by physician name (also alphabetically ordered). And be sure to place your records in reverse chronological order, so that the most recent record from each physician is on top when you open to that doctor's tab. Your hospital records can go last.

5. The next tab is for your "Family Health History." See page 295 for this form and guidance on what it should include.

So, for example, if you have records you've collected from your ENTs, an internist, neurologists, and rheumatologists, you'd divide them in the following manner, using separate tabs.

Ear, Nose, and Throat
- Dr. Jones (after each doctor's name place all records from that doctor in reverse chronological order)
- Dr. Smith

Internal Medicine
- Dr. Adams

Neurology
- Dr. Fisher
- Dr. Jackson

Rheumatology
- Dr. Patel
- Dr. Robbins

6. Finally, any disks with imaging or other materials relevant to your care can be placed in the inside sleeve or pocket of your binder.

Bring this binder with you to physician consultations so that your doctors can review and make copies of your complete medical history for their own files. This binder is a crucial body of medical evidence about you. And it will give your physicians many of the important facts they need to know in order to help you live a longer, healthier life.

MEDICAL RECORDS

for

_____

Phone(s): _____

Email: _____

Emergency Contact: _____

MEDICAL SUMMARY

The first few pages of your records binder consist of your Medical Summary—an important document about YOU. This summary signals to your doctors that you are bringing your A-game to the consultation. Writing a Medical Summary is a crucial step when you're dealing with a newly diagnosed serious illness, a chronic issue that needs better management, or a mysterious condition that no one seems to be able to figure out. It provides your doctors with a snapshot of your health status, while highlighting medical events they may want to investigate further within your medical records binder.

A Medical Summary, whether you're making it for yourself or for a loved one, should include the following:

1. The patient's name and date of birth
2. Any known allergies
3. A few sentences about the patient's current health as it relates to the answers they are seeking

For example:

> *This sixty-seven-year-old patient has had eye irritation (redness, dryness, discharge) since February 2015. Symptoms began at the end of a cold/flu and have not abated. He's received no relief after several rounds of antibiotic treatments and is seeking help.*

4. A few sentences about any past conditions or surgeries, as well as current coexisting conditions. For example:

> *Patient has mild psoriasis; hyperlipidemia; positive hepatitis B status but asymptomatic and not being treated; underwent knee replacement surgery*

in 2011. No known previous eye problems reported. Is not taking any prescribed medications. Occasionally takes an OTC multivitamin supplement. General good health.

5. Next, comes a chronological narrative of the current problem and steps the patient has taken to solve it, including what worked and what didn't. For example:

2/2015: Patient developed a serious cold or flu, which persisted for a week. Over the course of a few months, other family members came down with similar cold/flu symptoms that ended with an eye infection—but their symptoms cleared up after a week and patient's did not. By late February, patient developed more serious redness, tearing, and discharge in both eyes equally.

3/9/2015: Visited internist. Diagnosed with conjunctivitis and prescribed **Maxitrol***, 3.5 mg drops (every four hours for seven days). Eyes did not get better.*

4/1/2015: Visited ophthalmologist. Diagnosed with conjunctivitis and allergies and began new prescriptions:

- **FML Forte** *.25% eye drops (1 drop 4x day)*
- **Gatifloxicin** *.5% eye drops (1 drop 4x day)*
- **Bacitracin** *500 units/gm (apply to both eyes at bedtime)*

5/2015: Patient reports no relief after the above treatment round, in fact his eyes feel much worse (more inflammation and dryness).

And so on, until you arrive at the present time.

Deciding the time to write a Medical Summary will depend on your health status. If you're generally well and have no serious problems, just complete numbers 1 to 3. When a health problem arises, make your summary more detailed to give specialists the clues they need to get you to a successful diagnosis and treatment sooner and more efficiently.

MEDICAL RECORDS WORKSHEET

These forms can help you begin the process of collecting your medical records. Call the office of your Primary Care Physician (PCP) and request a copy of your medical files, either for pick up, regular mail, or email if they are able to send digital copies.

PRIMARY CARE

My PCP: _____

Primary Contact Info (email/phone): _____

_____

File Request Date and Method: _____

Comments: _____

_____

_____

File Received Date: _____

Previous PCP: _____

Primary Contact Info (email/phone): _____

_____

File Request Date and Method: _____

Comments: _____

_____

_____

File Received Date: _____

Call the offices of other specialists and hospitals that have cared for you in the past ten years—especially for any surgical procedures or major medical events—and request a copy of your complete medical records.

SPECIALIST CARE

Doctor #1: _____

Primary Contact Info (email/phone): _____

_____

File Request Date and Method: _____

Comments: _____

_____

_____

File Received Date: _____

Doctor #2: _____

Primary Contact Info (email/phone): _____

_____

File Request Date and Method _____

Comments: _____

_____

_____

File Received Date: _____

Doctor #3: _____

Primary Contact Info (email/phone): _____

_____

File Request Date and Method: _____

Comments: _____

_____

_____

File Received Date: _____

Doctor #4: _____

Primary Contact Info (email/phone): _____

_____

File Request Date and Method _____

Comments: _____

_____

_____

File Received Date: _____

HOSPITALS

Hospital #1: _____

Primary Contact Info (email/phone): _____

_____

File Request Date and Method: _____

Comments: _____

_____

_____

File Received Date: _____

Hospital #2: _____

Primary Contact Info (email/phone): _____

_____

File Request Date and Method: _____

Comments: _____

_____

_____

File Received Date: _____

Hospital #3: _____

Primary Contact Info (email/phone): _____

_____

File Request Date and Method: _____

Comments: _____

_____

_____

File Received Date: _____

FAMILY HEALTH HISTORY

A health history based on the collective memories of your closest relatives can give your physicians the information they need to better prevent and treat potential illness. At a minimum, plot the serious medical problems of parents and siblings—the closer the relation, the more significant the information. Use that information to complete the Family Health History below.

I. MY PARENTS

1. If alive, what is their current and historical health status? (Any significant diseases, such as diabetes, cancer, heart disease, autoimmune disorders, etc.?):

_____

_____

_____

_____

_____

2. If deceased, what is the date, age, and cause of death?

_____

_____

_____

_____

_____

3. Any known inherited genetic disorders, mysterious conditions or symptoms, or allergies? (For example: positive for BRCA mutation, unexplained anemia, penicillin or peanut allergies, etc.)

_____

_____

_____

_____

_____

II. MY SIBLINGS

1. If alive, what is their current and historical health status? (Any significant diseases, such as diabetes, cancer, heart disease, autoimmune disorders, etc.?):

_____

_____

_____

_____

_____

2. If deceased, what is the date, age, and cause of death?

_____

_____

_____

_____

3. Any known inherited genetic disorders, mysterious conditions or symptoms, or allergies?

_____

_____

_____

_____

III. MY GRANDPARENTS AND GREAT-GRANDPARENTS

1. If alive, what is their current and historical health status? (Any significant diseases, such as diabetes, cancer, heart disease, autoimmune disorders, etc?):

_____

_____

_____

_____

_____

2. If deceased, what is the date, age, and cause of death?

_____

_____

_____

_____

_____

3. Any known inherited genetic disorders, mysterious conditions or symptoms, or allergies?

_____

_____

_____

_____

_____

IV. MY OTHER BLOOD RELATIVES

1. If alive, what is their current and historical health status? (Any significant diseases, such as diabetes, cancer, heart disease, autoimmune disorders, etc.?):

    _____

    _____

    _____

    _____

    _____

2. If deceased, what is the date, age, and cause of death?

    _____

    _____

    _____

    _____

    _____

3. Any known inherited genetic disorders, mysterious conditions or symptoms, or allergies?

    _____

    _____

    _____

    _____

    _____

EMERGENCY INFORMATION

Copy and fill out this emergency form for everyone in your family. At a minimum, create an inventory of the most pertinent medical details and keep this information in your purse or wallet—because that's the first place a medical responder will look during an emergency.

My name: _____

Please contact (name/phone): _____

_____

My primary care physician (name/phone): _____

_____

My allergies: _____

_____

My medical conditions and major surgeries: _____

_____

_____

_____

_____

Medications I'm taking: _____

_____

_____

_____

My other doctors (cardiologist, oncologist, etc.) who should be notified are (name/phone): _____

_____

_____

_____

Additional emergency info: _____

_____

_____

_____

STANDARD HIPAA RELEASE FORM

Medical Information Release (HIPAA Release Form) for:
Name: _____
Date of Birth: _____/_____/_____

HEALTH INFORMATION TO BE DISCLOSED
(CHECK ALL THAT APPLY):

[ ] I authorize the release of my complete health record (including records relating to mental health care, communicable diseases, HIV or AIDS, and treatment of alcohol or drug abuse).

OR

[ ] I authorize the release of my complete health record with the exception of the following information:
    [ ] Mental health records
    [ ] Communicable diseases (including HIV and AIDS)
    [ ] Alcohol/drug abuse treatment
    [ ] Other (please specify): _____

Recipient of Information (I authorize the release of this information to):
[ ] Me
[ ] Spouse
[ ] Children
[ ] Other (please specify): _____

This Release of Information will remain in effect until _____/_____/_____, or when terminated by me in writing.

For messages, please call:

[ ] My home: _____

[ ] My work: _____

[ ] My cell: _____

If unable to reach me:

[ ] You may leave a detailed message.

[ ] Please leave a message asking me to return your call.

[ ] _____

The best time to reach me is (day) _____

between (time)_____ and _____.

Signed: _____ Date: _____

Witness: _____ Date: _____

MY PILL INVENTORY

Adverse drug reactions are dangerous. By maintaining an up-to-date list of the medications, vitamins and/or supplements, and OTC pills you're taking, you're helping your caregivers to keep your medication schedule on track and giving your doctors the information they need to pinpoint potential problems and prevent harmful drug interactions.

PRESCRIPTIONS

Brand Name: _____

Generic: _____

Dosage: I take ____ (amount, e.g., 10 mg) ____times per day/week/other

This pill looks like: _____ (example: "small blue oval")

I take this for: _____

Doctor(s) who prescribed it: _____

Approximate date I started taking this: _____

Brand Name: _____

Generic: _____

Dosage: I take ____ (amount, e.g., 10 mg) ____times per day/week/other

This pill looks like: _____ (example: "small blue oval")

I take this for: _____

Doctor(s) who prescribed it: _____

Approximate date I started taking this: _____

Brand Name: _____

Generic: _____

Dosage: I take ____ (amount, e.g., 10 mg) ____times per day/week/other

This pill looks like: _____ (example: "small blue oval")

I take this for: _____

Doctor(s) who prescribed it: _____

Approximate date I started taking this: _____

Brand Name: _____

Generic: _____

Dosage: I take _____ (amount, e.g., 10 mg) _____times per day/week/other

This pill looks like: _____ (example: "small blue oval")

I take this for: _____

Doctor(s) who prescribed it: _____

Approximate date I started taking this: _____

Brand Name: _____

Generic: _____

Dosage: I take _____ (amount, e.g., 10 mg) _____times per day/week/other

This pill looks like: _____ (example: "small blue oval")

I take this for: _____

Doctor(s) who prescribed it: _____

Approximate date I started taking this: _____

Brand Name: _____

Generic: _____

Dosage: I take _____ (amount, e.g., 10 mg) _____times per day/week/other

This pill looks like: _____ (example: "small blue oval")

I take this for: _____

Doctor(s) who prescribed it: _____

Approximate date I started taking this: _____

Brand Name: _____

Generic: _____

Dosage: I take _____ (amount, e.g., 10 mg) _____times per day/week/other

This pill looks like: _____ (example: "small blue oval")

I take this for: _____

Doctor(s) who prescribed it: _____

Approximate date I started taking this: _____

Brand Name: _____

Generic: _____

Dosage: I take _____ (amount, e.g., 10 mg) _____times per day/week/other

This pill looks like: _____ (example: "small blue oval")

I take this for: _____

Doctor(s) who prescribed it: _____

Approximate date I started taking this: _____

OVER-THE-COUNTER MEDICATIONS

Brand Name: _____

Dosage: I take _____ (amount, e.g., 10 mg) _____times per day/week/other

This pill looks like: _____ (example: "small blue oval")

I take this for: _____

Doctor(s) who prescribed it: _____

Approximate date I started taking this: _____

Brand Name: _____

Dosage: I take _____ (amount, e.g., 10 mg) _____times per day/week/other

This pill looks like: _____ (example: "small blue oval")

I take this for: _____

Doctor(s) who prescribed it: _____

Approximate date I started taking this: _____

Brand Name: _____

Dosage: I take _____ (amount, e.g., 10 mg) _____times per day/week/other

This pill looks like: _____ (example: "small blue oval")

I take this for: _____

Doctor(s) who prescribed it: _____

Approximate date I started taking this: _____

Brand Name: _____

Dosage: I take _____ (amount, e.g., 10 mg) _____times per day/week/other

This pill looks like: _____ (example: "small blue oval")

I take this for: _____

Doctor(s) who prescribed it: _____

Approximate date I started taking this: _____

VITAMINS/SUPPLEMENTS

Name: _____

Dosage: I take _____ (amount, e.g., 10 mg) _____times per day/week/other

This pill looks like: _____ (example: "small blue oval")

I take this for: _____

Doctor(s) who prescribed it: _____

Approximate date I started taking this: _____

Name: _____

Dosage: I take _____ (amount, e.g., 10 mg) _____times per day/week/other

This pill looks like: _____ (example: "small blue oval")

I take this for: _____

Doctor(s) who prescribed it: _____

Approximate date I started taking this: _____

Name: _____

Dosage: I take _____ (amount, e.g., 10 mg) _____times per day/week/other

This pill looks like: _____ (example: "small blue oval")

I take this for: _____

Doctor(s) who prescribed it: _____

Approximate date I started taking this: _____

Name: _____

Dosage: I take _____ (amount, e.g., 10 mg) _____times per day/week/other

This pill looks like: _____ (example: "small blue oval")

I take this for: _____

Doctor(s) who prescribed it: _____

Approximate date I started taking this: _____

THE SIX WEBSITES YOU NEED TO KNOW ABOUT FOR SERIOUS ILLNESSES

Whether you've been newly diagnosed with a serious disease, struggling for some time with a chronic condition, or found yourself suddenly playing the role of quarterback for a loved one—you're going to need some online-reference starting points. Here are six websites you can rely on. Check out www.PatientsPlaybook.com for more websites and helpful resources for specific disease and health care problems.

1. NATIONAL COMPREHENSIVE CANCER NETWORK (NCCN)
For a diagnosis of cancer, www.nccn.org/patients offers patient-friendly treatment guidelines, video libraries, patient-advocacy resources, and practical information to supplement the advice you receive from your doctors.

2. NATIONAL CANCER INSTITUTE (NCI) AT THE NATIONAL INSTITUTES OF HEALTH
The website www.cancer.gov provides a wealth of comprehensive information about cancer screening, prognosis, and treatments, as well as government-funded research efforts. Patients and caregivers can direct their cancer-related questions, in English or Spanish, to information specialists at a toll-free number or via live-chat assistance.

3. PUBMED
At www.pubmed.org, a website from the U.S. National Library of Medicine at the National Institutes of Health, you can find abstracts (and sometimes entire articles) of peer-reviewed, published findings on any medical topic. Though the reading can be dense, as you dig deeper and come to understand the language of your condition, you will become infinitely more competent in your dealings with physicians and caregivers.

4. CERTIFICATION MATTERS

As part of your search for a specialist, it's important to check credentials. At www.certificationmatters.org, a website of the American Board of Medical Specialties, you can type in a physician's name to find out whether he or she is board certified in the specialty and if their certification is up-to-date.

5. DOCINFO

A website of the Federation of State Medical Boards, www.docinfo.org is the place to go to learn more about whether a doctor is actively licensed to practice in your state and if he or she has had any disciplinary actions.

6. EXPERTSCAPE

Type the name of your disease into www.expertscape.com, a physician-created search engine, and you'll find a list of authors, ranked via various proprietary algorithms, including the number and depth of scientific papers they've written. Here, you can browse through the latest research findings from the world's top minds on your illness. Or you can use Expertscape for its original purpose: To help you find an expert with whom you may want to consult. The search engine lets you easily view the names and affiliations of experts at specific hospitals and geographic areas. An invaluable tool.

NOTES

INTRODUCTION: HOW TO SAVE A LIFE

3 **Churg-Strauss Syndrome typically**: The websites of nonprofit disease organizations are a good place to begin your research. If you have a rare disease, as Catherine did, it's often easier to find the right organizations because there will be so few to choose from. In Catherine's case, the Churg-Strauss Syndrome Association (**http://www.cssassociation.org**) was an excellent resource.

5 **prednisone, a corticosteroid**: Prednisone is a very effective and widely used corticosteroid that really helps people who are suffering from allergies, autoimmune disorders, and other conditions. But the side effects are, unfortunately, bothersome to many. The Johns Hopkins Vasculitis Center has helpful information about what to expect if you start taking prednisone, at **http://bit.ly/YufVKU.**

5 **Wegener's is a**: See "Granulomatosis with Polyangiitis (Wegener's)," American College of Rheumatology, updated June 2012, **http://bit.ly/1DE4jlz.**

7 **a groundbreaking . . . report**: L. T. Kohn, J. M. Corrigan, and M. S. Donaldson, *To Err Is Human: Building a Safer Health System* (Washington, D.C.: Institute of Medicine/National Academies Press, 2000), **http://bit.ly/Yug54Z.**

7 **at least 44,000 and up to 98,000 people**: The IOM extrapolated these figures from the 33.6 million hospital admissions recorded in 1997. The National Center for Health Statistics reported 2.3 million total deaths in the United States in 1997 (**http://1.usa.gov/1G2gGxy**). This means that medical error was ranked fifth (assuming 98,000 deaths) or eighth (assuming 44,000 deaths) among all causes of death that year.

7 **A year later, in a 2000 *Journal***: Barbara Starfield, in her excellent commentary—"Is U.S. Health Really the Best in the World?" *JAMA* 284, no. 4 (July 2000): 483–85, **http://bit.ly/1BR59MI**—observes that the 225,000-deaths-per-year figure (which she concedes was likely an underestimate) makes "iatrogenic causes" (inadvertent errors induced by a medical practitioner, treatment, or diagnostic procedure) the third leading cause of death in the United States.

7 **That's akin to a jumbo jet**: Many have cited the jumbo-jet-crash analogy as a way to bring our medical error crisis into sharp focus. But patient safety expert Dr. Lucian L. Leape may have

been the earliest and most noted physician to employ it in a December 21, 1994, article that predated even the IOM report. See "Error in Medicine," *JAMA* 272, no. 23 (1994): 1851–57, **http://bit.ly/1wAdB0L**.

7 **And it makes medical error the third leading**: In 2013, the most recent statistics available, heart disease was the cause of 611,105 deaths in the United States; cancer caused 584,881; and chronic lower respiratory diseases led to 149,205. See "Leading Causes of Death," CDC, updated February 6, 2015, **http://1.usa.gov/1uLT1IN**.

7 **These startling reports, picked up**: As Lucian L. Leape and Donald Berwick noted in their comprehensive assessment of heath care safety, the IOM report "galvanized a dramatically expanded level of conversation and concern" on a subject that was previously ignored and misunderstood, making it "a frequent focus for journalists, health care leaders and concerned citizens." See Leape and Berwick, "Five Years After *To Err Is Human*: What Have We Learned?," *JAMA* 293, no. 19 (May 2005): 2384–90, **http://bit.ly/1p2Fs43**.

7 **the Patient Safety and Quality . . . Act**: The Patient Safety and Quality Improvement Act of 2005, Public Law 109-41, 109th Congress, July 2005, **http://1.usa.gov/1op6TEM**.

7 **the creation of patient safety organizations**: For more on the role and function of patient safety organizations, see the Agency for Healthcare Research and Quality's "About the PSO Program: A Brief History of the Program," **http://1.usa.gov/1EXoIpq**.

7 **Numerous hospitals incorporated checklists**: A. Gawande, "The Checklist," *New Yorker*, December 10, 2007, **http://nyr.kr/1uiS4JK**.

7 **they spent millions of dollars**: S. Silow-Carroll, J. N. Edwards, and D. Rodin, *Using Electronic Health Records to Improve Quality and Efficiency: The Experience of Leading Hospitals*, Commonwealth Fund, publication no. 1608 (July 2012), **http://bit.ly/1Bq93Mh**.

7 **Sleep-deprived residents'**: A.B. Blum et al., "Implementing the 2009 Institute of Medicine Recommendations on Resident Physician Work Hours, Supervision, and Safety," *Nature of Science and Sleep* 24, no. 3 (June 2011): 1–39, **http://1.usa.gov/1qBXBds**. See also J. Gold, "New Rules Provide Relief for Sleep-Deprived Medical Residents," *Kaiser Health News*, July 2001, **http://bit.ly/WESEUI**.

7 **"Despite all the focus on patient safety"**: *More Than 1,000 Preventable Deaths a Day Is Too Many: The Need to Improve Patient Safety: Hearing Before the U.S. Senate Subcommittee on Primary Health and Aging*, 113th Cong. (2014) (statement of Dr. Ashish Jha, M.D., M.P.H., professor of Health Policy and Management, Harvard School of Public Health), **http://1.usa.gov/1sdcDGE**.

7 *More Than 1,000 Preventable Deaths a Day*: Ibid.

8 **losing his teenage son**: James recounts the tragic event in *A Sea of Broken Hearts: Patient Rights in a Dangerous, Profit-Driven Health Care System* (Bloomington, Ind.: AuthorHouse, 2007).

8 **vowed to take a closer look**: J. T. James, "A New, Evidence-Based Estimate of Patient Harms Associated with Hospital Care," *Journal of Patient Safety* 9, no. 3 (September 2013): 122–28, **http://1.usa.gov/1r1QGqe**.

8 **Dr. Michael Wechsler**: Dr. Wechsler is now the director of the asthma program at National Jewish Health in Denver. See his web page, **http://bit.ly/YVXqiO**.

10 **A typical primary care physician**: According to researchers at Duke University, a PCP would need to spend 21.7 hours per day to provide all the recommended acute, chronic, and preventive care for a patient panel of 2,500 (i.e., a doctor's total number of patients). Researchers at UC San Francisco used the Duke studies as a starting point to determine optimal panel size for PCPs who delegated some of their workload to nonphysicians (medical assistants, registered nurses, etc.). Under the most ambitious delegation model (whereby doctors handed over about 77 percent of preventive care tasks), a doctor could still reasonably care for a panel of only 1,947 patients. Unfortunately, the

average PCP panel size is about 2,300. For more, see J. Altschuler et al., "Estimating a Reasonable Patient Panel Size for Primary Care Physicians with Team-Based Task Delegation," *Annals of Family Medicine* 10 (September–October 2012): 396–400, **http://bit.ly/1opLNGg**.

10 **receiving lower reimbursements**: In a 2012 survey of 1,303 U.S. physicians—33 percent of whom were primary care doctors—the national average reimbursement rate for an existing patient's office visit ranged from $20 to $86, depending on the complexity of interaction. That's about half of what doctors received in 2006 ($39 to $177). See "Year-to-Year Comparison of Average Commercial Reimbursement," UBM Medica Network Physicians Practice 2012 Fee Schedule Survey Data, January 31, 2013, **http://bit.ly/1wfsJjd**.

10 **In 2007 the IOM estimated**: P. Aspden et al., *Preventing Medication Errors* (Washington, D.C.: Institute of Medicine/National Academies Press, 2007), **http://bit.ly/1uiU5W4**. But patients can proactively work to avoid mistakes. See "20 Tips to Help Prevent Medical Errors: Patient Fact Sheet," Agency for Healthcare Research and Quality, **http://1.usa.gov/1nJuAHZ**.

11 **when actor Dennis Quaid**: See Oprah Winfrey and Dr. Mehmet Oz, "Medical Mistakes: Dr. Oz Talks to Actor Dennis Quaid," *Oprah Winfrey Show*, June 10, 2009, **http://bit.ly/1zFL12F**; and "Dennis Quaid Recounts Twins' Drug Ordeal," *60 Minutes*, CBS News, March 13, 2008; the updated August 22, 2008, version is at **http://cbsn.ws/ZXs0bu**. Some details here about the Hep-Lock/heparin mix-up in the Quaids' case are from Jacob Goldstein, "Baxter's Other Heparin Problem: Dennis Quaid," *Wall Street Journal*, March 14, 2008, **http://on.wsj.com/134xinA**. Facts about the twins' recovery and the family's realization that theirs was not an uncommon problem were also noted in Kathleen Doheny's "How Are the Quaid Twins Doing?" WebMD, September–October 2008, **http://bit.ly/1uHsKeA**.

11 **the bottle labels, which looked very similar**: The Hep-Lock and heparin bottles looked so similar, in fact, that the drug maker had recently redesigned the heparin vials to prevent this very problem from occurring. But it hadn't recalled the old vials, which is what the Quaid twins received. See "Dennis Quaid Recounts Twins' Drug Ordeal," *60 Minutes*, CBS News, **http://cbsn.ws/ZXs0bu**.

15 **Dr. Robert H. Brook**: Dr. Brook currently holds the Distinguished Chair in Health Care Services at RAND Corporation, **http://bit.ly/1uuMmna**.

15 **when it came to coronary artery bypass**: C. M. Winslow et al., "The Appropriateness of Performing Coronary Artery Bypass Surgery," *JAMA* 260, no. 4 (July 22–29, 1988): 505–9.

16 **a 2013 investigative series**: "Paying Till It Hurts," Elisabeth Rosenthal's multipart series, began with a searing report on the inexplicably disparate (and expensive) cost of a routine colonoscopy: "The $2.7 Trillion Medical Bill: Colonoscopies Explain Why U.S. Leads the World in Health Expenditures," *New York Times*, June 1, 2013. The series has since delved into pregnancy ("American Way of Birth, Costliest in the World," June 30, 2013), joint replacement ("In Need of a New Hip, but Priced Out of the U.S.," August 3, 2013), diabetes ("Even Small Medical Advances Can Mean Big Jumps in Bills," April 5, 2014), and other common conditions and procedures for which comparative information about quality and prices are not readily available to patients before they make health care decisions. See also Steven Brill, "Bitter Pill: Why Medical Bills Are Killing Us," *Time*, April 4, 2013.

16 **the Patient Protection and Affordable Care Act**: Patient Protection and Affordable Care Act, "About the Law," U.S. Department of Health and Human Services, **http://1.usa.gov/1opbC9r**.

16 **It guarantees that health insurance companies can no longer**: The law makes some exceptions for plans that have been grandfathered in. Also, some plans may be able to enforce annual and lifetime limits on spending for health care services that are not considered "essential." For specifics, see "Lifetime & Annual Limits," **http://1.usa.gov/1yVVghN**, and "About the Law," **http://1.usa.gov/1opbC9r**.

17 **Millions of previously uninsured**: According to analysis of health insurance enrollments, 9.3 million more people had health care coverage in March 2014, lowering the uninsured rate from 20.5 percent to 15.8 percent. See K. G. Carman, and C. Eibner, "Changes in Health Insurance

Enrollment Since 2013: Evidence from the RAND Health Reform Opinion Study," RAND Corporation, April 8, 2014, **http://bit.ly/19YXMK4**.

17 **Baby boomers are**: According to the Association of American Medical Colleges, the United States is on course toward a major physician shortage: we have 45,000 fewer primary care doctors and 46,000 fewer specialists than we will need to care for an aging population by 2020. See "GME Funding: How to Fix the Doctor Shortage," Association of American Medical Colleges, **http://bit .ly/1tIgcqu**. Some of this shortage can, and should, be offset by an increased reliance on nurse practitioners and other nonphysician providers, who can serve as part of a patient's total care team.

CHAPTER 1. WHY HAVING THE RIGHT PRIMARY CARE PHYSICIAN WILL CHANGE YOUR LIFE

23 **"frozen shoulder"**: "Diseases and Conditions: Frozen Shoulder," Mayo Clinic, April 28, 2011, **http://mayocl.in/ZXOfhJ**.

23 **Dr. Robert R. Simon**: Dr. Simon, who serves as medical director of Private Health Management (**http://bit.ly/1K8E0KK**), is probably best known as the founder and chairman of International Medical Corps (IMC), a global humanitarian organization that sets up medical clinics in war-torn regions. You can learn more about Dr. Simon and IMC at **http://bit.ly/1CqZkoe**.

25 **Up to 30 percent of psoriasis**: According to the National Psoriasis Foundation, **http://bit .ly/1qCY7Y8**. See also the American College of Rheumatology, **http://bit.ly/1BrnfXq**.

25 **Dr. Philip Mease**: Dr. Mease's bio is available at Swedish Medical Center, **http://bit .ly/1Bqe8Eq**.

29 **depression nearly doubles your risk of a stroke**: Mental health absolutely influences physical health. Australian researchers studied 10,457 women, who had no history of stroke, over a twelve-year period to discover that those with chronic depression nearly doubled their risk of having a stroke. Those findings confirm an earlier, 2011 study, of 81,000 women over a six-year period, in which Harvard researchers discovered a 29 percent risk of stroke in women who were currently depressed or had a history of depression. See C. A. Jackson, and G. D. Mishra, "Depression and Risk of Stroke in Midaged Women: A Prospective Longitudinal Study," *Stroke* 44 (May 16, 2013): 1555–60, **http:// bit.ly/1pY3Ov0**; and A. Pan et al., "Depression and the Risk of Stroke Morbidity and Mortality: A Meta-analysis and Systematic Review," *JAMA* 306, no. 11 (September 21, 2011): 1241–49, **http:// 1.usa.gov/1uzxT9w**.

29 **that 23 percent of stroke victims suffer**: PTSD is common among people who have endured wartime combat, potentially fatal accidents, and serious medical events, like heart attacks. But researchers at Columbia University found that one in four stroke and ministroke (transient ischemic attack) victims also developed PTSD within a year of the stroke event. See D. Edmondson et al., "Prevalence of PTSD in Survivors of Stroke and Transient Ischemic Attack: A Meta-Analytic Review," *PLoS ONE*. June 19, 2013, **http://bit.ly/1s00ve5**.

29 **but bacterial meningitis?**: For more on the risk factors, warning signs, and treatment of meningitis, see "Meningitis," CDC, **http://1.usa.gov/ZjIJpy**.

30 **Dr. Eugene Sayfie**: Dr. Sayfie's bio can be found on the website of the University of Miami's Miller School of Medicine, at **http://bit.ly/1qtk510**.

31 **Dr. Steven W. Tabak**: Dr. Tabak's bio can be found at the website of the Cardiovascular Medical Group of Southern California, **http://bit.ly/1EAatZe**.

CHAPTER 2: HOW TO FIND THE BEST PRIMARY CARE PHYSICIAN FOR YOU

39 **four hundred men and women**: S. U. Rehman et al., "What to Wear Today? Effect of Doctor's Attire on the Trust and Confidence of Patients," *American Journal of Medicine* 118, no. 11 (November 2005): 1279–86, abstract at **http://1.usa.gov/XpCOOj**.

41 **Dr. Philip M. Bretsky**: More about Dr. Bretsky and his practice, Santa Monica Primary Care, can be found at **http://bit.ly/1Kp2wpU**.

42 **HMO vs. PPO**: Unfortunately, health insurance has become very complex, and the insurers don't do a good job of explaining what care is covered and which physicians and practices are in-network. Selecting the right insurance plan is an art that's beyond the scope of this book, but *Consumer Reports* regularly publishes informative articles on the topic, including "How to Pick a Health Insurance Plan: The Three Most Important Questions You Need to Ask," updated September 2014 and available free at **http://bit.ly/Zn3ZL9**. The Henry J. Kaiser Family Foundation has a helpful consumer resources website for individuals who are shopping for coverage through the Affordable Care Act's insurance marketplace; see "Understanding Health Insurance," **http://bit.ly/14e4DMV**. Finally, if you have a complex health care coverage issue and need private counsel, Healthcare Navigation—**http://bit .ly/1CbkGHC**—is a firm that I've come to rely on for clients who need professional advocacy.

42 **In return, you get a wider selection**: Some PPOs have developed "narrow" networks, with fewer hospitals and physicians, in an attempt to offer lower-cost insurance in the new health care exchanges. However, the vast majority of patients with PPO coverage still have very broad access. An editorial in *The New York Times* has also taken on this issue, dubbing it, "The Phony 'Narrow Network' Scare," July 24, 2014.

43 **a family practice physician rather than**: The most important factor is finding a doctor with whom you can develop a strong, enduring relationship. To learn more about the differences between family practice physicians and medical internists, see the American College of Physicians' "What's an Internist?" brief at **http://bit.ly/1uBfLgk**, and the American Academy of Family Physicians' "Family Medicine Specialty," **http://bit.ly/1BGWmgc**, and "Family Medicine Facts," **http://bit .ly/1q8H23n**.

43 **seen by a hospitalist**: Hospitalists are becoming ever more present in health care. The challenge as a patient is to make sure your PCP is being kept in the loop, too. For interesting perspectives see Jane Gross, "New Breed of Specialist Steps in for Family Doctor," *New York Times*, May 26, 2010; and Paula Span, "Do Hospitalists Save Money?" *New York Times*, August 12, 2011.

49 **the data show that 7 percent**: In 7 percent of the times in which there are "clinically meaning-ful" results (code for "something is wrong"), they *do not* get reported back to the patient—that's one in fourteen patients. In practices that use a combination of paper and electronic health records, the rate can be as high as one in four. See L. P. Casalino et al., "Frequency of Failure to Inform Patients of Clinically Significant Outpatient Test Results," *Archives of Internal Medicine* 169, no. 12 (2009): 1123–29. You can read Weill Cornell Medical College's press release on the study at **http://bit.ly /Znjcf0**.

49 **things like mammograms, colonoscopies, PSA tests**: For information about how, when, and why to screen for certain cancers, good resources are the relevant medical-specialty societies; the American Cancer Society's "Guidelines for the Early Detection of Cancer," **http://bit.ly/1uEiXqw**; and "Recommendations for Primary Care Practice," U.S. Preventive Services Task Force, **http://bit .ly/1xD0s4z**. When their recommendations converge, it's comforting, but in some cases (such as for PSA testing and mammography) there may be dissonance. That's when it's even more important to discuss screening guidelines with your internist.

50 **financially penalized if they are spending too much time**: As physicians know, it's not pos-sible to care for a patient—especially one with chronic conditions—in fifteen minutes or less. And yet that's what many are being asked to do. Take the case of Dr. Janis Finer, a PCP in Tulsa, Oklahoma,

who was forced to make patients schedule another visit if they had more issues to discuss than she could fit into the allotted eleven minutes. Or Phoenix PCP Dr. Lawrence Gassner, who switched to a concierge model because he couldn't take another sleepless night of worry about whether he had missed important problems with patients because he had to cut their time short. Their stories are recounted in Roni Caryn Rabin and Kaiser Health News, "A Growing Number of Primary Care Doctors Are Burning Out. How Does This Affect Patients?," *Washington Post*, March 31, 2014.

51 **moving to direct-pay**: This isn't just based on my own observations. In a 2012 survey of more than 13,000 American physicians (35 percent of whom were PCPs), nearly 8 percent of PCPs said they planned to switch to a concierge-style practice in the next one to three years. *A Survey of America's Physicians: Practice Patterns and Perspectives*, Physicians Foundation, September 2012, p. 29, **http://bit.ly/1tZmYrO**. For an arresting account, see Devin Leonard, "Is Concierge Medicine the Future of Health Care?" *Bloomberg Business*, November 29, 2012.

51 **spending the extra money on a private PCP**: Some say that concierge medicine is heavy on service—and that's about it. In other words, you get more attention and the furniture is nicer, but you're not necessarily going to be healthier. See Paul Sullivan, "Dealing with Doctors Who Only Take Cash," *New York Times*, November 23, 2012. But the bottom line is that the retainer physicians charge enables them to spend the time needed to provide the type of care and support that patients—especially those with multiple or complex problems—really need.

52 **Dr. Bryan J. Arling**: Dr. Arling, a full-time faculty member at George Washington University School of Medicine and Health Sciences, doesn't keep a website, but a simple Internet search will produce his contact information.

56 **80 percent cited "patient relationships"**: *A Survey of America's Physicians: Practice Patterns and Perspectives,* Physicians Foundation, September 2012, p. 21, **http://bit.ly/1tZmYrO**.

57 **finding and developing a strong bond with a PCP**: I'm a data collector—the more information I can glean, the better. If you're similar and would like more advice from experts on how to pick a PCP, I recommend "What Is the Biggest Mistake Patients Make When Picking a Primary-Care Doctor?" *Wall Street Journal,* February 27, 2014; and results from a survey of 660 PCPs, "What Doctors Wish Their Patients Knew," *Consumer Reports*, updated February 2011, **http://bit.ly/1u49bww**.

CHAPTER 3. THREE THINGS YOU CAN DO RIGHT NOW TO BE BETTER PREPARED

63 **Dr. Michael H. Rosove**: For more about Dr. Rosove, visit his page at the UCLA Jonsson Comprehensive Cancer Center, **http://bit.ly/1zYlLDy**.

64 **"I think Amanda has hereditary spherocytosis"**: For more on this condition, see G. Gonzalez and E. C. Besa, "Hereditary Spherocytosis," *Medscape*, updated July 16, 2014, **http://bit.ly/1uRXOsh**. A short video, "How Hereditary Spherocytosis Causes Anemia," posted May 10, 2011, can be viewed at Oncology Tube, **http://bit.ly/1qKWt8p**.

65 **Dr. Carrie Carter**: More about Dr. Carter can be found at the website of her practice, E. Barrow Medical Group, **http://bit.ly/Xyo7c2**.

66 **In a yearlong study called OpenNotes**: See T. Delbanco et al., "Inviting Patients to Read Their Doctors' Notes: A Quasi-experimental Study and a Look Ahead," *Annals of Internal Medicine* 157, no. 7 (2012): 461–470, **http://bit.ly/1JpVsZf**; and J. Walker et al., "U.S. Experience with Doctors and Patients Sharing Clinical Notes," *BMJ*, 350 (February 2015): g7785, **http://bmj.co/1NbvzBU**.

67 **under federal privacy laws**: Learn more about HIPAA laws and your rights as a patient at "Protecting Your Privacy & Security: Your Health Information Rights," HealthIT.gov, updated February 4, 2013, **http://bit.ly/1wDWA7S**. If you experience resistance to your request, be firm: As one health information expert notes, "When hospitals talk about HIPAA or charge for releasing records what they're really saying is, 'I don't want to do this and I have to find an excuse.'" See Elisabeth Rosenthal,

"Medical Records: Top Secret," *New York Times*, November 9, 2014. More comprehensive information about HIPAA is available at "Understanding Health Information Privacy," U.S. Department of Health and Human Services, **http://1.usa.gov/XiyAHZ**.

67 **pay for the cost of copying**: See "Your Medical Records," U.S. Department of Health and Human Services, **http://1.usa.gov/1uHCfLZ**. Charges vary by state. For instance, Texas caps paper copies of your medical records at $25 for the first twenty pages and then 50 cents per page for every copy thereafter (**http://bit.ly/1o3EiF9**); in Vermont, it's a flat five-dollar fee or no more than 50 cents per page, whichever is greater (**http://bit.ly/1D6vF8N**).

67 **State laws govern how long**: For instance, the Arizona Medical Board (**http://bit.ly/1yi0LYY**) requires that physicians keep records for at least six years from the date of the patient's visit; the New Jersey State Board of Medical Examiners (**http://bit.ly/1yi0LrQ**) mandates seven years of retention.

68 **HIPAA Privacy Authorization forms**: Caring.com, a wonderful resource for caregivers, has a standard release at **http://bit.ly/1wqAwuI**.

70 **Don't be surprised if you discover**: Coded doctor slang is a mostly extinct practice, but one London physician charted more than two hundred examples of slang that physicians have used about patients (GLM = Good Looking Mum) and colleagues (Freud Squad = Psychiatrists). See "Doctor Slang Is a Dying Art," *BBC News Online*, August 18, 2003; and "Decoding 28 Medical Slang Terms," *Discovery Health*, **http://bit.ly/1mbSTTC**. Beyond the colorful insults, you may find codes that are just useful shorthand, for instance CBC for "complete blood count" or R/O for "rule out" (as in, "The next step is to rule out a suspected disease"). See William C. Shiel and Jay W. Marks, "Common Medical Abbreviations & Terms," Medicine.net, reviewed February 13, 2015, **http://bit.ly/1tpv7Fc**.

72 **the problem always seems to be on the other side**: Even worse is when medical institutions wrongly cite HIPAA to delay, misinform, or intentionally obfuscate, as reported in Charles Ornstein, "Are Patient Privacy Laws Being Misused to Protect Medical Centers?" *ProPublica*, July 24, 2014, **http://bit.ly/1mfAFjM**.

72 **Dr. Gail J. Roboz**: You can read more about Dr. Roboz at the Weill Cornell Physicians website, **http://bit.ly/1o43XNZ**.

CHAPTER 4: DEVELOP A SUPPORT TEAM

77 **it's up to you to coordinate your care**: Because no one else is doing it! This is "the dirty little secret about health care," notes Harvard health policy analyst Dr. Lucian L. Leape, in Roni Caryn Rabin's excellent "Health Care's 'Dirty Little Secret': No One May Be Coordinating Care," *Washington Post*, April 30, 2013.

78 **Dr. Sheldon Elman**: You can read more about Dr. Elman and Medisys at **http://bit.ly/1tpCeg4**.

78 **It used to be that primary care physicians**: A New York internist recently wrote about playing the quarterback for a seventy-year-old patient, Mr. K., who had kidney disease. As Dr. Matthew J. Press explained, in the 80 days from discovery of a tumor to surgery, Mr. K. had 5 procedures, was cared for by 11 additional doctors, and had 11 office visits. Dr. Press counted 32 e-mails and 8 phone calls with other doctors about Mr. K. and had 12 communications with the patient or his wife. On the busiest day, Dr. Press had 6 different communications. Let me assure you, this tally represents the most *basic* level of care coordination, but the majority of internists do not have time to provide even that. As Dr. Press attested, "I was able to play the role I did in Mr. K.'s care largely because, as a clinician-researcher, I had a patient panel about one tenth the size of the average primary care panel." Matthew J. Press, "Instant Replay: A Quarterback's View of Care Coordination," *New England Journal of Medicine* 371 (August 7, 2014): 489–91, **http://bit.ly/1pkKisl**.

78 **But the majority simply don't have the time**: Nor does it pay to take on this role. Medicare only recently began reimbursing physicians for care coordination of chronically ill patients—and at

press time that fee was $42 a month. Robert Pear, "Medicare to Start Paying Doctors Who Coordinate Needs of Chronically Ill Patients," *New York Times*, August 16, 2014.

79 **Studies show that when a family member**: Patients were more likely to understand their PCP's advice and discuss difficult topics when a companion participated in the visit, according to A. Rosland, "Family and Friend Participation in Primary Care Visits of Patients with Diabetes or Heart Failure: Patient and Physician Determinants and Experiences," *Medical Care* 49, no. 1 (January 2011): 37–45, **http://1.usa.gov/YVQFNM**. And a majority of patients and their physicians felt that having a patient-companion in the room improved communication and understanding, in L. M. Schilling, "The Third Person in the Room: Frequency, Role, and Influence of Companions During Primary Care Medical Encounters," *Journal of Family Practice* 51, no. 8 (August 2002): 685–90, **http://1.usa.gov/1NKYNpg**.

79 **when the patient is elderly**: J. L. Wolff et al., "An Exploration of Patient and Family Engagement in Routine Primary Care Visits," *Health Expectations*, October 29, 2012, **http://1.usa.gov/1ATwjAh**.

79 **Under HIPAA, as long as you do not object**: See "Family Members and Friends," U.S. Department of Health and Human Services, **http://1.usa.gov/ZsfuRn**.

CHAPTER 5. OVERTREATMENT CAN BE AS DANGEROUS AS UNDERTREATMENT

89 **they could do a coronary angiogram**: The American Heart Association website (**http://www.heart.org**) has more information, plus videos that provide a visual reference for coronary angiograms and many of the most common cardiac procedures and conditions. See "Watch, Learn, and Live," American Heart Association, **http://bit.ly/1wtHpeA**. See also "Coronary Angioplasty and Stents," Mayo Clinic, **http://mayocl.in/1uLBe5m**.

93 **a bronchoscopy procedure**: For more detail, see "Bronchoscopy," Johns Hopkins Medicine Health Library, **http://bit.ly/1mjWOh3**.

93 **video-assisted thoracoscopic surgery (VATS)**: For more on the history and results of this minimally invasive procedure developed at Cedars-Sinai, see the hospital's "Video-Assisted Thoracoscopic Surgery (VATS)," **http://bit.ly/1u56UVD**.

94 **Dr. Robert McKenna, Jr.**: Dr. McKenna's bio and publications are available at the Cedars-Sinai website, **http://bit.ly/1wKcIVm**.

94 **He explained the VATS process**: We knew that Jim would get the best outcome this time, because Dr. McKenna and his colleagues had introduced and pioneered the VATS procedure in 1992 and performed it on thousands of patients since. For more, see interview with Dr. McKenna, "With Tiny Incisions, Video Cameras, Surgeons Pioneer Chest Procedures That Are Less Painful, Faster to Heal, Studies Show," Cedars-Sinai, **http://bit.ly/1rhJWZc**.

94 **called hypersensitivity pneumonitis**: The U.S. Department of Health and Human Services' National Heart, Lung, and Blood Institute provides extensive information about this disease at "What Is Hypersensitivity Pneumonitis?" **http://1.usa.gov/1qPsc8j**.

96 **the United States spends $2.7 trillion a year**: H. Moses et al., "The Anatomy of Health Care in the United States," *JAMA* 310, no. 18 (November 13, 2013): 1947–64, **http://bit.ly/1vFyEyg**. See also Elizabeth Rosenthal, "The $2.7 Trillion Medical Bill: Colonoscopies Explain Why U.S. Leads the World in Health Expenditures," *New York Times*, June 1, 2013.

96 **About 30 percent of that—roughly $750 billion**: "If the care in every state were of the quality delivered by the highest-performing state, an estimated 75,000 fewer deaths would have occurred across the country in 2005. Current waste diverts resources from productive use, resulting in an estimated $750 billion loss in 2009." See *Best Care at Lower Cost: The Path to Continuously Learning Health Care in America (2013)* (Washington, D.C.: Institute of Medicine/National Academies Press,

2012), available as a free download at **http://bit.ly/1mmi9qk**. The Kaiser Health News Daily Report lists interesting articles across the Web (some sites require registration) devoted to this topic at **http://bit.ly/1mmftZU**.

96 **Heart catheterizations with stents**: This reflects the most recent numbers from the 2010 CDC/NCHS National Hospital Discharge Survey. See "Inpatient Surgery," CDC, **http://1.usa .gov/1uOIsWs**.

96 **But that number has been on the decline**: In 2009 there were 644,240 hospital stays that included the implantation of a cardiac stent; the rate of the procedure rose steadily from 1999 to 2006 (by 61 percent), then declined sharply between 2006 and 2009 (by 27 percent), according to an April 2012 analysis by D. I. Auerbach, J. L. Maeda, and C. Steiner, "Hospital Stays with Cardiac Stents, 2009," Agency for Healthcare Research and Quality, Healthcare Cost and Utilization Project, Statistical Brief no. 128, **http://1.usa.gov/1wOlvWy**.

96 **researchers found that the procedure didn't prevent**: This is from the Clinical Outcomes Utilizing Revascularization and Aggressive Drug Evaluation, or COURAGE, trial, which sparked nationwide debate about our overstenting epidemic. Its authors (all twenty-three of them) noted that in 2004 more than 1 million coronary stent procedures were performed in the United States—the majority of them elective surgeries in patients whose heart disease was stable. See W. E. Boden et al., "Optimal Medical Therapy with or without PCI for Stable Coronary Disease," *New England Journal of Medicine* 356, no. 15 (April 12, 2007): 1503–16, **http://bit.ly/1wx9WA6**.
Although surgical stenting can alleviate angina symptoms in patients with stable heart disease, the COURAGE trial (and numerous additional studies since) have shown that it does not *prevent* heart attack or death when compared to medical therapy (i.e., a reduction in risk factors and lifestyle interventions) alone. But most patients don't know this. Researchers interviewed 1,000 patients with stable heart disease who were undergoing stenting voluntarily at one of ten different centers. They discovered that most patients substantially overestimated the benefits of the surgery (88 percent thought it would prevent a heart attack) and its urgency (20 percent deemed it an emergency). In other words, too many patients wrongly believed that they needed stents *now* to save their lives. The researchers also found that the informed-consent process was all over the map—some institutions provided educational materials, but most didn't. Only one center provided a consent form a day prior to surgery; the rest were put in front of the patient the day of the procedure. See F. Kureshi et al., "Variation in Patients' Perceptions of Elective Percutaneous Coronary Intervention in Stable Coronary Artery Disease: Cross Sectional Study," *BMJ* 349 (September 8, 2014): g5309, **http://bit.ly/1wxfWJ1**.
Which is not to say that elective stenting simply for symptom relief is bad medicine. In a thoughtful essay, Dr. Lisa Rosenbaum writes about a case in which she tried to be a hero to a suffering patient by *not* inserting stents—only to realize she had needlessly prolonged his pain. In other words, hewing to the maxim that it's *always* wrong to stent patients with stable coronary disease is sometimes . . . also wrong. Lisa Rosenbaum, "When Is a Medical Treatment Unnecessary?," *New Yorker*, October 23, 2013.

96 **only half of 144,000 nonemergency**: P. S Chan et al., "Appropriateness of Percutaneous Coronary Intervention," *JAMA* 306, no. 1 (July 6, 2011): 53–61, **http://1.usa.gov/1p4l8zc**.

96 **finding a tumor and recommending**: A staggering example was recently discovered in South Korea. In 1999 the government initiated a health-screening initiative to help catch and cure cancer. Although it wasn't a part of the program, many doctors and hospitals offered a simple and inexpensive ultrasound test to screen for thyroid cancer. Practically overnight, thyroid cancer became the most diagnosed cancer in that country—a fifteenfold increase in the last two decades, according to a *New England Journal of Medicine* study. Despite this intensive screening and treatment, however, the death rate from thyroid cancer didn't change. Which led researchers to believe that many people were being diagnosed and treated for a disease that wasn't likely to kill them or even cause serious symptoms while they were alive. As one of the paper's coauthors noted, South Korea had suffered from an "epidemic of diagnosis," which begat "an epidemic of treatment." See H. Gilbert Welch, "An

Epidemic of Thyroid Cancer?," *New York Times*, November 6, 2014. See also H. S. Ahn, H. J. Kim, and H. G. Welch, "Korea's Thyroid-Cancer 'Epidemic'—Screening and Overdiagnosis," *New England Journal of Medicine* 371, no. 19 (November 6, 2014): 1765–67, **http://bit.ly/1ElVX2r**; and Gina Kolata, "Study Points to Overdiagnosis of Thyroid Cancer," *New York Times*, November 6, 2014.

97 **To help doctors and patients better communicate**: See *Choosing Wisely: An Initiative of the ABIM Foundation*, "Lists," **http://bit.ly/1B0bkwl**.

98 **Stents are a huge moneymaker**: Anahad O'Connor, "Heart Stents Still Overused, Experts Say," *New York Times*, August 15, 2013.

98 **Medicare has spent tens of billions**: According to a report from the Senate Finance Committee, Medicare Part A paid an estimated $25.7 billion for about 1.9 million hospital stays, where the patient's principal diagnosis was heart-related and the patient received a cardiac stent, from fiscal year 2004 to 2009; during 2005–9, Medicare Part B paid $1.3 billion for nearly 250,000 procedures. See "Baucus, Grassley Outline Millions of Wasted Taxpayer Dollars, Examine Reports of Hundreds of Improper Cardiac Stent Implantations," U.S. Senate Committee on Finance, press release, December 6, 2010, **http://1.usa.gov/1tm2vYM**.

A 2013 *Bloomberg* investigation estimated that Americans had spent $110 billion on stents over the last decade. (That figure was developed from a combination of data sources including the Healthcare Cost and Utilization Project maintained by the Agency for Healthcare Research and Quality, outpatient stent information collected by a private research company, and data from the Society for Cardiovascular Angiography and Interventions, as well as Medicare figures.) "Cardiologists get paid less than $250 to talk to patients about stents' risks and alternative measures, and an average of four times that fee for putting in a stent," *Bloomberg* reporters noted in this frightening three-part series about the overuse—and frank abuse—of stenting procedures by U.S. hospitals and doctors. The articles were based on a review of thousands of pages of court documents and regulatory filings, as well as interviews with several dozen doctors, patients, and family members. See Peter Waldman, David Armstrong, and Sydney P. Freedberg, "Deaths Linked to Cardiac Stents Rise as Overuse Seen," *Bloomberg*, September 26, 2013, **http://bloom.bg/XQQqCt**.

98 **investigations were slowly made public**: Waldman, Armstrong, and Freedberg, "Deaths Linked." See also the third part of this series: Sydney P. Freedberg, "Mother Dies Amid Abuses in $110 Billion U.S. Stent Assembly Line," *Bloomberg*, October 9, 2013, **http://bloom.bg/1o9AvGg**.

98 **the "full-metal jacket" treatment**: Waldman, Armstrong, and Freedberg, "Deaths Linked."

98 **can have *more* to do with your zip code**: Is geography destiny when it comes to health care? The Dartmouth Atlas of Health Care's online library has a plethora of fascinating reports (e.g., "Trends in Cancer Care at the End of Life," and "Tracking the Care of Patients with Severe Chronic Illness") that attempt to answer this question in all its complexity. See "Publications: Atlases & Reports," Dartmouth Atlas of Health Care, **http://bit.ly/1pm0CJx**.

98 **There's no better data**: One point to be drawn from the Dartmouth data is that frequent and aggressive treatment doesn't always lead to better outcomes. But what accounts for the differences in procedure rate? According to the authors, "where there are more hospital beds per capita, more people will be admitted (and readmitted more frequently) than in areas where there are fewer beds per capita. . . . Similarly, where there are more specialist physicians per capita, there are more visits and revisits." But variation can also be related to the practice style of an area's hospitals and physicians, meaning *when* and *how often* they advocate for more aggressive and/or unnecessary treatments. For more, see "Tools: FAQ," Dartmouth Atlas of Health Care, **http://bit.ly/1r7pslx**.

99 **patients in Casper, Wyoming, were seven**: S. Brownlee et al., *Improving Patient Decision-Making in Health Care: A 2012 Dartmouth Atlas Report Highlighting the New England Region* (Washington, D.C.: Dartmouth Institute for Health Policy and Clinical Practice, 2012), p. 20, **http://bit.ly/1mmD5x0**.

99 **women over sixty-five in Grand Forks**: Ibid., p. 10.

99 **When the researchers looked at elective stenting**: Ibid., p. 16.

99 **a consequence of the doctor shortage in Hawaii**: Researchers at the John A. Burns School of Medicine at the University of Hawaii Mānoa posit that the physician shortage will only get worse as aged doctors retire, leaving the state about 1,448 physicians shy by 2020. See "Medical School Researchers Report Physician Workforce Shortage Worsening," University of Hawaii System, press release, April 19, 2013, **http://bit.ly/1o9DfUg**.

99 **Depending on what hospital you went to**: The data are based on a Dartmouth Atlas of Health Care custom report, input by the author using 2010 as the year, Jim's region, and "Inpatient Percutaneous Interventions (PCI) per 1,000 Medicare Enrollees" as the procedure.

101 **About 332,000 hip replacements**: This reflects the most recent numbers from the 2010 CDC/NCHS National Hospital Discharge Survey. See "Inpatient Surgery," CDC, **http://1.usa .gov/1uOIsWs**.

101 **Knees are replaced at more than**: Ibid.

101 **made by five companies that have**: Elizabeth Rosenthal, "In Need of a New Hip, but Priced Out of the U.S.," *New York Times*, August 3, 2013.

101 **probably costs about $350**: Ibid.

101 **the final hospital bill could range from $11,000**: J. A. Rosenthal, X. Lu, and P. Cram, "Availability of Consumer Prices from U.S. Hospitals for a Common Surgical Procedure," *JAMA Internal Medicine* 173, no. 6 (March 25, 2013): 427–32, **http://bit.ly/1AVUM86**.

101 **Dallas doctors performed 3.2 hip replacements**: The data are based on a Dartmouth Atlas of Health Care custom report, input by the author using 2010 as the year, Dallas as the region, and "Inpatient Hip Replacement per 1,000 Medicare Enrollees" as the procedure.

102 **Dr. Michael H. Huo**: For more about Dr. Huo, see the website of the University of Texas Southwestern Medical Center, **http://bit.ly/1ukN9dW**.

103 **Orthopedic surgeons and cardiologists are consistently**: Leslie Kane and Carol Peckham, "*Medscape* Physician Compensation Report 2014," *Medscape*, April 15, 2014, **http://bit.ly/ YZM2Cw**.

103 **The problem is compounded when Medicare is paying**: And sometimes it amounts to outright fraud, as evidenced by a report that studied newly released Medicare data: John Carreyrou, Christopher S. Stewart, and Rob Barry, "Taxpayers Face Big Medicare Tab for Unusual Doctor Billings," *Wall Street Journal*, June 9, 2014.
   In 2014, as part of an effort to make health care spending more transparent, the Obama administration began releasing 2012 Medicare data reports at the Centers for Medicare and Medicaid Services website. See "Medicare Provider Utilization and Payment Data: Physician and Other Supplier," **http://go.cms.gov/1o9EWRz**. Shortly afterward *ProPublica* followed the money in an informative investigative series, "Examining Medicare," which also provided readers with tools to get a sense of the average Medicare reimbursements their own doctors received in 2012, compared to others in the same state and specialty. See "Examining Medicare," *ProPublica*, **http://bit.ly/1sbmPSe**; and Lena Groeger, Charles Ornstein, and Ryann Grochowski Jones, "Treatment Tracker: The Doctors and Services in Medicare Part B," *ProPublica*, May 15, 2014, **http://bit.ly/1uPoFpK**.

103 **Further, we don't recognize that the real currency**: In fact, when *USA Today* did an investigation on paid malpractice claims, they found that 10 to 20 percent of common surgeries weren't even needed. See Peter Eisler and Barbara Hansen, "Doctors Perform Thousands of Unnecessary Surgeries," *USA Today*, June 30, 2013, **http://usat.ly/1r7Gro2**.

103 **Dr. Michael Davidson**: Dr. Davidson's bio is at the University of Chicago School of Medicine's website, **http://bit.ly/1AW0yXf**.

CHAPTER 6. HOW TO FIND AND INTERVIEW THE MEDICAL EXPERTS YOU NEED

107 **something called otosclerosis**: Throughout this chapter, I delve into the best ways to do focused research on a topic using the most sophisticated websites and practices. However, if you are simply in need of basic information on otosclerosis, its causes, symptoms, and treatments, you could begin at the National Institute on Deafness and Other Communication Disorders' "Otosclerosis" page, **http://1.usa.gov/1schnP0**. See also "Hearing and Balance Disorders: Otosclerosis," American Hearing Research Foundation, **http://bit.ly/1wzK5Yc**; and "What You Should Know About Otosclerosis," American Academy of Otolaryngology–Head and Neck Surgery, **http://bit.ly/1sJK3Jw**.

109 **More than sixty thousand medical articles are published**: This number was extrapolated from the most recent Medline indexing figures. (Medline is a database of more than 21 million references to biomedical articles, searchable at PubMed.) To wit, there were 734,052 articles indexed in Medline in 2013; and 376,312 in 1993. See the National Institutes of Health's U.S. National Library of Medicine, Medline/PubMed Resources, "Detailed Indexing Statistics, 1965–2013," **http://1.usa.gov/1mswCB2**. However, the PubMed/Medline database is *very* selective and covers only a portion of the biomedical publishing universe, which, by one estimate, amounted to about 1.35 million scientific articles published in 2006 alone. See B. C. Bjork, A. Roos, and M. Lauri, "Scientific Journal Publishing: Yearly Volume and Open Access Availability," *Information Research* 14, no. 1 (March 1, 2009), **http://bit.ly/1xXcMjZ**.

110 **There is no insurance reimbursement code for studying**: This conundrum underscores the terrible riptide physicians are caught in: they want to serve patients who are sick, anxious, and need their attention, but they don't have as much time as they'd like, in part because they must comply with the complex reimbursement rules and regulations. Fee-for-service physicians get paid based on "CPT codes," of which there are a gazillion, but none that provide payment for researching the literature to find out how best to treat a patient. There are, by the way, whole industries built around this increasingly rigid process. Just to give you a flavor, here's a typical question posted at the SuperCoder.com readers' questions blog (**http://bit.ly/1rbn8ZL**)—this is the kind of mind-numbing minutiae that your doctor and her staff are dealing with on a regular basis:

Question: *The patient is seen in the hospital for a 410.31, and then is discharged. The patient is scheduled to be seen in the office for a follow-up visit. For this follow-up visit, which is less than eight weeks from the myocardial infarction, is it appropriate to use the fifth digit of "2" on the MI (410.32), or would you still use 410.31?*

Answer: You should use 410.32 (*Acute myocardial infarction of inferoposterior wall; subsequent episode of care*) for this follow-up visit. ICD-9 notes with the 410.xx fifth digit options state that you should "use fifth-digit 2 to designate an episode of care following the initial episode when the patient is admitted for further observation, evaluation or treatment for a myocardial infarction that has received initial treatment, but is still less than eight weeks old." You should report 410.31 (*Acute myocardial infarction of inferoposterior wall; initial episode of care*) only during the initial episode of care. The fifth digit "1" applies until the patient is discharged, regardless of where the cardiologist provides the care. Notes in the ICD-9 manual clarify that you use "1" for the first episode of care, "regardless of the number of times a patient may be transferred during the initial episode of care." If documentation doesn't specify the episode of care (initial or subsequent), you should use fifth digit "0" (*Episode of care unspecified*). If the patient returns more than eight weeks after the infarction, you should use 414.8 (*Other specified forms of chronic ischemic heart disease*). Notes with this code specify it is appropriate for "any condition classifiable to 410 specified as chronic, or presenting with symptoms after eight weeks from date of infarction."

111 **When you are ready to dig deeper**: Information about the breadth and scope of PubMed can be found at the NIH's U.S. National Library of Medicine's Fact Sheet, **http://1.usa.gov/1rqujyK**.

111 **Dr. George Wilding**: More about Dr. Wilding is available at the website of the University of Wisconsin School of Medicine and Public Health, **http://bit.ly/1Dnigrl**.

114 **Dr. William Lippy**: For more about Dr. Lippy and his practice, The Lippy Group, see **http://bit.ly/1C68A2p**.

114 **Dr. Herbert Silverstein**: More about The Silverstein Institute is available at **http://bit.ly/1v9lvwj**; for more on Dr. Silverstein's work with the American Academy of Otolaryngology, see **http://bit.ly/1rs5SB8**.

114 **he had more than two hundred articles in PubMed**: Although we did a search of Dr. Silverstein's articles on PubMed prior to Rachel's interview, the doctor and his colleagues also keep a running tally of their published articles online; that signals to patients how focused they are on this condition. See "About: Publications," Silverstein Institute, **http://bit.ly/XOXYp6**.

116 **Dr. Robert Udelsman**: For more about Dr. Udelsman, see the Yale School of Medicine's website, **http://bit.ly/1wH0SbL**.

116 **Harvard researchers wanted to find out if patients who**: M. L. McCrum et al., "Beyond Volume: Does Hospital Complexity Matter? An Analysis of Inpatient Surgical Mortality in the United States," *Medical Care* 52, no. 3 (March 2014): 235–42, **http://bit.ly/1E1dq2P**.

117 **A few years ago, when Walmart was looking**: For more information on this program, see Margot Sanger-Katz, "Wal-Mart's Super-Counterintuitive Health Care Plan," *National Journal*, May 23, 2013; Larry Husten, "Free Cardiac and Spine Surgery for Walmart Employees at Six Hospitals," Forbes.com, October 12, 2012; Richard Pollock, "Surprise! Walmart Health Plan Is Cheaper, Offers More Coverage Than Obamacare," *Washington Examiner*, January 7, 2014; "Walmart, Lowe's and Pacific Business Group on Health Announce a First of Its Kind National Employers Centers of Excellence Network," Walmart News Archive, press release, October 8, 2013, **http://bit.ly/XYfdVj**; and "Walmart Expands Health Benefits to Cover Heart and Spine Surgeries at No Cost to Associates," Walmart News Archive, press release, October 11, 2012, **http://bit.ly/ZDiiex**.

117 **Home improvement chain Lowe's**: See "Walmart, Lowe's and Pacific Business Group on Health Announce a First of Its Kind National Employers Centers of Excellence Network," Walmart News Archive, press release, October 8, 2013, **http://bit.ly/XYfdVj**; and "Executive Interview: David Lansky," *Journal of Healthcare Contracting*, March 6, 2014, **http://bit.ly/1x2N3Yr**.

117 **Beverage and snack food giant PepsiCo**: See Andrea K. Walker, "PepsiCo to Pay for Employee Surgeries at Hopkins," *Baltimore Sun*, December 11, 2011, **http://bit.ly/1sVgy7v**; and "Johns Hopkins Medicine to Offer PepsiCo Employees New Travel Surgery Benefit," John Hopkins Medicine, press release, December 8, 2011, **http://bit.ly/1x2P4DL**.

124 **Dr. Marc Selner**: Find out more about Dr. Selner and his practice at **http://bit.ly/ZDtyHP**.

CHAPTER 7. EMERGENCY ROOM 101

140 **The doctor showed Tracey her X-rays**: For starting-point information on Central Cord Syndrome, see the American Association of Neurological Surgeons' brief, "Central Cord Syndrome," **http://bit.ly/1CtDCkX**.

141 **In those first few minutes, it can be difficult to decide**: For more extensive information and a list of symptoms and signs to help you decide when it's time to go to an ER or urgent care, see "When to Use the Emergency Room—Adult," from MedLine Plus, a website run by the U.S. National Library of Medicine and the National Institutes of Health, at **http://1.usa.gov/YlPVAF**.

144 **It's very difficult to break through the triage-style shuffling**: "In almost all cases of missed or delayed diagnoses essential pieces of information weren't available at the time the doctor made a decision," says Laura Landro, in "Hospitals Overhaul ERs to Reduce Mistakes," *Wall Street Journal*, May 10, 2011. Keeping your PCP in the information loop will help the hospital staff fill in any missing gaps in your medical history.

144 **an anterior cervical discectomy and fusion, or ACDF**: A video of this very complex surgery, being performed by neurosurgeon Dr. Ali Bydon of Johns Hopkins, can be seen at the school's neurology and neurosurgery video gallery, **http://bit.ly/1vatevV**.

145 **But when the risk involves never**: In a 2012 study of nearly fifty thousand patients who had surgery for spinal stenosis, researchers found that patients treated by very-low-volume surgeons (those who did fewer than 15 procedures over four years) had higher complication rates than patients treated by very-high-volume surgeons (those who performed more than 81 surgeries every four years). Just sixteen extra procedures a year gave these doctors a significant edge (and better outcomes for their patients) over their lower-volume counterparts. See H. H. Dasenbrock et al., "The Impact of Provider Volume on the Outcomes After Surgery for Lumbar Spinal Stenosis," *Neurosurgery* 70, no. 6 (June 2012): 346–53, **http://1.usa.gov/1t2JCKk**.

145 **Dr. Richard G. Fessler**: More on Dr. Fessler and his practice can be found at his website, **http://bit.ly/1uNnF4d**.

146 **these surveys are critical to the hospital**: In 2002 the Centers for Medicare and Medicaid Services teamed with the Agency for Healthcare Research and Quality to develop the Hospital Consumer Assessment of Healthcare Providers and Systems Survey (HCAHPS), which measures patient satisfaction after a hospital stay. Annual results are posted at Medicare's Hospital Compare website, **http://1.usa.gov/1uNKC7k**. Beginning in 2012, with the Affordable Care Act, these surveys became even more important to participating hospitals, as the results were factored into Medicare's incentive-pay reimbursement formula. More on this at the HCAHPS website, **http://bit.ly/1rkwbtV**.

148 **tape-recorded ninety-three encounters**: See K. V. Rhodes et al., "Resuscitating the Physician-Patient Relationship: Emergency Department Communication in an Academic Medical Center," *Annals of Emergency Medicine* 44, no. 3 (September 2004): 262–67, available at the University of Pennsylvania's Scholarly Commons, **http://bit.ly/1rwE7WB**.

Poor communication in the ER also leaves patients prone to medical error and greater potential for problems when they get home, according to one study in which nearly 80 percent of discharged patients didn't fully understand the treatment they had received or how to care for themselves upon release. See Laurie Tarkan, "ER Patients Often Left Confused After Visits," *New York Times*, September 15, 2008.

149 **Dr. C. Noel Bairey Merz**: More about Dr. Bairey Merz can be found at the Cedars-Sinai website, **http://bit.ly/1mHW4m0**.

149 **Heart disease is the number one killer of women**: See "About Heart Disease in Women," Go Red for Women, American Heart Association, **http://bit.ly/1yv2vtI**.

150 **But one-third of all women (and 10 percent of men)**: C. N. Bairey Merz et al., "Insights from the NHLBI-Sponsored Women's Ischemia Syndrome Evaluation (WISE) Study. Part II: Gender Differences in Presentation, Diagnosis, and Outcome with Regard to Gender-Based Pathophysiology of Atherosclerosis and Macrovascular and Microvascular Coronary Disease," *Journal of the American College of Cardiology* 47, no. 3 (February 7, 2006): S21–S29, **http://bit.ly/1BFt1AW**. See also C. Noel Bairey Merz, "The Single Biggest Health Threat Women Face," TEDTalk video, December 2011, **http://bit.ly/1uxltSb**.

150 **women tend to have more general aches**: Want to see the difference in how a female heart attack looks and feels? Comedian Elizabeth Banks gives a lifesaving performance in Go Red for Women's short video, "Just a Little Heart Attack," **http://bit.ly/1vquv21**.

150 **Every woman needs to be aware of the symptoms**: See "Symptoms of Heart Attack," Go Red for Women, American Heart Association, **http://bit.ly/11zq3m8**.

151 **what's called Against Medical Advice, or AMA**: About 1 percent of discharges in the United States are AMA, and physicians and hospitals face intense pressure to be sure they are done ethically. For a physician's perspective on this issue, see J. T. Berger, "Discharge Against Medical Advice:

Ethical Considerations and Professional Obligations," *Journal of Hospital Medicine* 3, no. 5 (2008): 403–8, http://bit.ly/1C7MKiG.

151 **your chances of surviving a coronary event**: Getting care within those first ninety minutes is imperative, but studies show that the *sooner* you can get balloon angioplasty started, the better. See S. S. Rathore et al., "Association of Door-to-Balloon Time and Mortality in Patients Admitted to Hospital with ST Elevation Myocardial Infarction: National Cohort Study," *BMJ* (May 19, 2009): 338:b1807, http://bit.ly/1rkztgO.

152 **check online with the American Board of Medical Specialties**: The ABMS provides a patient-friendly website (http://www.certificationmatters.org) to check on a specialist's certification. Registration (free) is required.

152 **annual Best Hospitals rankings**: For the most recent rankings, see "Best Hospitals," *U.S. News & World Report*, http://bit.ly/1mzq5V9.

152 **designations for a trauma center's ability**: See "Verified Trauma Centers FAQs," American College of Surgeons, September 30, 2009, http://bit.ly/1t3c2UB; and "Access to Trauma Care," CDC, http://1.usa.gov/1rz20OP.

153 **The difference in care infants receive at a pediatric ER**: Of the 119 million emergency room visits in the United States in 2006, almost 20 percent were for children; yet according to a 2002 hospital survey, only 6 percent of emergency departments have all the recommended pediatric supplies and equipment. See the American Academy of Pediatrics Committee on Pediatric Emergency Medicine, the American College of Emergency Physicians Pediatric Committee, and the Emergency Nurses Association Pediatric Committee, "Joint Policy Statement—Guidelines for Care of Children in the Emergency Department," *Annals of Emergency Medicine* 54, no. 4 (October 2009): 543–52, http://bit.ly/1u6ry6w. In a 2009 follow-up, researchers surveyed a random sample of ERs and found that little improvement had been made in our nation's emergency pediatric care capabilities. A. F. Sullivan et al., "National Survey of Pediatric Services Available in U.S. Emergency Departments," *International Journal of Emergency Medicine*. 61, no. 1 (April 24, 2013): 13, http://bit.ly/1wRqoLE.

154 **If the tests confirmed jaundice**: For in-depth information on jaundice signs, symptoms, and treatment, see Ronald J. Wong and Vinod K. Bhutani, "Patient Information: Jaundice in Newborn Infants (Beyond the Basics)," UpToDate.com, http://bit.ly/YHhVi3.

159 **The ombudsman explained that hospitals are prohibited**: For more on the Emergency Medical Treatment and Labor Act of 1986, see "EMTALA," American College of Emergency Physicians, http://bit.ly/1pCPvMi.

CHAPTER 8. PATIENT, M.D.

167 **diagnosed with primary hyperparathyroidism**: For more on this condition, including its causes, risks, and treatments, see G. E. Fuleihan, "Patient Information: Primary Hyperparathyroidism (Beyond the Basics)," UpToDate.com, updated February 18, 2014, http://bit.ly/1tcl2Xw; and "Hyperparathyroidism (Primary)," Yale School of Medicine, http://bit.ly/1tcDwHs.

168 **There was zero chance that a bisphosphonate**: For patients who have no symptoms or who cannot risk having surgery, then monitoring and managing the disease (with treatments that may include a bisphosphonate) is certainly an option. But that was not the case here. "All patients with biochemically confirmed primary hyperparathyroidism (PHPT) who have specific symptoms or signs of their disease should undergo surgical treatment," according to J. P. Bilezikian, A. A. Khan, and J. T. Potts, "Guidelines for the Management of Asymptomatic Primary Hyperparathyroidism: Summary Statement from the Third International Workshop," *Journal of Clinical Endocrinology & Metabolism* 94, no. 2 (February 2009): 335–39, http://1.usa.gov/1pCVTDf.

168 **Dr. John P. Bilezikian**: For more on Dr. Bilezikian, see his Columbia University Department of Medicine faculty page at http://bit.ly/1roreQA.

169 **He's also a lead author in the longest case study**: The conclusion of this study? That the disease continues to progress—and cause further bone-mineral density loss—in patients who did not have surgery. See M. R. Rubin et al., "The Natural History of Primary Hyperparathyroidism with or without Parathyroid Surgery After 15 Years," *Journal of Clinical Endocrinology and Metabolism* 93, no. 9 (September 2008): 3462–70, http://1.usa.gov/1uxtM01.

170 **Dr. Robert Udelsman**: Dr. Udelsman's bio is at the Yale School of Medicine website, http://bit.ly/1wH0SbL.

170 **pioneered an approach to parathyroid surgery**: In a paper presented in December 2001 at the 113th Annual Session of the Southern Surgical Association, Dr. Udelsman described a groundbreaking study of 656 primary hyperparathyroid patients who underwent surgery. He found that the 255 patients who received new-at-the-time, minimally invasive surgery (which included intraoperative testing) enjoyed "a 50 percent reduction in operating time, a sevenfold reduction in length of hospital stay, and a mean cost savings of $2,693 per procedure," compared to those who underwent the older method, with no testing. His pioneering work helped make this technique the globally accepted gold standard of practice for parathyroid surgery. See R. Udelsman, "Six Hundred Fifty-Six Consecutive Explorations for Primary Hyperparathyroidism," *Annals of Surgery* 235, no. 5 (May 2002): 665–72, http://1.usa.gov/ZlUewX.

171 **published an incredible study**: Ibid.

172 **That would have meant more surgery**: The most common cause of redo surgeries for my condition? Missed bad glands. See A. Agarwal and R. Pradhan, "Failed Parathyroidectomy: The Road Ahead," *Indian Journal of Endocrinology and Metabolism* 16, no. 2 (December 2012): S221–S223, http://1.usa.gov/1nCa2qm. And my risk of failure would have been even greater had I gone to a low-volume surgeon. See H. Chen et al., "Operative Failures after Parathyroidectomy for Hyperparathyroidism: The Influence of Surgical Volume," *Annals of Surgery* 252, no. 4 (October 2010): 691–95, http://1.usa.gov/1uXNb74.

CHAPTER 9. STEP 1—IMMERSION

177 **idiopathic acquired angioedema**: Basic information on angioedema can be found at "Angioedema," MedlinePlus, http://1.usa.gov/YOJ7vh. For a more in-depth clinical review, see A. P. Kaplan, "Angioedema," *World Allergy Organization Journal* 1, no. 6 (June 2008): 103–13, http://1.usa.gov/1vuDu2b.

177 **lupus, a chronic autoimmune disease**: P. H. Schur, "Patient information: Systemic Lupus Erythematosus (SLE) (Beyond the Basics)," UpToDate.com, updated May 13, 2014, http://bit.ly/1own6bJ; "What is Lupus?," National Institute of Arthritis and Musculoskeletal and Skin Diseases, http://1.usa.gov/1qSIiIp; and "Frequently Asked Questions," Lupus Foundation of America, http://bit.ly/1DX0Q4G.

177 **something called polysorbate 80, an inactive ingredient**: It's also known as Tween 80 and can be found in numerous cosmetic products, medical prep solutions, and even whipped dessert products. See "Food Additive Status List," U.S. Food and Drug Administration, http://1.usa.gov/1vsMd31; and "Polysorbate 80: Excipient (Pharmacologically Inactive Substance)," Drugs.com, http://bit.ly/1MvzCbW.

181 **"For instance, with psoriatic arthritis"**: Even psoriasis sufferers face many potential comorbidities, such as cardiovascular disease, obesity, diabetes, and depression, as well as psoriatic arthritis. See W. P. Gulliver, "Importance of Screening for Comorbidities in Psoriasis Patients," *Expert Review of Dermatology* 3, no. 2 (2008): 133–35, http://bit.ly/1uoEeWF.

184 **Eric had prostate cancer**: The Prostate Cancer Foundation (PCF), the world's largest philanthropic source of research funding for the disease, is a tremendous resource of information for patients and their families. For more, see http://www.pcf.org. If you are at the beginning of a prostate cancer immersion journey, PCF has a plethora of guides to help keep you and your family steady:

see its "Prostate Cancer Guides and Books," **http://bit.ly/1mRC68x**; its in-depth information in "Clinical Trials," **http://bit.ly/1oAPAkC**; and its information on "Treatment Options," **http://bit.ly/1uC7ZEK**. Review them once you have a firm diagnosis and are ready to collect information about therapies.

184 **the second most common cause of cancer death**: There were an estimated 233,000 new cases of prostate cancer in 2014. See "SEER Stat Fact Sheets: Prostate Cancer," National Cancer Institute, posted April 2014, **http://1.usa.gov/1pp6hj2**. But while prostate cancer is the most *common* diagnosed cancer among men, more men will die from lung cancer. See "Cancer Among Men," CDC, updated September 2, 2014, **http://1.usa.gov/1qT3qyn**.

184 **But while one in seven men will be diagnosed**: The median age of diagnosis is sixty-six. See "How Many Men Get Prostate Cancer?," American Cancer Society, revised September 12, 2014, **http://bit.ly/1rrMN2P**.

184 **In fact, about 2.5 million Americans are alive**: Ibid.

184 **There are several different initial courses**: For more on treatment options, questions to ask your doctors, and issues to consider when making treatment decisions, see "Newly Diagnosed," Prostate Cancer Foundation, **http://bit.ly/1CFmOaP**.

185 **Dr. Mark Kawachi**: Dr. Kawachi's bio is at the City of Hope website, **http://bit.ly/1mNo7R7**.

185 **but what if the reading had not been accurate?**: In a study to determine the value of second opinions, researchers analyzed the results of 855 men who were originally diagnosed with prostate cancer and were considering radical prostatectomy. After independent readings, there were major discrepancies in the Gleason scores in 124 cases (or 14.5 percent): 57 (6.7 percent) were upgraded; 67 (7.8 percent) were downgraded. And in 11 cases, a second opinion found that the cells were only atypical (meaning not abnormal enough to call it cancer) or benign with no cancer. See F. Brimo, L. Schultz, and J. I. Epstein, "The Value of Mandatory Second Opinion Pathology Review of Prostate Needle Biopsy Interpretation Before Radical Prostatectomy," *Journal of Urology* 184, no. 1 (July 2010): 126–30, **http://1.usa.gov/1pG7AJx**.

185 **Dr. Jonathan Epstein**: More on Dr. Epstein and his colleagues at the Johns Hopkins Pathology website, **http://bit.ly/1v6bWOi**. See also Janet Farrar Worthington, "Better Send It to Epstein," *Hopkins Medical News*, Fall 2002, **http://bit.ly/1thGZom**.

186 **In fact, thirty years ago prostate cancer surgery**: The side effects of surgery were, to many men, worse than the disease itself. That was before urologist Dr. Patrick Walsh, with the help of a retired urology professor in the Netherlands named Dr. Pietr Donker, discovered and developed a nerve-sparing technique that preserved sexual and urinary function for the majority of men who had surgery. To learn more, see Dr. Walsh interviewed by Charlie Rose, March 31, 2008, on Johns Hopkins's James Buchanan Brady Urological Institute website, **http://bit.ly/YU20Np**.

186 **Dr. Patrick Walsh**: Ibid. See also Dr. Walsh's bio on the Johns Hopkins Medicine website, **http://bit.ly/1yzqNHa**.

186 **he would heal faster with the robotic option**: Studies and anecdotal evidence in the last six years suggest that some surgeons were performing robotic surgery without proper training and credentialing, causing unnecessary harm to patients. See J. K. Parsons et al., "Diffusion of Surgical Innovations, Patient Safety, and Minimally Invasive Radical Prostatectomy," *JAMA Surgery* 149, no. 8 (August 1, 2014): 845–51, **http://bit.ly/YU2anW**; and Roni Caryn Rabin, "Salesmen in the Surgical Suite," *New York Times*, March 25, 2013. Which is why it's so important to be on the cutting—and not the bleeding—edge of new technologies. To protect yourself, ask potential surgeons, as Eric did, *How many times have you done this procedure?*; choose a doctor who spends the majority of his time on your specific disease and has a great deal of experience with the exact surgery or procedure you need; and have your treatment done at a hospital with the volume and resources to care for you if anything goes wrong.

188 **To start, he went to a general urologist**: In his case, he needed to be at a larger hospital with volume in prostate cancer treatment. For studies that support this, see L. M. Ellison et al., "The Effect of Hospital Volume on Cancer Control after Radical Prostatectomy," *Journal of Urology* 173, no. 6 (June 2005): 2094–98, **http://bit.ly/10lHS8r**; and D. A. Barocas et al., "Impact of Surgeon and Hospital Volume on Outcomes of Radical Prostatectomy," *Urologic Oncology* 28, no. 3 (May–June 2010): 243–50, **http://1.usa.gov/1CGnmgn**.

189 **Volume—that is, the number of times a surgeon has**: For an extensive review of volume studies, see Maria Hewitt, *Interpreting the Volume–Outcome Relationship in the Context of Health Care Quality: Workshop Summary* (Washington, D.C.: Institute of Medicine/National Academies Press, 2000), free download at **http://bit.ly/1wZxWMr**; and A. Elixhauser, C. Steiner, and F. Fraser, "Volume Thresholds and Hospital Characteristics in the United States," *Health Affairs* 22, no. 2 (March–April 2003): 167–77, **http://bit.ly/1xDdELS**.

190 **To test this idea—that a doctor's surgical volume**: For more on surgical volume with respect to prostatectomy, see A. J. Vickers et al., "The Surgical Learning Curve for Prostate Cancer Control After Radical Prostatectomy," *Journal of the National Cancer Institute* 99, no. 15 (August 1, 2007): 1171–77, **http://bit.ly/1v7m21n**. Note that procedures in which a surgeon only *assists* don't count as part of that doctor's volume, and the researchers in this study did not include them when calculating the total number of radical prostatectomies a surgeon had performed prior to each subject patient's operation.

190 **researchers studied the survival outcomes**: R. E. Bristow et al., "High-Volume Ovarian Cancer Care: Survival Impact and Disparities in Access for Advanced-Stage Disease," *Gynecologic Oncology* 132, no. 2 (February 2014): 403–10, **http://bit.ly/1rJErTc**.

191 **Although the chemo-first, surgery-second approach**: Recent studies show that men with *advanced* metastatic prostate cancer that is hormone-sensitive (or men who have a recurrence of the disease after surgery or radiation treatment but can still benefit from hormone therapy) will have better outcomes if they are treated with chemotherapy *combined* with hormone therapy *early* rather than later—but that's a small population of patients, and it was not Patrick's presentation. See "NIH-Funded Study Shows Increased Survival in Men with Metastatic Prostate Cancer Who Receive Chemotherapy When Starting Hormone Therapy," National Cancer Institute, press release, updated June 1, 2014, **http://1.usa.gov/YU35op**; and Andrew Pollack, "Study May Alter Approach to Prostate Cancer," *New York Times*, June 2, 2014. For more information on treatment options at different stages of the disease, see "Treatment Options," Prostate Cancer Foundation, **http://bit.ly/1uC7ZEK**.

191 **Dr. Peter T. Scardino**: More about Dr. Scardino is available at the Memorial Sloan Kettering Cancer Center website, **http://bit.ly/1CGwMso**.

191 **the study that found better outcomes for prostate**: Vickers et al., "Surgical Learning Curve for Prostate Cancer Control after Radical Prostatectomy."

192 **but this was a difficult and risky procedure**: Patients had, on average, a 1.5 times higher risk of mortality when they had esophageal cancer surgery at a low-volume hospital than at a high-volume hospital, according to Elixhauser, Steiner, and Fraser, "Volume Thresholds and Hospital Characteristics."

192 **You want to be at an institution where the experience**: Ibid. See also M. L. McCrum et al., "Beyond Volume: Does Hospital Complexity Matter? An Analysis of Inpatient Surgical Mortality in the United States," *Medical Care* 52, no. 3 (March 2014): 235–42, **http://bit.ly/1E1dq2P**.

193 **staffed by full-time, board-certified intensivists**: Having intensivists on staff may help reduce complications and shorten a patient's length of stay, according to K. Kumar et al., "The Benefits of 24/7 In-House Intensivist Coverage for Prolonged-Stay Cardiac Surgery Patients," *Journal of Thoracic and Cardiovascular Surgery* 148, no. 1 (July 2014): 290–97, **http://bit.ly/YU3t6m**; and U. P. Iyegha et al., "Intensivists Improve Outcomes and Compliance with Process Measures in Critically Ill Patients," *Journal of the American College of Surgeons* 216, no. 3 (March 2013): 363–72, **http://bit.ly/1xDpntN**.

193 **Dr. Anthony D'Amico**: Dr. D'Amico's profile is at the Dana-Farber Cancer Institute website, **http://bit.ly/1vyQfc5**.

194 **"especially the ones that have a Level I trauma center"**: See "Verified Trauma Centers FAQ," American College of Surgeons, September 30, 2009, **http://bit.ly/1t3c2UB**; and "Access to Trauma Care," CDC, **http://1.usa.gov/1rz2OOP**.

CHAPTER 10. STEP 2—DIAGNOSIS

197 **A 2015 report from the Institute of Medicine**: "Postmortem examination research spanning decades has shown that diagnostic errors contribute to approximately 10 percent of patient deaths," according to *Improving Diagnosis in Healthcare*, "Report in Brief" (Washington, D.C.: Institute of Medicine/National Academies Press, 2015), **http://bit.ly/2b9fr4d**.

197 **missed diagnoses alone may lead to 40,000 to 80,000**: "Autopsy studies consistently find undiagnosed disease as the cause of death in 10 percent to 20 percent of patients, of whom half could have been successfully treated. Applied to current U.S. hospital mortality, this yields 40,000 to 80,000 preventable deaths annually from missed diagnoses alone," according to L. L. Leape, D. M. Berwick, and D. W. Bates, "Counting Deaths Due to Medical Error—Reply," *JAMA*. 288, no. 19 (November 20, 2002): 2404–5, **http://bit.ly/1sRMqQm**. These 2002 figures have been cited in some two dozen papers; to name a couple of recent examples: A. S. Saber Tehrani et al., "25-Year Summary of US Malpractice Claims for Diagnostic Errors 1986–2010: An Analysis from the National Practitioner Data Bank," *BMJ Quality & Safety* 22, no. 8 (2013): 672–80, **http://bit.ly/YUPNZf**; and M. L. Graber, R. M. Wachter, and C. K. Cassel, "Bringing Diagnosis into the Quality and Safety Equations," *JAMA* 308, no. 12 (September 26, 2012): 1211–12, **http://bit.ly/1sPWlWQ**. But in arriving at these estimates, Dr. Leape and his colleagues cite a now decades-old study of patients who died in a teaching hospital in Switzerland in 1972, 1982, and 1992: K. Sonderegger-Iseli et al., "Diagnostic Errors in Three Medical Eras: A Necropsy Study," *Lancet* 355, no. 9220 (June 10, 2000): 2027–31, **http://bit.ly/Z1ks7f**.

Most patient safety leaders believe that 40,000 to 80,000 deaths a year due to diagnostic error is a very low estimate—and that coming to a precise and current figure is not easy. Diagnostic error is examined through very different prisms (via autopsy reports, paid malpractice claims, or hospitals' self-reporting), which leads to variable results—from as low as 1 percent to as high as 55 percent in certain diseases and patient groups. See L. Zwaan, G. D. Schiff, and H. Singh, "Advancing the Research Agenda for Diagnostic Error Reduction," *BMJ Quality and Safety* 22, no. S2 (October 2013): ii52–ii57, **http://1.usa.gov/ZBGJti**.

In an exhaustive 2008 review of diagnostic error studies, researchers noted what I think is the most important take-away point, "[While] the exact frequency may be difficult to determine precisely, it is clear that an extensive and ever-growing literature confirms that diagnostic errors exist at non-trivial and sometimes alarming rates." Their study also offers an interesting breakdown of diagnostic mistakes by disease, gleaned from select papers: for instance, a rate of 21 percent missed breast cancers in one study; a delayed or inaccurate diagnosis in 69 percent of patients with bipolar disorders in another. See E. S. Berner and M. L. Graber, "Overconfidence as a Cause of Diagnostic Error in Medicine," *American Journal of Medicine* 121, no. 5 (May 2008): S2–S23, **http://bit.ly/1x4vMLn**.

198 **The figure doubles to 80, 000 to 160,000 patients annually**: As its authors noted, the data they examined reflect only *paid* claims for serious, diagnostic-related harms. Many more mistakes go unrecognized and/or unreported, and claims are never filed. See A. S. Saber Tehrani et al., "25-Year Summary of US Malpractice Claims for Diagnostic Errors 1986–2010: An Analysis from the National Practitioner Data Bank," *BMJ Quality & Safety* 22, no. 8 (2013): 672–80, **http://bit.ly/YUPNZf**.

199 **Dr. Neda Pakdaman**: More about Dr. Pakdaman is available at the Stanford School of Medicine website, **http://stanford.io/YUP89X**.

200 **And yet that's what most people do**: In fact, 70 percent of Americans are so confident in their doctor's advice that they don't feel the need to do additional research or get a second opinion, according to a November 2010 Gallup Health and Healthcare Survey. That's an increase from 2002, when it was 64 percent. And it made no difference if the respondent had a graduate degree or had

barely finished high school—blind trust reigned at all educational levels. See Frank Newport, "Most Americans Take Doctor's Advice Without Second Opinion," Gallup.com, December 2, 2010, **http://bit.ly/1veuqfJ**.

Doctors are also guilty of sometimes being overly confident in their own advice. According to a survey of four hundred cancer specialists, 60 percent estimated that misdiagnoses happen 0 to 10 percent of the time—which runs counter to published studies estimating error rates as high as 44 percent for some cancers. See "Exploring Diagnostic Accuracy in Cancer," National Coalition on Health Care, Best Doctors, January 2013, **http://bit.ly/ZxdEio**.

200 **asked to make a risky financial decision**: J. B. Engelmann et al., "Expert Financial Advice Neurobiologically 'Offloads' Financial Decision-Making Under Risk," *PLoS ONE*. 4, no. 3 (March 24, 2009): e4957, **http://bit.ly/1pu9uxO**; and Noreena Hertz, "Why We Make Bad Decisions," *New York Times*, October 20, 2013.

201 **Researchers interested in learning more about the rate**: H. Singh et al., "Errors in Cancer Diagnosis: Current Understanding and Future Directions," *Journal of Clinical Oncology* 25, no. 31 (November 1, 2007): 5009–18, **http://bit.ly/1tl70mu**. As the authors of the study noted, literature on diagnostic error rates for cancer is fairly scarce; most analysis in this realm relies on malpractice claims and autopsy studies.

201 **missed breast cancer was one of the most frequent**: Ibid. The authors cited rankings on breast and skin cancer (as the first- and second-most-error-prone diagnoses) from D. B. Troxel, "Pitfalls in the Diagnosis of Malignant Melanoma: Findings of a Risk Management Panel Study," *American Journal of Surgical Pathology*, 27, no. 9 (September 2003): 1278–83. A free online version of this study can be also found at The Doctors Company website, **http://bit.ly/1x499a0**.

201 **an alarming 2006 white paper**: "Why Current Breast Pathology Practices Must Be Evaluated," Susan G. Komen for the Cure White Paper, Komen.org, June 2006, **http://sgk.mn/1vyCxUW**.

201 **the medical value of second opinions**: See interview with MD Anderson's Thomas Feeley in Laura Landro, "What If the Doctor Is Wrong?" *Wall Street Journal*, January 17, 2012.

201 **How do diagnostic flubs happen?**:The factors cited are based on my own observations as well as the anecdotal evidence shared by clients, colleagues, and physicians. For additional insights, see Laura Landro, "The Biggest Mistakes Doctors Make," *Wall Street Journal*, November 17, 2013, which has helpful sidebars on (1) common biases, and (2) steps to take to prevent errors (sourced from Dalhousie University and *BMJ Quality and Safety*, respectively). Internist Kevin Pho also has an informative website, KevinMD.com, where he shares the collective posts and opinions of practitioner bloggers as well as an array of patient-friendly posts on diagnostic error and patient safety, **http://bit.ly/1rHjSWf**.

202 **742 patients who got a second opinion**: And these second-opinion disagreements actually prompted a change in clinical management for 32 of the 742 patients—or more specifically, a change of course for patients who had tissues examined from their thyroids (13 cases), necks (soft tissue and lymph node, 9 cases), salivary glands (2 cases), livers (2 cases), and other lymph nodes, pancreas, lung, breast, kidney/adrenal, and mediastinum (one case each), according to P. E. Bomeisl, S. Alam, and P. E. Wakely, "Interinstitutional Consultation in Fine-Needle Aspiration Cytopathology: A Study of 742 Cases," *Cancer Cytopathology* 117, no. 4 (August 25, 2009): 237–46, **http://bit.ly/1tlfv0U**.

202 **a lab technician's ability to accurately interpret**: T. M. Elsheikh et al., "Does the Time of Day or Weekday Affect Screening Accuracy?" *Cancer Cytopathology* 118, no. 1 (February 25, 2010): 41–46, **http://1.usa.gov/1C8WKGN**.

203 **Health insurers regularly cover second opinions**: For a medically necessary procedure that a doctor is recommending, some plans require a second opinion, while others will pay simply if the patient asks. See "How to Find a Doctor or Treatment Facility If You Have Cancer," National Cancer Institute, **http://1.usa.gov/1r4pLZR**. For patients with Medicare, 80 percent of the cost of a second opinion is covered; if the second differs from the first, Medicare pays for 80 percent of

a third opinion. See "Your Medicare Coverage: Second Surgical Opinions," Medicare.gov, **http://1.usa.gov/1uhjvDP**.

204 **Another way to protect yourself from diagnostic error**: Laura Landro, "The Biggest Mistakes Doctors Make," *Wall Street Journal*, November 17, 2013.

206 **How to question your diagnosis**: For additional resources, see the nonprofit National Patient Safety Foundation's "Checklist for Getting the Right Diagnosis," at **http://bit.ly/1GIXa9B**. The Society to Improve Diagnosis in Medicine houses the latest research on diagnostic error, as well as excellent educational resources for patients, at **http://bit.ly/YV3U0a**.

CHAPTER 11. STEP 3—TREATMENT

213 **Marissa had had an unremarkable freckle**: Marissa's mole didn't appear troubling until years later, when it became bigger and darker—which should have set off alarm bells for her dermatologist and her PCP. There were about 76,100 new cases of melanoma in the United States in 2014, and about 9,710 melanoma deaths, according to the National Cancer Institute (NCI). NCI's helpful "What Does Melanoma Look Like?" (**http://1.usa.gov/1xi49i1**) is a primer on the ABCDEs of detection. "Common Moles, Dysplastic Nevi, and Risk of Melanoma" (**http://1.usa.gov/1oK7O3a**) includes helpful comparison photos of cancerous and benign blemishes. See also NCI's patient-friendly "Melanoma" page, **http://1.usa.gov/Z9YEpP**; the advanced version for health professionals is at **http://1.usa.gov/1rdC0mU**.

214 **It might be cancerous**: There are several different kinds of skin cancer. Basal cell carcinoma is the most common form (an estimated 2.8 million cases are diagnosed annually in the United States), but it is rarely fatal. Squamous cell carcinoma is the second most common (700,000 cases a year), but only about 2 percent of patients die from it. Melanoma is the least common skin cancer (about 76,100 cases were diagnosed in 2014, and an estimated 73,870 in 2015), yet it is the most deadly: one person dies of melanoma every hour. For more information on appearance, prognosis, and treatment options, see "Skin Cancer Facts" (**http://bit.ly/1s5gTJ0**), and "Skin Cancer Information" (**http://bit.ly/1xXc2wz**) at the Skin Cancer Foundation's website, and "Cancer Facts & Figures 2015," a report from the American Cancer Society (**http://bit.ly/1ydSvdg**).

214 **trained in something called Mohs surgery**: For specific details about Mohs surgery, see the American College of Mohs Surgery's "About Mohs Surgery" page, **http://bit.ly/1GIYGbQ**.

214 **wasn't convinced that Mohs was the correct**: It's important to remember that there are a range of treatment options for skin cancers, so you really need to get an expert opinion on your pathology and the therapies that would be best for your condition and its presentation. NCI offers information at "General Information About Skin Cancer," Health Professional Version, **http://1.usa.gov/1uScXgI**.

215 **Dr. Erica H. Lee**: More about Dr. Lee is available at the Memorial Sloan Kettering Cancer Center website, **http://bit.ly/1vJ1iPb**.

216 **Pathology is an art**: You don't want to take chances when it comes to skin cancer: Get an expert opinion. In a 2002 paper that looked at pathology results from 5,136 skin cancer patients, researchers found that 559 patients (11 percent) had diagnoses that were significantly different on second opinion. Of these, 439 patients (almost 9 percent of the total) had the severity of their diagnosis either upgraded or downgraded in ways that resulted in a significant impact on their treatment and prognosis. In addition, 120 patients (2.3 percent) had a total change in diagnosis from malignant to benign or vice versa. See K. S. McGinnis et al., "Pathology Review of Cases Presenting to a Multidisciplinary Pigmented Lesion Clinic," *JAMA Dermatology* 138, no. 5 (May 2002): 617–21, **http://bit.ly/1vJ2VMO**.

216 **looked to be between Stage I and Stage II**: For more information on treatment guidelines and how melanoma is staged (p. 26), see the National Comprehensive Cancer Network's Guidelines for Patients, "Melanoma," version 1.2014, **http://bit.ly/ZPnE6R**.

217 **With back pain, for example**: See R. Chou et al., "Diagnosis and Treatment of Low Back Pain: A Joint Clinical Practice Guideline from the American College of Physicians and the American Pain Society," *Annals of Internal Medicine* 147, no. 7 (October 2, 2007): 478–91, **http://bit.ly/1EmOAw7**.

219 **glioblastoma, a very aggressive brain tumor**: Glioblastomas (the type of brain tumor that killed Senator Edward Kennedy) and malignant gliomas are the most common types of malignant brain tumors, with about 17,000 new diagnoses annually. See A. Omuro and L. M. DeAngelis, "Glioblastoma and Other Malignant Gliomas: A Clinical Review," *JAMA*. 310, no. 17 (November 6, 2013): 1842–50, **http://bit.ly/1yI8zDu**. They are extremely difficult to treat, and the prognosis is poor. (The median survival rate is nine months, or up to sixteen months for patients who receive surgery and chemo-radiation.) But as with any serious condition, there's a bell curve for survival outcomes, and some patients do beat the odds and live much longer. In fact, half of the patients who survive four years will survive four more. See W. L. Bi and R. Beroukhim, "Beating the Odds: Extreme Long-Term Survival with Glioblastoma," *Journal of Neuro-Oncology* 16, no. 9 (September 2014): 1159–60, **http://bit .ly/1yIezMC**; and one UC San Francisco patient's incredible story, Victoria Colliver, "Survival Odds Increase for Brain Tumor," *San Francisco Chronicle*, December 25, 2012, **http://bit.ly/1xXSSql**.

219 *a meningioma, . . . a very slow-growing tumor*: For detailed information on meningioma, see Helen A. Shih, "Patient Information: Meningioma (Beyond the Basics)," UpToDate.com, updated July 22, 2013, **http://bit.ly/ZPqskB**. See also the Brain Science Foundation's "Meningioma" page, **http://bit.ly/1CPZWFy**.

225 **a candidate for stereotactic radiation therapy**: See the American Association of Neurological Surgeons' "Meningiomas" patient information page, updated June 2012, **http://bit.ly/1xj9yW5**; D. Kondziolka, J. C. Flickinger, and L. Dade Lunsford, "Clinical Research in Stereotactic Radiosurgery: Lessons Learned from Over 10,000 Cases," *Neurological Research* 33, no. 8 (October 1, 2011): 792–802, **http://bit.ly/1EXq3tb**; and "Stereotactic Radiosurgery Overview," International RadioSurgery Association, **http://bit.ly/ZjjW4m**.

226 **if the radiation didn't work, or the tumor came back**: When active surveillance is no longer a viable option, surgery is typically the next choice—barring any major risk factors—because the complete removal of the tumor lowers the rate of recurrence. However, there is no one-size-fits-all therapy, and patients should try to understand the pros and cons of a treatment plan within the context of their *specific* condition: in other words, what are the known results for patients who have your disease profile? For more on meningioma treatment, see "Meningioma Treatment Options," Brain Science Foundation, **http://bit.ly/ZrnyBw**.

226 **chance of developing radiation-induced cancer**: I found fewer than two dozen reported cases of it in a recent review of the literature, but the factors that lead to secondary malignancies are not well understood. Several papers conclude that while the risk of radiation-induced disease is small, patients must be informed of *all* potential complications. See M. Abedalthagafi and A. Bakhshwon, "Radiation-Induced Glioma Following Cyberknife Treatment of Metastatic Renal Cell Carcinoma: A Case Report," *Journal of Medical Case Reports* 6, no. 271 (2012), **http://1.usa.gov/1nc8QJy**; A. Balasubramaniam et al., "Glioblastoma Multiforme after Stereotactic Radiotherapy for Acoustic Neuroma: Case Report and Review of the Literature," *Journal of Neuro-Oncology* 4 (October 2007): 447–53, **http://1.usa.gov/ZsgMM7**; and Rodney C. Diaz, "Gamma Knife and Other Stereotactic Radiotherapies for Acoustic Neuroma," *MedScape*, updated September 23, 2013, **http://bit .ly/1vLnfgA**.

228 **mother had taken diethylstilbestrol, or DES**: "Fact Sheet: Diethylstilbestrol (DES) and Cancer," National Cancer Institute, reviewed October 5, 2011, **http://1.usa.gov/1vLBnFC**.

228 **Five to ten million children were exposed**: "DES Exposure: Questions and Answers—What is DES?," American Cancer Society, revised February 18, 2014, **http://bit.ly/1sb6201**.

228 **"the numbers show it's a low risk"**: Secondary malignancies, if they occur at all, typically arise within five to ten years posttreatment. Of the sixteen reported cases of radiation-induced malignancies that Georgetown University Hospital researchers examined, nine patients were under the age of

forty at the time of radiation. See M. Abedalthagafi and A. Bakhshwon, "Radiation-Induced Glioma Following Cyberknife Treatment of Metastatic Renal Cell Carcinoma: A Case Report," *Journal of Medical Case Reports* 6, no. 271 (2012), http://1.usa.gov/1nc8QJy.

230 **For the first time ever, when you are**: In 2012 the *New England Journal of Medicine* celebrated its two hundredth anniversary with a special series of articles that looked at the history and rapidly changing future of medicine in America. Biomedical discoveries will only accelerate, an NEJM editorial noted, as precision medicine allows practitioners to view a patient's condition from molecular, genetic, and organ-based perspectives. See *NEJM's* two hundredth anniversary Articles database, at http://bit.ly/1vNNaVL. Further evidence of progress: life expectancy rates in the United States reached an all-time high of 78.8 years in 2012, while death rates reached a record low of 732.8 per 100,000 people. See J. Q. Xu et al., "Mortality in the United States, 2012," National Center for Health Statistics, data brief no. 168, October 2014, http://1.usa.gov/1pRf51h.

230 **In 1964, for instance, the five-year survival**: The most common type of leukemia in children and adolescents is acute lymphoblastic leukemia (ALL). Between 2003 and 2009, the most recent stats available, the five-year survival rate for ALL patients was 91.7 percent for adolescents under fifteen years, and 92.6 percent for children under five years. See the Leukemia and Lymphoma Society's "Facts Spring 2014," p. 11, revised April 2014, http://bit.ly/ZsjhOV. See also "Cancer in Children and Adolescents," National Cancer Institute, reviewed May 12, 2014, http://1.usa.gov/ZcviXK.

230 **with the help of a daily multidrug cocktail**: For more information on the drugs that are used to fight HIV and AIDS, see Sarah Moughty, "20 Years After HIV Announcement, Magic Johnson Emphasizes: 'I Am Not Cured,'" November 7, 2011, *Frontline* at PBS.org, http://to.pbs .org/1oOyHTr; "The Virus: Fighting Back," *Frontline* at PBS.org, http://to.pbs.org/Zsk4Pi; and Allison Samuels, "Magic Johnson: 20 Years of Living with HIV," *Newsweek*, May 15, 2011.

230 **Immunotherapy, for example, is an exciting**: For an excellent overview, see Jennifer Couzin-Frankel, "Breakthough of the Year: Cancer Immunotherapy," *Science* 6165, no. 342 (December 20, 2013): 1432–33, http://bit.ly/1DYV94f; and Ron Winslow, "Cancer's Super-Survivors: How the Promise of Immunotherapy Is Transforming Oncology," *Wall Street Journal*, December 4, 2014.

231 **In fact, whenever we take on a cancer client**: This targeted-therapy approach, which tackles cancer on a genetic level, has shifted the way we talk about cancers. See Anne Eisenberg, "Variations on a Gene, and Tools to Find Them," *New York Times*, April 28, 2013. See also "Cancer Biology & Biomarkers," Caris Molecular Intelligence, http://bit.ly/1qrFrGw; and "FAQs: Patients," Foundation-One, http://bit.ly/1w3TRRw.

231 **In some cases, there are already drugs on the market**: For a list of FDA-approved drugs, see "Targeted Cancer Therapies," National Cancer Institute, reviewed April 25, 2014, http://1.usa .gov/1rhsb7n. See also "Cancer Biology & Biomarkers," Caris Molecular Intelligence, http://bit .ly/1b4S1f1.

231 **his cancer had an EGFR mutation**: Tarceva is the brand name of a drug called erlotinib, which has been approved for treatment of non-small-cell lung cancer and of advanced pancreatic cancer in some patients. See "FDA Approves First Companion Diagnostic to Detect Gene Mutation Associated with a Type of Lung Cancer—New Use for Tarceva Also Approved," FDA, news release, May 14, 2013, http://1.usa.gov/1qjkopt; and "Erlotinib," FDA, updated April 19, 2010, http:// 1.usa.gov/1vOV6nV.

231 **HER2-targeting Herceptin for some types of breast cancers**: See "Targeted Agents Active Against HER2-Positive Breast Cancer: Questions and Answers," National Cancer Institute, updated June 1, 2014, http://1.usa.gov/1vNsImS; and "Tumor Characteristics," Komen.org, updated October 23, 2013, http://sgk.mn/1oZcGRZ.

231 **for late-stage papillary thyroid cancer**: For more on this disease, its staging, prognosis, and treatments, see "Thyroid Cancer Treatment," National Cancer Institute, patient version, http:// 1.usa.gov/1CVNmob; health professional version, http://1.usa.gov/1rm1Xkm.

231 **BRAF mutation, which is relatively common**: BRAF mutations may be found in melanoma, thyroid cancer, and colorectal cancer. For more on the detection of BRAF-gene defects, see Sherilyn Alvaran Tuazon, "BRAF Gene Mutation Tests," *Medscape*, updated December 12, 2012, **http://bit .ly/1sgAPso**.

231 **Zelboraf, had just been approved**: "FDA Approves Zelboraf and Companion Diagnostic Test for Late-Stage Skin Cancer—Second Melanoma Drug Approved This Year That Improves Overall Survival," FDA, news release, August 17, 2011, **http://1.usa.gov/1y7NEZh**.

232 **But Matthew was using this brand-new**: Off-label drug use to treat cancer—and the side effects of cancer therapies—is common and perfectly legal: Once the FDA approves a drug, doctors can prescribe it for any purpose that makes sense for the patient. The challenge is getting insurance companies to cover it if the use is novel. Individual cases vary, and you should always check with your insurance company. See "Cancer Drug Information: Off-Label Drug Use in Cancer Treatment," National Cancer Institute, posted January 1, 2014, **http://1.usa.gov/Zevw0B**.

232 **What do you do in a situation like this?**: In cases when patients want to try a drug that's *not* yet FDA-approved and when, for various reasons, they cannot enter the drug's clinical trials or simply get access to the treatment, they can apply for expanded access, or "compassionate use." See "Expanded Access: Information for Patients," FDA, updated September 15, 2014, **http://1.usa.gov /ZtkoNJ**. See also Darshak Sanghavi, "How Dying Patients Get Access to Experimental Drugs," *New York Times Magazine*, November 3, 2013.

233 **His bridge ended up being a short one, about four months**: An early clinical trial of Zelboraf (vemurafenib) in three patients with papillary thyroid cancer showed more promising results. They enjoyed 11.4 months, 13.2 months, and 11.7 months of stable disease—and in some cases a reduction in lesions—before the drug stopped working. But as with any drug, there can be serious side effects, and more research still needs to be done on larger groups of patients to truly gauge Zelboraf's efficacy for patients with papillary thyroid cancer. See K. B. Kim et al., "Clinical Responses to Vemurafenib in Patients with Metastatic Papillary Thyroid Cancer Harboring BRAFV600E Mutation," *Thyroid* 23, no. 10 (October 2013): 1277–83, **http://1.usa.gov/1vRq9kN**. See also S. M. Ali et al., "Extended Antitumor Response of a *BRAF* V600E Papillary Thyroid Carcinoma to Vemurafenib," *Case Reports in Oncology* 7, no. 2 (May–August 2014): 343–48, **http://1.usa.gov/1s0DqVM**.

233 **But we know that the trajectory of benefit**: The anecdotal evidence is vast, but take, for instance, the phenomenon of "exceptional responders"—cancer patients who defy the statistics, surprising their doctors and researchers, when their tumors shrink and they respond well to drugs that don't work for the majority of clinical trial participants. In one study, researchers at Memorial Sloan Kettering wanted to find out if everolimus, a drug that's traditionally used on kidney and breast cancer patients, could also work for bladder cancer. Of the forty-five patients who got the drug, only two responded. But their results were dramatic. One patient who was thought to have had less than a year to live saw her tumors disappear. Another patient appeared to be completely cured—her cancer did not come back even after she stopped taking the drug. Researchers at Dana-Farber got similar results in a study of everolimus for anaplastic thyroid cancer. It worked for only one patient, but her tumors shrank and didn't return for eighteen months. When they profiled her cancer, they discovered a genetic mutation—it was sensitive to everolimus—that also existed in the bladder cancer patients who responded. See Gina Kolata, "Finding Clues in Genes of 'Exceptional Responders,'" *New York Times*, October 8, 2014.

The National Cancer Institute has since begun an Exceptional Responders Initiative (see **http:// 1.usa.gov/1xNEelN**), to seek out similar cases that may help us better understand the molecular underpinnings of these seemingly unique positive responses to treatment.

233 **especially if there's a chance it will make a difference**: When patients ask: *How much time do I have left?*, physicians are often at a loss for words, because, "the range of what is reasonably possible is just so wide," wrote Dr. Paul Kalanithi in his excellent op-ed, "How Long Have I Got Left?," *New York Times*, January 26, 2014. In May 2013, in his mid-thirties, when he was chief resident in neurological surgery at Stanford University, Dr. Kalanithi was diagnosed with Stage IV non-small-cell

lung cancer. He figured he had a few months left. But then he started taking Tarceva to target the EGFR mutation in his cancer. His tumors shrank, and his health dramatically improved. "I might die within two years, or I might make it to ten," he wrote in the *Times*. "If you add in the uncertainty based on new therapies available in two or three years, that range may be completely different." Dr. Kalanithi took it one bridge at a time, gradually continuing to work, write, and teach. In July 2014, he and his wife welcomed a daughter. Shortly before his death on March 9, 2015, at the age of 37, he wrote an essay in *Stanford Medicine* (**http://stanford.io/1aoe8gs**), in which he tells his daughter, "You filled a dying man's days with a sated joy . . . In this time, right now, that is an enormous thing." The extra time his therapy provided surely made a difference in his and his family's life.

234 **Don't be upset if you get some resistance**: Large institutions that embrace research and precision medicine often are more open to this kind of technology. For instance, it's becoming protocol at such top hospitals as Memorial Sloan Kettering and Dana-Farber. See Drew Armstrong, "Cancer Hospitals Make Gene Tests a New Standard for Care," *Bloomberg*, June 2, 2014, **http://bloom.bg/1vWjxzi**.

234 **FDA-sanctioned clinical trials**: The U.S. National Library of Medicine's FAQ page has some starting-point information about the different phases of clinical trials, how to search the **ClinicalTrials.gov** website, the benefits and risks of participating in a trial, and the ways you are protected as a participant. See "FAQ: ClinicalTrials.gov Questions," **http://1.usa.gov/1vPg3z9**. See also "A Guide to Understanding Clinical Trials," American Heart Association, **http://bit.ly/1qu2Vea**; and "Clinical Trials," American Cancer Society, **http://bit.ly/1EBzp0C**.

235 **Call the leading disease-research foundations**: A number of disease-specific philanthropies are *very* focused on clinical trials research and are doing an excellent job connecting patients to the right trials. For instance, the Pancreatic Cancer Action Network (**http://www.pancan.org**) offers free, confidential, and personalized clinical trial searches. The Cystic Fibrosis Foundation (**http://www.cff.org**) has its own trials-search database. Faster Cures (**http://www.fastercures.org**), a Milken Institute center that aims to speed medical research, has a clinical trials matching website, EmergingMed Navigator (**http://www.emergingmed.com**), which helps patients identify cancer trials that match their needs.

237 **was diagnosed with acute myeloid leukemia**: Adult acute myeloid leukemia is a cancer of the blood and bone marrow. For detailed information, see the National Cancer Institute's "Adult Acute Myeloid Leukemia Treatment" page, **http://1.usa.gov/1BKNLNd**. See also the American Cancer Society's "Leukemia—Acute Myeloid (Myelogenous)," revised February 7, 2014, **http://bit.ly/14HxIRB**.

238 **woman with advanced bladder cancer**: Bladder cancer is the sixth most common cancer in the United States, and men are three times more likely to be diagnosed with it than women. For treatment guidelines and basic information about staging, symptoms, and prognosis, see "Bladder Cancer Treatment," National Cancer Institute, modified August 13, 2014, **http://1.usa.gov/1q9ygU2**.

239 **Because Joan's cancer appeared to be very aggressive**: There were many moving parts to Joan's care, and numerous debates among her physicians about the best regimen for her disease, but in the end she opted to try a combined chemotherapy regimen of gemcitabine plus cisplatin. Patients commonly have four cycles (sometimes fewer), but because Joan was responding so well—and the family wanted to be aggressive—she had six cycles. The literature on this treatment is evolving, and it's important to do contemporary research on any drugs you are considering, but one often-cited, early study on this therapy is A. Dash et al., "A Role for Neoadjuvant Gemcitabine Plus Cisplatin in Muscle-Invasive Urothelial Carcinoma of the Bladder: A Retrospective Experience," *Cancer* 113, no. 9 (November 1, 2008): 2471–77, **http://1.usa.gov/1AhShgp**.

240 **One way of making your wishes explicit**: Caring Connections (**http://www.caringinfo.org**) is a great place for practical information about planning and preparing for end-of-life considerations. The Conversation Project (**http://www.theconversationproject.org**) helps caregivers initiate thoughtful discussions about a loved one's end-of-life wishes. AARP has a helpful "Caregiving

Resource Center" website that focuses on legal and financial issues (**http://bit.ly/1EF1bsS**). And the American Cancer Society's "Nearing the End of Life" page provides resources for caregivers and cancer patients who are facing a fatal illness (**http://bit.ly/1vXYy1n**). You also may wish to seek private legal advice. Dr. Ira Byock (**http://irabyock.org**), a leading expert on palliative care and improving care at the end of life, has written several very helpful books, including *Dying Well* and *The Four Things That Matter*, for more guidance on how to help someone facing an end-of-life situation. Dr. Atul Gawande's *Being Mortal* uses powerful personal stories to illuminate how our modern medical system commonly mishandles end-of-life issues.

CHAPTER 12. STEP 4—COORDINATION

245 **Willie King, a fifty-one-year-old**: Information about Willie King's case is widely available online. The facts from the retelling here are primarily from four sources: Robert M. Wachter and Kaveh G. Shojania's excellent book, *Internal Bleeding: The Truth Behind America's Terrifying Epidemic of Medical Mistakes*, 2nd ed. (New York: Rugged Land, 2005), pp. 121–25; "Doctor Who Cut Off Wrong Leg Is Defended by Colleagues," *New York Times*, September 17, 1995; Pat Leisner, "Surgeon Says It Was Too Late to Stop Amputation on Wrong Leg," Associated Press, September 14, 1995, **http://bit .ly/1wubAlb**; and "Hospital Settles Case of Amputation Error," *New York Times*, May 12, 1995.

246 **Called a never-event**: The phrase was coined in 2001 by Dr. Ken Kizer, the founding president and CEO of the National Quality Forum, to refer to medical errors that are shockingly bad. The Agency for Healthcare Research and Quality keeps a backgrounder on never-events, along with an updated compendium of articles and essays on serious medical error, at "Never Events: Background," Patient Safety Network, **http://1.usa.gov/1vY3JNX**.

In 2007 the Centers for Medicare and Medicaid Services (CMS) announced that it would no longer pay for additional costs associated with preventable errors, including never-events. Many private insurers have adopted similar policies. By 2009, CMS stopped paying for any costs associated with wrong-site surgeries. See "Never Events: Background," Patient Safety Network, **http://1.usa .gov/1vY3JNX**. Before these policy changes, a hospital could potentially charge patients for revision surgeries due to medical error it caused. See S. Eappen et al., "Relationship Between Occurrence of Surgical Complications and Hospital Finances," *JAMA* 309, no. 15 (April 17, 2013): 1599–606, **http://bit.ly/1sIt1Qj**.

246 **Today, if he were to walk into a hospital**: Safety measures continue to evolve, and some hospitals adhere to them better than others. The Patient Safety Network website (**http://1.usa.gov /1tp4BgM**) has more information and research about medical error, as well as links to classic articles about the way doctors and institutions have changed protocols. One notable example is Atul Gawande, "The Checklist," *New Yorker*, December 10, 2007, in which he introduced the work of Peter Pronovost, the Johns Hopkins physician who dramatically reduced errors and infection rates in Michigan's ICUs simply by instituting checklists.

246 **Thankfully, never-events like King's botched**: Researchers who analyzed information from nearly three million operations between 1985 and 2004 found just forty reported wrong-site surgeries, in M. R. Kwaan et al., "Incidence, Patterns, and Prevention of Wrong-Site Surgery," *Archives of Surgery* 141, no. 4 (April 1, 2006): 353–58, **http://bit.ly/1xLwdL8**.

Though uncommon, never-events (also called sentinel events) are still potentially catastrophic to patients. But it's difficult to truly gauge the rate of occurrence nationwide, when only twenty-six states, plus Washington, D.C., voluntarily report never-events to the Joint Commission (an independent health care accrediting organization). However, the most recent data suggest that these incidents are on the downswing. See the Joint Commission's "Topics: Sentinel Event" page, **http:// bit.ly/1w4I9Xh**; and R. K. Michaels et al., "Achieving the National Quality Forum's 'Never Events': Prevention of Wrong Site, Wrong Procedure, and Wrong Patient Operations," *Annals of Surgery* 245, no. 4 (April 2007): 526–32, **http://1.usa.gov/ZBtKHq**.

246 **two decades' worth (from 1990 to 2010)**: W. T. Mehtsun et al., "Surgical Never Events in the United States," *Surgery* 153, no. 4 (April 2013): 465–72, **http://1.usa.gov/1z5ikMc**.

246 **in the case of one Canadian woman who didn't**: Wachter and Shojania, *Internal Bleeding*, pp. 135–36.

246 **The next most common never-events included**: Kwaan et al., "Incidence, Patterns, and Prevention."

247 **Coordination is especially important**: For more on this, see Agency for Healthcare Research and Quality, *National Healthcare Quality Report, 2013*, publication no. 14-0005 (Rockville, Md., 2013), chap. 7, http://1.usa.gov/1weFzhg.

252 **Some 40 percent of the 5.8 million car crashes**: U.S. Department of Transportation, National Highway Traffic Safety Administration, *Crash Factors in Intersection-Related Crashes: An On-Scene Perspective*, report no. DOT HS 811 366, September 2010, http://1.usa.gov/1MuJcXb. Figures are based on data collected from 2005 to 2007 via the National Motor Vehicle Crash Causation Survey.

256 **prevent hospital-acquired conditions**: For more information on hospital-acquired conditions, see Agency for Healthcare Research and Quality, *National Healthcare Quality Report, 2013*, publication no. 14-0005 (Rockville, Md., 2013), chap. 4, http://1.usa.gov/19eznAL.

256 **they occur in about 12 out of every 100 patients**: According to a December 2014 report, estimates for 2013 showed a 9 percent decline in the rate of hospital-acquired conditions (HACs) from 2012 to 2013, and a 17 percent decline, from 145 to 121 HACs per 1,000 discharges, from 2010 to 2013. See Agency for Healthcare Research and Quality, *Efforts to Improve Patient Safety Result in 1.3 Million Fewer Patient Harms*, publication no. 15-0011-EF (Rockville, Md., 2014), http://1.usa.gov/1pOVKDC. For more ways to prevent HACs, see "Preventing Infections in the Hospital," National Patient Safety Foundation, http://bit.ly/1L2sDXp; and *Consumer Reports'* "Your Hospital Survival Guide," which has helpful actions to take before, during, and after your stay, at http://bit .ly/1sUGYur.

258 **nearly one-fifth of Medicare patients discharged**: S. F. Jencks, M. V. Williams, and E. A. Coleman, "Rehospitalizations Among Patients in the Medicare Fee-for-Service Program," *New England Journal of Medicine* 360, no. 14 (April 2, 2009): 1418–28, http://bit.ly/1wfMu9V. Yale cardiologist Dr. Harlan Krumholz also cites these figures—and provides some insightful observations on the prevention of unplanned rehospitalizations—in "Post-Hospital Syndrome—a Condition of Generalized Risk," *New England Journal of Medicine* 368, no. 2 (January 10, 2013): 100–102, http://1.usa.gov/1tOHSqq.

258 **Called posthospital syndrome**: Krumholz, "Post-Hospital Syndrome."

261 **The National Patient Safety Foundation**: See "Pharmacy Safety and Service," National Patient Safety Foundation, http://bit.ly/1NLljx5.

CHAPTER 13. COMPETENCE AND COURAGE

269 **In October 2003, during a CT scan of his kidneys**: Walter Isaacson, *Steve Jobs* (New York: Simon and Schuster, 2011), pp. 452–56, 476.

269 **"Incidental findings"—things that show up**: Incidental findings happen so often, doctors have dubbed them "incidentalomas," and it's important to get an expert opinion if your doctors find one. But keep in mind that very often they are nothing at all. In fact, when the department of radiology at the Mayo Clinic examined imaging records of 1,426 patients, 567 (40 percent) had incidental findings, but just 35 people (6.2 percent) needed follow-up clinical actions such as second opinions, biopsies, more diagnostics, and so on. See N. M. Orme et al., "Incidental Findings in Imaging Research: Evaluating Incidence, Benefit, and Burden," *Archives of Internal Medicine* 170, no. 17 (September 27, 2010): 1525–32, http://bit.ly/1t1eBLh.

269 **a pancreatic neuroendocrine tumor**: Jobs refused surgery and resorted to the kind of magical thinking that worked for him in his professional life. But this was a foolish decision. See Alison G.

Walton, "Steve Jobs' Cancer Treatment Regrets," Forbes.com, October 24, 2011, **http://onforb .es/1y8ykZt**; and "Pancreatic Cancer Treatment: Treatment Options Overview," National Cancer Institute, **http://1.usa.gov/11Tv5KY**.

270 **Despite the urging of his physicians, friends**: Isaacson, *Steve Jobs*.

270 **Instead, he tried to heal himself with diet**: Ibid.

270 **His surgeons found three liver metastases**: Ibid.

270 **John T. James, the founder of Patient Safety**: *More Than 1,000 Preventable Deaths a Day Is Too Many: The Need to Improve Patient Safety: Hearing Before the U.S. Senate Subcommittee on Primary Health and Aging*, 113th Cong. (July 17, 2014) (testimony of John T. James), video and transcripts at **http://1.usa.gov/1sdcDGE**.

270 **his exhaustive study, which revealed that preventable harm**: J. T. James, "A New, Evidence-Based Estimate of Patient Harms Associated with Hospital Care," *Journal of Patient Safety* 9, no. 3 (September 2013): 122–28, **http://1.usa.gov/1r1QGqe**.

270 **At nineteen, Alex collapsed during a run**: James retells the events in *A Sea of Broken Hearts: Patient Rights in a Dangerous, Profit-Driven Health Care System* (Bloomington, Ind.: AuthorHouse, 2007), and at his website, **http://www.PatientSafetyAmerica.com**.

ONE FINAL THOUGHT

273 **Elie Wiesel, the Nobel**: See "Elie Wiesel," Elie Wiesel Foundation for Humanity, **http://bit .ly/1wrpneG**.

273 **"I say to myself, since I did survive"**: "Patt Morrison Asks: Elie Wiesel, History's Witness," *Los Angeles Times*, April 24, 2013.

INDEX

A

AARP, 333n
acute lymphoblastic leukemia (ALL), 331n
Adam (patient), 153–9
Affordable Care Act of 2010, 313n, 322n
Against Medical Advice (AMA), 151, 322n
Agency for Healthcare Research and Quality, 110–11, 318n, 322n, 334n, 335n
AIDS, deaths from, 7
allergens, 94–5
Allow Natural Death (AND), 241
alopecia (hair loss), 120
Amanda (patient), 63–4, 176
ambulances, 142–4, 162
American Academy of Pediatrics, 97
American Board of Internal Medicine, 97
American Board of Medical Specialties, 41, 132, 152
American Cancer Society, 334n
American College of Surgeons (ACOS), 97, 152
American Heart Association, 150, 316n
American Journal of Medicine, 39
American Society of Clinical Oncology, 97
amputations, 245–6
Andrea (patient), 262–3
anemia, 63–4, 198, 204

Angela (patient's mother), 153–9
angina, 96, 317n
angioedema, 177–8, 179
angiograms, 89, 90, 92
angioplasty, 91
anterior cervical discectomy and fusion (ACDF), 144–5
appcrawlr.com, 262
Arling, Bryan J., 52–3, 59, 209, 240–1, 314n
arrhythmia, x–xi
arthritis, 22
artificial hip replacement, 100, 101, 236
artificial knee replacements, 101
Association of American Medical Colleges, 312n
asthma, 4, 141–2, 161
auditory loss, 107–9

B

back surgery, 99
Bairey Merz, C. Noel, 149
balloon angioplasty, 31
Baltimore, Md., 115
Barbra Streisand Women's Heart Center, 149
basal cell carcinoma, 329n

Bates, D. W., 327*n*
Being Mortal (Gawande), 334*n*
below-the-knee amputation (BKA surgery),
    245
Ben (patient), 29–31
Benadryl, 179
Berwick, Donald, 310*n*
Bilezikian, John P., 168–70, 171
biliblankets, 155
bipolar disorder, 13
bisphosphonate, 168, 323*n*
Black, Keith, 117
bladder cancer, 238–9, 333*n*
blood-bacterial infection, 156
blood-oxygen saturation levels, 92
blood thinners, 91, 92
blood transfusions, 237
Bloomberg, 318*n*
Boston, Mass., 58
BRAF mutations, 231–2, 332*n*
brain tumors, 330*n*
    see also glioblastomas
breast cancer, 99, 201
    deaths from, 7
Bretsky, Philip M., 41, 44–5, 48
Brigham and Women's Hospital, 8, 193
Britt, Gregg, 232
bronchoscopy procedures, 93, 96
Brook, Robert H., 15
Buchenwald concentration camp, 273
Buffington, Kimberly, 11
bunions, 123–4
Byock, Ira, 334*n*

C

calcium, 167, 168, 173
California, 89, 93–4, 190
California, University of:
    at Los Angeles, 63
    at San Diego, 178
    at San Francisco, 310*n*
    San Francisco Medical Center, 93
Canada, 78
cancer, 200–1, 243, 249, 269–70
    death statistics of, 310*n*
    diagnostic errors related to, 201, 327*n*
    off-label drug use for treatment of, 332*n*
    radiation-induced, 330*n*
    targeted therapy for, 231
    tumor profiling and, 232–4, 243
    see also specific types of cancer

Cancer Cytopathology, 202
Carbone Cancer Center, 111, 130
car crashes, 7, 252
cardiologists, 103
cardiovascular disease, 324*n*
Caring Connections, 240, 333*n*
Caris Life Sciences, 231
Carter, Carrie L., 60–1, 65, 110
Carter administration, 12
Casper, Wyo., 99
Catherine (patient), 3–7, 8–10, 33, 70, 79,
    121, 176, 309*n*
Cedars-Sinai Medical Center, 11, 31, 93, 94,
    149, 208
    Thoracic Surgery and Trauma Program at, 94
Cedars-Sinai Medical Network, 117
Centers for Medicare & Medicaid Services
    (CMS), 319*n*, 322*n*, 334*n*
Central Cord Syndrome, 140
CertificationMatters.org, 41
cervical spinal cord injury, 140
Chalifour, Martin, 194
Chandler (patient's father), 175, 177–9, 184,
    202
chemotherapy, 188, 191, 198, 231, 237, 239,
    248, 263, 326*n*, 333*n*
Chicago, Ill., 23, 58
Chicago, University of, School of Medicine
    at, 103
childhood leukemia, 230, 331*n*
cholesterol, 89
Choosing Wisely, 97, 104, 133
chronic conditions, monitoring of, 180–3, 195
chronic eosinophilic pneumonia, 9
chronic hepatitis B, 248
chronic lower respiratory diseases, 310*n*
Churg-Strauss Syndrome, 3–4, 6, 8–9, 79, 176
Churg-Strauss Syndrome Association, 8, 121
cisplatin, 333*n*
City of Hope National Medical Center, 185
Claire (patient), 198, 202
clean hands, 257
Cleveland, Ohio, 237
Cleveland Clinic, 117, 207
Clinical Outcomes Utilizing Revascularization
    and Aggressive Drug Evaluation
    (COURAGE), 317*n*
clinical trials, 234–6, 332*n*–33*n*
    exceptional responders and, 332*n*
clinicaltrials.gov, 132, 235, 236
coded doctor slang, 315*n*
colonoscopy, 16

Columbia University, 312*n*
  College of Physicians and Surgeons at, 169
coming alongside, 274
communication, 252, 253, 266, 316*n*
  during medical emergencies, 147–50, 322*n*
  medical errors and, 147, 322*n*
  PCP's style of, 55–6
  treatment decisions and, 97
  see also coordination
competence, 9, 17, 102, 103, 104–5, 106,
    136, 221, 269–71
concierge-style medical practices, 51, 314*n*
Congress, U.S., 7, 12, 270
Connecticut, 116
connective tissue disorders, 24
Consumer Reports, 313*n*, 314*n*, 335*n*
Conversation Project, 333*n*
coordination, 5, 173, 221, 245–67
  communication and, 97, 252, 253, 266
  conductor for care and, 249–50, 266
  during course of treatment, 247–52
  helper for, 248, 253, 254, 266
  hospital discharge orders and, 258
  at intersections of care, 247, 252–3,
    266–7
  medication scheduling and, 261–2
  mistakes in, 11, 245–7
  multiple doctors and, 26–7, 77, 249, 252
  multiple medications and, 9, 248
  to prevent hospital-acquired conditions,
    256–8, 267
  reconnecting with friends and, 262–5, 267
  safety during hospital stays and, 254–8
  support team for, *see* support teams
  ten things to ask before hospital discharge,
    259–61, 267
cornea transplant, 102
Cornell University, 72
coronary angiogram, 89, 90
coronary artery bypass graft surgeries, 15
corticosteroid, 5, 309*n*
courage, 4, 9, 17, 52, 99, 100, 102, 103,
    104–5, 106, 126, 158, 162, 197, 221,
    269–71
Cronkite, Walter, 17
cytotechnologists, 203

D

Dallas, Tex., 65, 100, 101, 110
D'Amico, Anthony V., 57–8, 193, 201
Dana (patient), 199, 202

Dana-Farber Cancer Institute, 186, 193,
    327*n*, 332*n*, 333*n*
Dartmouth Atlas of Health Care, 98, 101,
    104, 318*n*, 319*n*
Dartmouth Institute for Health Policy and
    Clinical Practice, 98
data collection:
  separating decision making from,
    226–9
  staying neutral and, 227
  see also research
Davidson, Michael H., 103, 207
Debbie (patient), 120–1
depression, 13–14, 29, 168, 312*n*, 324*n*
diabetes, 245
diagnosis, x, 173, 197–212, 221
  delayed, 198
  how to question, 206
  overdiagnosis and, 96, 318*n*
  as relying on human judgment, 202–3
  second opinions for, *see* second opinions
diagnostic errors, 7, 21–6, 197–206, 327*n*,
    328*n*
  cancer-related, 201, 328*n*
  confirmation bias and, 204
  deaths due to, 327*n*
  factors influencing, 201
  see also medical errors
diethylstilbestrol (DES), 228
direct-pay models, 51, 314*n*
Donker, Pietr, 325*n*
Do Not Resuscitate (DNR), 241
Drugs.com, 120
Duarte, Calif., 185
Duke University, 310*n*
Dying Well (Byock), 334*n*

E

earache, 29–31
ear disorders, 107–8
EGFR mutations, 331*n*, 333*n*
Eisenhower, Dwight D., 270
electroshock therapy, 14
Elman, Sheldon, 78, 130, 182–3, 200, 225
Elyria, Ohio, 99
emergency departments:
  communication in, 147–50, 158, 322*n*
  pediatric expertise of, 153–6, 158–9, 163,
    323*n*
Emory University, 200
endocrine diseases, 167

end-of-life issues, 240–1, 243, 333n–34n
Ephron, Nora, 73
epilepsy, 121
Epstein, Jonathan, 185
Eric (patient), 184–8, 202, 219
erlotinib (Tarceva), 231, 331n, 333n
esophageal cancer, 192
everolimus, 332n
exceptional responders, 332n
experts, see specialists
Expertscape, 113, 132, 135, 176

F
fainting, 139–40
Federation of State Medical Boards, 41
Fellow of the American Academy of
      Emergency Medicine (F.A.A.E.M.),
      152
Fellow of the American College of Emergency
      Physicians (F.A.C.E.P.), 152
Fessler, Richard G., 145, 146–7
Finer, Janis, 313n–14n
Food and Drug Administration (FDA), U.S.,
      133, 183, 232, 234, 324n
Foundation Medicine, 231
Four Things That Matter, The (Byock), 334n
friendships and relationships, 262–5, 267
functional MRI, 200, 228–9

G
Gallup Health and Healthcare Survey,
      327n–28n
Gamma Knife radiosurgery (stereotactic
      radiation therapy), 225–6, 228
gangrene, 245
Gassner, Lawrence, 314n
Gavin (patient), 80
Gawande, Atul, 334n
Gelfand, Jeffrey A., 178
gemcitabine, 333n
genetics, 65
genomics, 233
Georgetown University Hospital, 330n–31n
George Washington University, School of
      Medicine and Health Services, 314n
Gleason score, 184, 185
glioblastomas, 219, 330n
Google Scholar, 132
Gordon, Tom, 117

Grand Forks, N. Dak., 98
Greene, Dr., 251
Guardant Health, 231
Gynecologic Oncology, 190

H
hair loss (alopecia), 120
Hal (patient), 237
Haley (patient), 39–45, 48
Hannah (patient's sister), 252–3
Harvard Medical School, 57, 193
Harvard University, 8, 116, 178, 201
      School of Public Health at, 7
Hawaii, 99
Hawaii, University of, at Mānoa, 319n
Health and Human Services Department
      (HHS), U.S., 12, 222, 243
health care advance directive, 240, 243
Healthcare Cost and Utilization Project,
      317n, 318n
health care costs, 96, 98
Healthcare Navigation, 313n
health care reform, 16–17, 270
health insurance, 16, 115, 136, 151, 232,
      311n, 313n, 320n
      finding physicians in one's network, 40, 42
      meet-and-greets covered by, 44
      physicians reimbursed by, 10, 17, 44, 50–1,
      294n
      for Walmart employees, 117
Health Insurance Portability and
      Accountability Act of 1996 (HIPAA), 67,
      74, 79, 314n–15n, 316n
health maintenance organizations (HMOs), 42
hearing loss, 107–9
heart, as intricately connected to lungs, 94
heart attacks, 90, 140, 149–50
      in men vs. women, 150, 163
      stents and, 96
      symptoms of, 150, 163
heart catheterizations, 96
heart disease, 31, 163
      death statistics of, 7, 149–50, 310n
hematology, 63–4
Henry J. Kaiser Family Foundation, 313n
heparin, 11, 311n
hepatitis, 63, 248
Hep-Lock, 11, 311n
Herceptin, 231
hip replacements, 100, 101, 236

HIV, 230
holistic medicine, 102, 269–70
Holocaust, 273
Honolulu, Hawaii, 99
hormone therapy, 326*n*
hospice care, 17
hospital-acquired conditions (HACs), 256–8, 267, 335*n*
Hospital Consumer Assessment of Healthcare Providers and Systems Survey (HCAHPS), 322*n*
hospital discharges, 148, 258
    against medical advice (AMA), 322*n*
    ten things to ask before, 259–61, 267
hospitalists, 43–4, 254, 313*n*
hospitals:
    on-call administrators in, 146, 162
    preventable harm in, 270
    small-community vs. large academic medical center, 116–17, 136, 192–4
    transfers between, 150–1
    trauma center ratings for, 152–3
    see also emergency departments
hospital stays:
    discharge orders and, 148, 258
    medical information for, 254–5, 267
    medical intersections and, 266–7
    organizational information for, 255, 267
    personal information for, 255–6, 267
    safety and coordination during, 254–8
    ten things to ask before discharge, 259–61, 267
Huo, Michael H., 102
hypersensitivity pneumonitis, 94–5

I

idiopathic acquired angioedema, 177
immersion, 173, 175–95, 201, 221
    decision making and, 185
    important parts of, 176
    questions to research, 185–7
    revisiting medical records and, 176
    three things to do, 189
    see also data collection; research
immunosuppressants, 178, 179
immunotherapy, 230
Imuran, 179
incidental findings, 335*n*
Institute of Medicine (IOM), 7, 8, 10, 96, 309*n*, 310*n*, 311*n*

Intensive Case Management, 13, 78, 172–3, 174, 197, 221, 247, 271
    see also coordination; diagnosis; immersion; treatment
International Medical Corps (IMC), 141, 312*n*
Isaacson, Walter, 270

J

Jack (patient's son-in-law), 263–4
James, Alex, 270
James, John T., 270
Jane (patient's sister), 139–40, 145–6
jaundice, 64, 153, 154, 155, 158
Jenna (patient), 265
Jennifer (patient), 21–7, 31, 33, 47, 66, 78–9, 141, 176
Jessica (patient), 175, 177–9, 180, 184
Jha, Ashish, 7, 8
Jim (patient), 89–96, 97–8, 99, 200, 265, 316*n*
Joan (patient), 238–9, 333*n*
Jobs, Steve, 269–70, 335*n*–36*n*
John A. Burns School of Medicine, 319*n*
Johns Hopkins Hospital, 185, 186
Johns Hopkins School of Medicine, 7, 79, 117, 197–8, 220, 322*n*
Johnson, Magic, 230
Joint Commission, 334*n*
Jonathan (patient), 252–3
Jonsson Comprehensive Cancer Center, 63
Journal of Patient Safety, 8
Journal of the American Medical Association (*JAMA*), 7, 96, 135
Jules Stein Eye Institute, 102
Justice Department, U.S., 98

K

K, Mr. (patient), 315*n*
Kaiser Permanente, 42
Kalanithi, Paul, 332*n*–33*n*
Kalunian, Kenneth C., 178
Kawachi, Mark, 185, 187
Kelly (patient's daughter), 264
Kennedy, Edward, 330*n*
KevinMD.com, 328*n*
kidney cancer, 198–9
kidneys, 269
kidney stones, 269

King, Willie, 245–6
Kizer, Ken, 334n
knee replacements, 101

L

Leape, Lucian L., 309n, 310n, 315n
Lee, Erica H., 215–16
Lenox Hill Hospital, 14–15
leukemia, 230, 237, 331n, 333n
Lippy, William, 114
lithium, 14
liver, 64
Loestrin, 120
Logan, Bruce D., 57, 178
Long Island, N.Y., 188
Los Angeles, Calif., 9, 24, 58, 93–4, 102, 208
Los Angeles Philharmonic, 194
low blood pressure, 147
Lowe's, 117
lung cancer, 325n, 331n, 333n
lung disease, 92
lung function, 94, 95
lungs:
    allergens and, 94–5
    as intricately connected to heart, 94
lupus, 177–9
Lyme disease, 52
lymph nodes, 64

M

Madison, Wis., 111
malignant brain tumors, 330n
malignant gliomas, 330n
malpractice:
    claims of, 97, 198, 319n, 327n, 328n
    oncology claims of, 201
    see also diagnostic errors; medical errors
Marissa (patient), 213–16, 219, 263,
    329n
mastectomies, 99
Matthew (patient), 231–3
Mayo Clinic, 111, 117, 133, 207, 335n
McKenna, Robert, Jr., 94, 316n
MD Anderson, 186, 201
Mease, Philip, 25, 26, 33, 129, 181,
    208
Medicaid, 16
medical emergencies, 139–64
    ambulances and, 142–4, 162
    communication during, 147–50

decision to call 911 during, 141–4,
    161
and forgetting who's in charge, 159–60
medical information for, 67, 71–2,
    148–9, 162
mistakes made within first 24 hours of,
    141–60
wrong hospitals and, 150–9
medical errors, 245–7, 270–1, 308n
    as cause of death, 7–8, 309n–10n
    communication and, 147, 322n
    iatrogenic causes of, 309n
    medication error, 10–12, 54
    patient safety protocols for avoiding, 246,
        247, 271, 334n
    by PCPs, 54–5
    "retained foreign body," 246
    wrong patients, 247
    wrong procedures, 245–7
    wrong-site surgery, 246, 334n
    see also diagnostic errors; never-events
medical negligence, 270
medical records, 27, 72
    immersion and, 176
    for preparedness, 12, 65, 66, 68–9, 70,
        74, 75
    retention of, 315n
Medical Summary, 248, 250–1, 266
Medicare, x, 16, 53, 98, 101, 103, 136,
    192, 195, 258, 315n–16n, 318n, 319n,
    322n, 328n, 329n, 334n, 335n
medication errors, 10–12, 54
medication scheduling, 261–2
Medisys, 78
Medline, 132, 320n
Medline Plus, 134
melanoma, 201, 216, 219, 231, 263,
    303n
Memorial Sloan Kettering, 188–9, 191,
    215–16, 326n, 329n, 332n, 333n
meningioma, 219, 220, 224, 226, 330n
meningitis, 29
mental health, as influence on physical health,
    312n
Miami, University of, Miller School of
    Medicine at, 30–31
Michael (patient's father), 120
Milken, Michael, 12
Minnesota, 109
Mohs surgery, 214, 216
More Than 1,000 Preventable Deaths a Day
    Is Too Many: The Need to Improve

Patient Safety (congressional hearing), 7–8
myeloid leukemia, 237

N

NantHealth, 231
NASA, 270
National Cancer Institute (NCI), 131, 176, 325*n*, 326*n*, 328*n*, 329*n*, 330*n*, 331*n*, 332*n*, 333*n*, 336*n*
National Center for Health Statistics, 309*n*, 331*n*
National Comprehensive Cancer Network (NCCN), 176, 222–3, 243
National Guideline Clearinghouse, 222
National Institutes of Health (NIH), 111, 120, 133–4, 179, 235
    Drug Information Portal, 120, 133
National Jewish Health, 310*n*
National Library of Medicine, U.S., 111
National Patient Safety Foundation, 261
National Quality Forum, 334*n*
natural cures, 269–70
neoadjuvant chemotherapy, 191
never-events, 245–7, 334*n*, 335*n*
New England Journal of Medicine, 135, 258, 315*n*, 317*n*, 318*n*, 331*n*, 335*n*
New York, N.Y., 14, 72, 100, 188, 215
New York–Presbyterian Hospital, 72, 168
New York Times, 14, 16, 101, 311*n*, 313*n*, 314*n*, 315*n*, 316*n*, 318*n*, 319*n*, 322*n*, 325*n*, 326*n*, 328*n*, 331*n*, 332*n*, 334*n*
Nicole (patient), 37–8
No-Mistake Zone, 114, 123, 127, 171, 172, 217–18, 242
Northwestern University, 145, 146

O

Obama, Barack, 270, 319*n*
Ohio, 117
ombudsman (patient advocate), 158–9
OncoPlexDx, 231
open-heart surgery, 14
OpenNotes, 66–7
Oprah Winfrey Show, 12
orthopedic surgeons, 103
otosclerosis, 107, 108
ovarian cancer, 190
overstenting, 96, 98, 99, 317*n*, 318*n*

overtreatment, 9, 89–106
    defensive medicine and, 97
    financial incentives of, 97–8
    Hawaii and, 99
    overdiagnosis and, 96
    unnecessary surgeries and, 15

P

Paget, Stephen A., 178
pain-management program, 21–2
Pakdaman, Neda, 199–200, 209–10, 248, 249
pancreatic neuroendocrine tumor, 269–70
papillary thyroid cancer, 231, 232, 331*n*, 332*n*
parathyroid glands, 167, 170–1
parathyroid hormone (PTH), 167, 170, 171–2
parathyroid surgery, 170–1, 192
patient advocate (ombudsman), 158–9
patient limitations, 140, 236–8
Patient Protection and Affordable Care Act of 2010, 16
patient safety, 246, 247, 271, 310*n*, 325*n*, 327*n*, 328*n*, 329*n*, 334*n*, 335*n*, 336*n*
Patient Safety America, 270
Patient Safety and Quality Improvement Act of 2005, 7
Patient Safety Network, 334*n*
PatientsPlaybook.com, 274
Patrick (patient), 188–9, 191–2, 265
Paula (patient), 261–2, 263
PCPs, *see* primary care physicians
Pennsylvania, 192
Pennsylvania, University of, 148, 192
PepsiCo, 117
Philadelphia, Pa., 192
Pho, Kevin, 328*n*
phototherapy, 155, 158
Physician Orders for Life-Sustaining Treatment (POLST) form, 240, 243
physicians:
    concierge-style practices of, 51, 314*n*
    and fee-for-service vs. direct-pay model, 51, 52–3, 320*n*
    financial incentives and, 98, 103
    how to cold-call, 128–31
    insurance reimbursement for, 10, 44, 50–1, 311*n*, 320*n*
    shortage of, 312*n*, 319*n*
    treatment time of, 37–8, 50, 51, 52–3, 60
    see also primary care physicians (PCPs); specialists

Pill Identifier, 133
plasma, 178
plasmapheresis, 178, 179
polysorbate 80, 177, 178, 179
posthospital syndrome, 258
postpartum depression, 13
post-traumatic stress disorder (PTSD), 29,
    312n
prednisone, 5, 94, 95, 179, 309n
preferred provider organizations (PPOs), 42,
    313n
preparedness, 19–164
    emergency information in, 67, 71–2, 74,
        148–9, 162
    family health history in, 12, 65, 70, 74
    finding and interviewing medical experts in,
        107–37
    medical records in, 12, 65, 66, 68–9, 70,
        74, 75
    medical summary in, 70
    overtreatment and, see overtreatment
    primary care physicians and, see primary
        care physicians (PCPs)
    rights and, 67, 74
    support team in, see support teams
    team leader in, 12, 81–5
    three steps for, 63–75
Press, Matthew J., 315n
primary care physicians (PCPs), 10, 37–62,
    310n–11n
    age of, 59
    communication style of, 55–6
    consulting with, before consulting
        specialists, 90–1, 106
    effective, importance of finding, 21–35
    medical errors by, 54–5
    meet-and-greets with, 44, 58
    private, 314n
    reasons to find new, 38–9, 54–6, 62
    relationship with, 12, 23, 28, 32, 35,
        46–7, 56
    three levels of partnership with, 32–4, 35
    three steps for finding, 40–6, 62
    and timely access to care, 55
    what to look for in, 46–50, 57–61, 62
    see also physicians
primary hyperparathyroidism (PHPT),
    167–72, 323n, 324n
Private Health Management, 12, 312n
Pronovost, Peter, 334n
ProPublica, 319n
prostate, 186

prostate cancer, 184–8, 202, 324n–25n
    metastatic, 326n
Prostate Cancer Foundation, 12, 184
prostatectomy, 185, 186, 190, 325n, 326n
prostate-specific antigen (PSA), 184, 188
psoriasis, 25
psoriatic arthritis, 25, 27
PubMed, 111, 112–13, 114, 121, 124, 125,
    132, 134, 168, 176, 181, 320n, 321n
pulmonology, 92–3

Q

quadriplegia, 144
Quaid, Dennis, 11–12
Quaid, Thomas Boone, 11, 311n
Quaid, Zoë Grace, 11, 311n
Question Builder, 110–11, 133

R

Rachel (patient), 107–9, 110, 111, 112–15,
    118, 119, 121, 124, 126, 176, 321n
radiation, 198, 330n–31n
radiation-induced cancer, 330n
RAND Health, 15
Reagan administration, 12
Red Cross, 63
Reeve, Christopher, 144
renal cell carcinoma, 198–9
renal pelvis cancer, 199
research, 109–12, 176
    to find specialists, 109, 110, 111, 121–2, 123
    sources for, 110–11, 132–5
    specific questions for, 110–11, 136
    see also data collection; immersion
"retained foreign body," 246
rheumatology, 24
Richard (patient's son), 100–1, 102, 105
Roberts, Robin, 73
robotic-assisted surgery, 186
Roboz, Gail J., 72–3, 77, 118, 194, 227
Rochester, Minn., 117
Rosenbaum, Lisa, 317n
Rosenthal, Elisabeth, 311n
Rosove, Michael H., 63–4
Rush University Medical Center, 23

S

Sally (patient), 100–2, 176, 236
Samantha (patient), 224–9, 238

Sandra (patient's wife), 90–1, 92, 93, 94–5
San Francisco, Calif., 99, 186
Sarasota, Fla., 114
Sayfie, Eugene J., 30–1, 32, 128, 207–8
Scardino, Peter T., ix–xi, 191
Seattle, Wash., 25, 117
secondary malignancies, 330n
second opinions, 202, 207–10, 325n,
 327n–28n
  for emergencies, 145–6
  for skin cancer, 328n, 329n
  from specialists, 9, 45
Selner, Marc, 124–5
Senate, U.S., Finance Committee of, 318n
Seth (patient's husband), 264
Setoodeh, Katy M., 24–5, 27, 33, 208–9
Silverstein, Herbert, 114, 119, 321n
Silverstein Institute and Ear Research
 Foundation, 114
Simon, Robert R., 23–4, 59–60, 141–6, 152,
 160, 161, 312n
sinus cancer, 198
skin cancer:
  second opinions for, 328n, 329n
  see also melanoma
sleeping pills, 147
Society for Cardiovascular Angiography and
 Interventions, 318n
Southern Surgical Association, 324n
South Korea, 317n
specialists, 90–3, 107–37
  consulting PCP before seeing, 90–1,
   106
  and favored treatment vs. appropriate
   treatment, 93, 97, 101
  finding, 109, 110, 111, 121–2, 123–4,
   134–5
  interviewing, 125–6, 136
  volume of surgeries and, 126, 187, 189,
   190, 322n, 324n, 326n
  see also physicians
specialist shuffle, 26–7
spherocytosis, 64
spinal stenosis, 322n
spinal surgery, 144–5
spleen, 63, 64
squamous cell carcinoma, 329n
Stanford Medicine, 333n
Stanford University, 199
  Concierge and Executive Medicine,
   199
stapes, 108, 109

Starfield, Barbara, 309n
statins, 89, 91
stents, 91, 92
  overuse of, 96, 98, 99, 317n, 318n
Stephanie (patient), 52–3
stereotactic radiation therapy (Gamma Knife
 radiosurgery), 225–6, 228
stroke, 29, 150, 312n
supplements, 73
support teams, 77–86, 243
  forms of support for, 80, 86
  leader of, 12, 78, 79–85, 86, 248, 253, 254,
   266
  sharing roles in, 79, 81–2
surgeons, volume of surgeries and, 126, 187,
 189, 190, 322n, 324n, 326n
surgery:
  geographical statistics on, 98–9
  revision, 116
  tumors and, 330n
  unnecessary, 15, 98, 101
  wrong-site, 246, 334n
  see also specific types of surgeries
Susan (patient), 264
Susan G. Komen for the Cure, 201
Swedish Medical Center, 25

T

Tabak, Steven W., 31–2, 58–9
Tampa, Fla., 245
Tarceva (erlotinib), 231, 331n, 333n
Taylor (patient), 250–2
technology, 234–5
Texas, University of, 201
  Southwestern Medical Center at,
   102
thyroid cancer, 231, 232, 317n–18n, 331n,
 332n
tinnitus, 109
To Err Is Human (IOM report), 7
Tommy (patient), 198–9, 204
Topamax, 120
Tracey (patient), 139–40, 141, 144–7, 150, 160
treatment, x, 173, 197, 213–43
  bridge as way to cure in, 230–4
  clear health goals and values in, 238–41
  clinical trials and, 234–5
  coordination and, 247–52
  disease progression and, 239–40
  end-of-life issues and, 240–1
  guidelines for, 222–3

treatment (*continued*)
    medical errors in, *see* medical errors
    patient limitations and, 140, 236–8
    questions to focus on, 214, 224–5, 235–6,
        238, 242
    separating data collection from decision
        making for, 226–9
    technology and, 234–6
    wealth and, 269, 270
    see also overtreatment
tumor profiling, 232–4, 243
tumors:
    secondary malignancies and, 330n
    surgery and, 330n
    see also brain tumors; cancer; *specific types*
        of tumors

U

Udelsman, Robert, 116, 122–3, 170–2, 192,
    193–4, 324n
Union, N.J., 14
UpToDate, 134
urgent care (walk-in clinics), 141, 142, 161
USA Today, 319n
U.S. News & World Report, 152

V

vemurafenib (Zelboraf), 231–3, 332n
video-assisted thoracoscopic surgery (VATS),
    93, 94, 97, 316n

Vietnam, 191
Virginia Mason Medical Center, 117

W

Wall Street Journal, 201
Walmart, 117
Walsh, Patrick, 186, 325n
Warren, Ohio, 114
Washington, University of, School of Medicine
    at, 25
WebMD, 111
Wechsler, Michael E., 8–9, 70, 121, 128–9,
    310n
Wegener's disease, 5–6
Weill Medical College, 72
Wiesel, Elie, 273
Wilding, George, 111, 130–1, 189, 233, 252
Winfrey, Oprah, 11
Wisconsin, University of, 111
Women's Guild Lung Institute, 94
World War II, 16
wrong-site surgery, 246

Y

Yale–New Haven Hospital, 116, 122, 170

Z

Zelboraf (vemurafenib), 231–3, 332n
Zuraw, Bruce L., 178